HOPE: PSYCHIATRY'S COMMITMENT

Papers Presented to Leo H. Bartemeier, M.D.
on the Occasion of His 75th Birthday

HOPE
Psychiatry's Commitment

Edited by

A. W. R. SIPE

Director of Family Services
Seton Psychiatric Institute

BRUNNER/MAZEL *Publishers* · New York

Published by
BRUNNER / MAZEL, INC.
80 East 11th Street, New York, N. Y. 10003

Library of Congress Catalog Card No. 71-113978

SBN 87630-027-1

MANUFACTURED IN THE UNITED STATES OF AMERICA

Acknowledgments

BY DEFINITION A *FESTSCHRIFT* is a cooperative venture. There were many besides the authors of the following chapters whose help was indispensable in the preparation of this volume. Two gracious ladies must be singled out especially—Marie Louise McHugh, because of her generous contribution and support, and Juanita H. Williams who as editorial assistant labored heroically through Minnesota cold, Baltimore heat and Illinois flood. Without them all of the ideas and efforts of the rest of us would have remained only good intentions.

Each of the contributors has a chance to state his debt to Dr. Bartemeier. There are others who wished to and have helped in other ways the preparation of this volume. Among them are the late Dr. John Rees of London, England, Rev. Eamonn O'Doherty of Dublin, Ireland, John Cardinal Krol of Philadelphia, Dr. John M. Dorsey of Wayne State University, Detroit, Dr. Hugh Stalker of Grosse Point Shores, Michigan.

Sister Ambrose Byrne, administrator of Seton Psychiatric Institute, encouraged this project from the beginning. Dr. Walter O. Jahrreisse, also of the Seton staff, read manuscript and was always available with wise and kindly direction. Dr. Nathan Schnaper and Dr. Waldemar H. Wenner are thanked for similar services. There are a host at St. John's Abbey, Collegeville, Minnesota, who helped in many ways. Chief among them is Abbot Baldwin Dworschak who extended his hospitality to several of us during a crucial period of work, and also Brothers Alan Reed, Michael Parrino, Vern Kronig and Cletus Connor who made us so comfortable we had to work.

In many ways it was Mrs. Frances Pond who bore the brunt of the "book in progress" by typing and retyping the manuscript, as well as the responsibility of keeping the priorities. She is a woman of endless patience whose occasional impatience was always helpful.

Contributors

A. RUSSELL ANDERSON, M.D. Private practice in psychoanalysis. Training analyst with Baltimore Psychoanalytic Institute and member of American Psychoanalytic Association.

WALTER E. BARTON, M.D., Medical Director, American Psychiatric Association, Washington, D.C. Clinical Professor of Psychiatry, Boston University School of Medicine.

HON. DAVID L. BAZELON, Chief Judge, United States Court of Appeals, Washington, D.C.

FRANCIS J. BRACELAND, M.D., Senior Consultant, Institute of Living, Hartford; Editor, *American Journal of Psychiatry;* Past President, American Psychiatric Association 1956-57.

EUGENE B. BRODY, M.D., Professor and Chairman, Department of Psychiatry, and Director, Psychiatric Institute, University of Maryland, Baltimore; Editor-in-Chief, *Journal of Nervous and Mental Disease.*

HENRY W. BROSIN, M.D., formerly Director and Chairman, Department of Psychiatry, University of Pittsburgh School of Medicine; Western Psychiatric Institute and Clinic, Pittsburgh; Past President, American Psychiatric Association 1967-68.

WALTER J. BURGHARDT, S.J., S.T.D. Professor of Historical Theology, Woodstock College, New York, N. Y.; Editor, *Theological Studies.*

JOEL ELKES, M.D., Henry Phipps Professor of Psychiatry, Director, Department of Psychiatry and Behavioral Sciences, Johns Hopkins University; Psychiatrist-in-Chief, Johns Hopkins Hospital.

DANA L. FARNSWORTH, M.D., Henry K. Oliver Professor of Hygiene, Director of University Health Services, Harvard; Member, American Medical Association Council on Mental Health (Chairman, 1967-69).

BERNARD H. HALL, M.D., Senior Clinical Consultant, The Menninger Foundation, Topeka.

J. COTTER HIRSCHBERG, M.D., Associate Director, Children's Division, The Menninger Clinic; Training and Supervising Analyst, and Supervisor in Child Analysis, Topeka Institute for Psychoanalysis.

M. RALPH KAUFMAN, M.D., Esther and Joseph Klingenstein Professor of Psychiatry; Chairman, Department of Psychiatry, Mount Sinai School of Medicine of The City University of New York.

LAWRENCE S. KUBIE, M.D., D.SC., Senior Associate in Research and Training, The Sheppard and Enoch Pratt Hospital, Towson, Maryland; Clinical Professor of Psychiatry, University of Maryland School of Medicine.

PAUL V. LEMKAU, M.D., Professor, Department of Mental Hygiene, The Johns Hopkins University School of Hygiene and Public Health, Baltimore.

DAVID M. LEVY, M.D., Consulting Psychiatrist, Department of Public Health, New York City; Honorary Consultant, New York State Psychiatric Institute.

PETER A. MARTIN, M.D., Clinical Professor of Psychiatry, University of Michigan Medical School and Wayne State University Medical School; in private practice of psychoanalysis in Detroit.

JULES H. MASSERMAN, M.D., Professor and Co-Chairman, Division of Psychiatry, Northwestern University Medical School, Chicago.

KARL MENNINGER, M.D., Founder and Chairman of the Board of Trustees, The Menninger Foundation, Topeka.

JOSEPH J. REIDY, M.D. In private practice of psychoanalysis; Assistant Professor, Pediatrics and Psychiatry, Johns Hopkins University School of Medicine; Consultant in Child Psychology, Seton Psychiatric Institute, Baltimore.

JOHN ROMANO, M.D., Distinguished University Professor of Psychiatry and Chairman, Department of Psychiatry, University of Rochester, School of Medicine and Dentistry; Psychiatrist-in-Chief, Strong Memorial Hospital, Rochester, New York.

HOWARD P. ROME, M.D., Senior Consultant, Professor of Psychiatry, Mayo Graduate School of Medicine; Past President, American Psychiatric Association 1965-66.

JOHN N. ROSEN, M.D., Trustee, Doylestown Foundation, Director of Training, Direct Psychoanalytic Institute; Chairman, Philadelphia Mental Health and Mental Retardation Advisory Board.

JONAS SALK, M.D., Fellow and Director, The Salk Institute, San Diego.

NATHAN SCHNAPER, M.D., Associate Clinical Professor of Psychiatry, University of Maryland Medical School; Consultant to U.S. Public Health Service, Baltimore; member of Baltimore Psychoanalytic Institute.

CARLOS A. SEGUIN, M.D., Chairman, Department of Psychological Science, University of San Marcos, Lima, Peru.

JOSEPH C. SOLOMON, M.D., Associate Clinical Professor of Psychiatry, University of California School of Medicine, San Francisco.

GENE L. USDIN, M.D., Director, Psychiatric Services, Touro Infirmary, New Orleans; Associate Professor, Clinical Psychiatry, Louisiana State University School of Medicine.

JOHN C. WHITEHORN, M.D., Professor Emeritus of Psychiatry, Johns Hopkins University, and Emeritus Psychiatrist-in-Chief, Johns Hopkins Hospital, Baltimore; Past President, American Psychiatric Association, 1950-51.

Table of Contents

Part IV—PSYCHIATRY'S COMMITMENT IN THE WORLD

Introduction

HOPE: PSYCHIATRY'S COMMITMENT is written in honor of Leo H. Bartemeier, M.D., who has lived 75 years and has practiced medicine for 50 of these years. A glance at the contributors to this volume will give some idea of the place Dr. Bartemeier holds in the field of psychiatry. The statements of his friends and colleagues which precede each chapter will offer the reader a glimpse of the measure of the man.

The greatness of a man is not measured by a list of his accomplishments or his friends, but by the qualities that inspired and are reflected in his life's labors and lifelong friendships. Those who know Dr. Bartemeier well are quick to point out that he is a man of unusual humanity. At the core of his humaneness is the quality of hope which marks, as Freud put it, *"Sein Arbeit und Liebe."*

A *Festschrift* poses special difficulties because the primary unity is the shared admiration, devotion or gratitude to a friend, teacher, or colleague. When one's students, friends, and colleagues represent as broad a spectrum as do Dr. Bartemeier's, one cannot look for homogeneity of thought and interest. Perhaps this is one of the values of this *Festschrift*, that it brings together a certain heterogeneity of thought —and even disharmony—without attempts at reconciliation or polemics.

A secondary unity, however, emerged from the essays—psychiatry's commitment to individuals, in the laboratory, to communities, and to the world. The hope which is so obviously part of Dr. Bartemeier's life work emerges in these essays as one of the positive forces of psychiatry's commitment. Hope is a necessary condition for any psychiatric intervention, whether in individual therapy or research, via community action in the present or for the future of man.

The essays in this volume represent the hopes and dreams of men who, like Dr. Bartemeier, have successfully merged scientific and humanistic concerns. The first part, *"Psychiatry's Commitment to the Individual,"* stresses some of the specific problems that afflict man: loneliness, "conditioned" love, the struggle for maturity, marital strife, the

xv

search for identity, and anger and despair culminating in self-destruction. The second part, *"Psychiatry's Commitment in the Laboratory,"* stresses the need for developing appropriate quantitative measurements for research purposes, and the necessity for discovering common denominators in antithetical theories about deviate behavior. The third part, *"Psychiatry's Commitment in the Community,"* explores practical means of salvaging man's fullest potential in either a religious—always an area of Dr. Bartemeier's deep concern—or secular environment. And the fourth, *"Psychiatry's Commitment to the World,"* implies psychiatry's obligation to and hope for the future.

Thus the contents of the book are concentrically arranged, with psychiatry's commitment to individuals occupying the inner circle, and psychiatry's broadest commitments and hope constituting the fourth parameter.

The intent of this book is to honor Dr. Bartemeier by contributing in some small measure to the strengthening of men's hopes.

A. W. R. SIPE

HOPE: PSYCHIATRY'S COMMITMENT

Part I

PSYCHIATRY'S COMMITMENT TO THE INDIVIDUAL

The miserable have no other medicine,
But only hope.

—SHAKESPEARE

Each man has his miseries. Most men have their hopes. Misery *per se* is not pathogenic, for suffering, guilt and death are universal realities. But suffering without meaning, guilt without redemption, and the prospect of death without understanding—all these paralyze and stultify the heart and mind of man.

Just so pathological suffering distorts reality because it blinds the sufferer to all but his miserable present and prevents him from employing his unutilized capabilities in the service of change.

The rational man involuntarily invokes hope in his battles, for hope, as Jurgen Moltmann points out, is realistic because it alone takes seriously the possibilities with which all reality is fraught. "It does not take things as they happen to stand or lie, but as progressing, moving things with the possibilities of change."

Hope is the healer.

Part I

Section One

SOME GENERAL PRINCIPLES OF TREATMENT

"Hope," writes Thornton Wilder in *The Eighth Day*, "(deep-grounded hope, not those sporadic cries and promptings wrung from us in extremity that more resemble despair) is a climate of the mind and an organ of apprehension." It is this climate of the mind and ability to apprehend reality that the patient seeks in order to relieve his loneliness and isolation. It is the hope of the psychiatrist—his climate of mind—which enables him to apprehend the dignity of each man.

Doctor Braceland considers loneliness a common human concern—and one that often comes to the psychiatrist's attention. Doctor Anderson writes about transference—one of the primary therapeutic tools in many forms of treatment. Attitudes of immaturity and maturity are outlined by Dr. Whitehorn. Doctor Hall discusses empathy—that indispensable quality of the therapist—especially as it affects the initial psychiatric interview. And Doctor Seguin speaks of love and its uniqueness in the interaction between doctor and patient.

1

FRANCIS J. BRACELAND, M.D.

It is a pleasure and an honor to be permitted to contribute to the Festschrift *which marks two anniversaries of a beloved colleague and friend who wears his honors as lightly as he does his years. His works and his character are inspirations to those who are privileged to know him.*

Character is never created by external advantage nor is it an inevitable accompaniment of birth, wealth, talent, or station. It comes only with personal endeavor and in the case of our revered colleague it is marked indelibly by his spiritual depth.

Fame is easy to acquire, but it is truly a fickle jade. To have given one's life to a cause and to be beloved for personal integrity and dedication to the welfare of persons sick and badly misunderstood is more lasting.

"Age," Bernard Baruch said, "is a number; a cipher for the records. A man can't retire his experience. He must use it. Experience achieves more with less energy and time."

As Leo Bartemeier celebrates his three-quarters of a century and his half century as a teacher, he must do so with understandable pride for it was an honorable and dedicated career, and he has won the love and affection of those whose lives he has touched. As he continues he should take heart in the example of some illustrious predecessors—King David and King Solomon:

But when old age crept over them
With many many qualms
King Solomon wrote the Proverbs
And King David wrote the Psalms.

Ad Multos Annos.

Loneliness—Man's Universal Plaint

As there is both good and bad society
there is also good and bad solitude.
St. Francis de Sales

A NEW PHILOSOPHY is abroad in the land—a destructive one that terrifies and divides the nation. It is a senseless phenomenon, ruinous in nature, settling nothing. Its memory, kept alive by the aftermath of heartache, lingers long afterward.

When we ask the historian whether there have been other times like these in our nation's history, he answers in the affirmative. George Rosen[1] notes that:

> Basically what is common to such periods is that they are at times when societies and their culture, or segments within them, are changed into something else; when the accustomed structure of order, power, beliefs, and meaning disintegrates and man confronts the inscrutable foe of the future not knowing what is to come.

That the accustomed structure of order, power, beliefs, and meaning has disintegrated today is everywhere evident, and that man, having jettisoned his spiritual moorings, is facing he "knows not what" *alone* is apparent. As each man sets out to face his future he will react in a fashion dependent not upon the old order or the new, indeterminate goals, but upon his background influences and the weight of external pressures upon him. More often than not he will contemplate the future without the safeguards which earlier sustained him and with a feeling of loneliness and isolation.

> For a crowd is not company and faces
> are but a gallery of pictures and talk
> but a tinkling cymbal where there is
> no love.
>
> EMERSON

The plaintive statement that someone feels lonely is commonly encountered. One hears it and reads it under various circumstances and in diverse places, and it is probable that everyone has experienced such feelings himself at some time or another. There is no universally accepted definition of loneliness, yet it is a significant, universal, emotional experience with far-reaching consequences for good or for evil. It is a strange and somewhat paradoxical phenomenon, for the monk alone in his cell is not lonely, while the man in the midst of a crowd is often wretchedly so. The Latin adage, *magna civitas, magna solitudo*, gives hint of the fact that there was knowledge of loneliness in the larger towns even in days of old. Loneliness has been called man's oldest theme and much of his poetry and literature is concerned with his efforts to break through its distressing bonds. It was the first thing God pronounced not good when He saw that man needed a companion, and today, even in this era of synthetic togetherness, the diagnosis is exactly the same as it was in the Garden of Eden. Loneliness is not good, but, strangely, some individuals are never less lonely than when they are alone.

One probably hears more about insecurity and loneliness today than twenty years ago, because of the disturbed state of our world as well as the imminent practicability of travel to other planets, where man will be both a stranger and an intruder. Having learned how to make this planet uninhabitable, man is now going off to see what he can do about colonizing the others. Despite his admittedly great technical successes, however, he is still seen by philosophical observers as assailed with and baffled by a corrosive loneliness—a worried victim of his own technological brilliance. His sense of aloneness is coupled with feelings of emptiness and both, in the last analysis, represent a form of basic anxiety.

Down through the years various writers have contemplated feelings of loneliness. Diderot thought it was only the bad man who was lonely; de Maupassant believed that all of us are always lonely. Chopin complained of being alone, alone, alone, even when he was surrounded. Thomas Wolfe saw the essence of human tragedy in loneliness, while Rogers thought that "through the wide world he only is alone who does not live for another." A number of modern writers are busy chronicling the loneliness of various misfits, drifters, beatniks, hippies, and rebels, whose isolation is often self-induced and of little value to mankind. Milton Bracker wrote of the loneliness of groups of drifters to be found in a modern big city. "Lacking internal resources to assuage that loneliness," he says, "they lurk in the arcades. Occasionally their frustrations and petty hostilities boil over in incidents of obscenity and menace, but the brief turmoil is apt to dissolve itself. It is like a sudden hiss of foam in a cave of the sea; its going is as mysterious as its coming." The same might be said of the turmoil on college campuses today.

The definitions of loneliness in the English language are broad and all inclusive. Often they include isolation somewhere in them. Actually the term "loneliness" has psychological connotations, while "isolation" hints at physical or psychic separation, voluntary or involuntary. Other languages have their own shades of meaning for various aspects of these phenomena, for some feelings of loneliness are normal and natural for all men, while others are pathologic to the point of mental disease. Solitude is something different; it is sought at times for retreat, for prayer, or creative thought and in this way it vivifies, but the irrational psychological withdrawal of the angry and the hurt is different, for it is of destructive nature.

Here we shall examine briefly the origins of loneliness, particularly of that form which separates a person from family or from those in the group with which he lives or works. In other words, we shall proceed upon the premise that all loneliness is relative and that psychic isolation can be just as destructive as physical isolation, and this will bring us to include the feelings of loneliness of people like you and me.

It will not surprise us to recognize, as we proceed, that we are often completely blind to the emotional feelings and needs of others, even as they are completely blind to ours, and it is possible for people to live in close proximity to one another and know nothing of their loneliness and the crises which they undergo. Such thoughts are not pleasant; in fact, the whole subject is unpleasant, and the contemplation of loneliness awakens heavy depressive feelings in the individual who undertakes it. This may account for the paucity of published material upon the subject. People who have experienced stark loneliness are hesitant to talk or write about it. Having once looked into that abyss, they want to forget about it.

We have known for a long time of some of the effects of isolation, but the subject came dramatically to the fore in recent years as the brain-washing techniques of the Chinese and Korean Communists were made known to us. Admiral Byrd, who had isolated himself in the Antarctic in the third decade of this century and nearly died before the experience was over, knew well the effect of isolation. For four years he could not bring himself to write about it, lest he make an "unseemly show" of his feelings. On one occasion he wrote in his diary: "Something, I don't know what, is getting me down. This would not seem important if I could only put my finger on the trouble, but I can't find any single thing to account for the mood. Yet, it has been here and tonight for the first time I must admit that the problem of keeping my mind on an even keel is a serious one." At another time he wrote that he was conscious only of the solitude of his own forlornness, and then again: "This morning I had to admit to myself that I was lonely. Try as I may, I find I can't take my loneliness casually; it is too big. But I must not dwell upon it, otherwise I am undone." He had been alone for 43 days, and it is probable that physical hardship was a factor in his difficulties.

As to sensory deprivation, we know that the psychological integrity of a person is critically dependent upon continuous meaningful contact with his outside surroundings. The various incoming stimuli serve to alert the individual's higher brain centers where the messages are sorted and evaluated. When these messages cease, the mind is, after a fashion, cut adrift and regresses; time seems to disappear; and the mind produces its own images, often in the form of hallucinations. A number of students, paid well to undergo experimental situations in which they were deprived of all external sensory stimuli, were unable to continue the experiment for long, and this is understandable, for most of us have a fear of utter loneliness and of complete isolation. Admiral Byrd had also commented upon this. "That is where the conflict arises," he said. "I don't think a man can do without sounds and smells and voices and touch any more than he can do without calcium and phosphorus." Hence, you see how simple, everyday things, which we often regard as annoying, are important for our well being, and it is important to keep this fact in mind. Fatigue, i.e., the deadly fatigue of the forced march or continuous round-the-clock interrogation, can produce the same type of vivid imagery as is seen in sensory deprivation, and it can be either bizarre or realistic. One can remember the haunted look seen in pictures of the men who had been brainwashed in the real sense of the term. It is a while before they can talk about it, and then they try to dissociate themselves from the memories of it and keep it a secret from others and sometimes from themselves.

There are two other forms of loneliness which we shall simply mention before we consider the background of the problem and speak of the everyday garden variety of the subject. The first is the loneliness of command, noteworthy here because it is the prototype of the loneliness of the executive. The second is the loneliness of the forgotten men, and, unfortunately, of some of the aged in this present culture. Their plight is important, for their numbers are fated to increase. The duty and the power to command the fate and the lives of others is a terrible responsibility. Whoever assumes it must dismiss all thoughts of his own comfort and ease, if he is to be sincere and not a hireling. The captain of the ship is the prototype; his word is law and the responsibilities for lives and cargo rest squarely upon him. He cannot share or delegate this responsibility; it is his alone, and in the discharge of his duty he remains alone. The head of any group is more often than not lonely. He sacrifices his freedom and he knows no eight hour day, no hours on and no hours off, and not infrequently he carries his responsibility most poignantly throughout the night. Often he cannot talk freely nor share his doubts or fears with his subordinates. The final decisions are his and, if he must talk, he must talk to disinterested parties.

Lincoln was alone and often lonely. He was reviled and abused while he lived, and then enshrined in people's hearts after his death. All of the presidents have made difficult decisions alone. Decisions had to be made when the problem reached their level. The importance of the decisions which the president has to make alone is far-reaching and frightening. Government officials are not the only ones who suffer from overwork and loneliness, however, for business and professional men often are similarly affected, though on a scale less world shaking. The welfare of countless others is dependent upon them. They are by no means free persons, and even though their power and prestige may be envied by subordinates, the price they pay for it is rarely considered.

The loneliness of the aging and aged in this culture is well known to all of us. The man who was a pillar of the community and a respected business man and father of the family finds himself with time on his hands and the wretched feeling of no longer being needed. There are poignant stories of this type of loneliness. I mention them here in order to comment upon recent work which indicates that, in addition to the culture pushing the man aside, the man growing old also frequently disengages himself emotionally from his surroundings and withdraws with an increasing preoccupation with self. As the aging process continues, the individual withdraws further and participates in the creation of his own shrinking environment. This lessened desire for esteem and approval helps explain the self-centered behavior which many of these people exhibit. It is becoming more and more evident that successful aging consists in continuing middle-aged activities, even though the tendency to disengage and withdraw is a strong one. This is very important for all of us to keep in mind.

Ancestry of Feelings of Loneliness

As in comparable phenomena, there are all shades and degrees of loneliness, from the mild fleeting feelings we experience due more often than not to our own hurt feelings when someone does not pay proper attention to us, to the more serious degrees we mentioned earlier—from the pique which we experience when we feel sorry for ourselves to the haunting essential loneliness which is in our very being, for it is part of the fundamental basis of our nature. Some psychiatrists believe that there are two major divisions of loneliness. The first is the primary or existential loneliness which we just mentioned. This only occasionally becomes pressing, for the interdependencies and activities of our daily lives keep us busy and keep us from dwelling upon it. The second type, we are told, is caused by the loss or threatened loss of a loved object or something which is essential to us. This can be a person, money, position, status, or any physical or emotionally-tinged possession. The loss of position and status lowers a man in his own eyes more than does the loss of money, and some believe that he never completely recovers from it.

Well, we have mentioned various types of loneliness, but how do we get that way? How do we develop that type of loneliness which separates us from our fellow men? Sullivan believes it has its inception in infancy and it is agreed that if the infant's needs for tenderness and love remain ungratified or are prematurely interrupted, the child may recoil and substitute fantasy satisfactions and become a lonely child. Investigators have demonstrated conclusively the fatal influence of the lack of love and warmth and tenderness in our earliest years. A need for loving, protective care, delicately adjusted to the immediate situations, is imperative if the child is to thrive emotionally. This need continues into childhood but then an additional need arises for the interest and participation of significant adults in the child's world. They are important to the child and the way they interact with him will have great influence in the future.

Then come the juvenile years and in them there is a need for compeers and playmates. The child belongs to the group, is comfortable in it, and he knows no prejudice except what is instilled in him. Companions become indispensable models for him and the child learns by imitation, trial, and error. There is a great need for acceptance, a dread of ostracism, a wanting to be like others and to wear whatever others wear. There is a great fear of being excluded from accepted significant groups and situations. Here is the nucleus. Here is where loneliness can get a head start if things go wrong. Here is the scene of the little tragedies which are burnt deeply into sensitive souls and leave their marks forever.

Sullivan says that early in life we develop a curious capacity to fear what might be injurious, and an incredible sensitivity to significant people. It is only in pre-adolescence that our profound need for dealings with others reaches such a proportion that even fear and anxiety do not have the power to stop our stumbling into situations which really in some measure simply typify a relief from loneliness. There is much wisdom in this observation. It explains why a child will even compromise standards to avoid being excluded and left alone.

Then comes adolescence and, in addition to all of the various physiological stirrings going on within as the adolescent tries to find his place in the scheme of things, there comes the need for intimate exchange, for friendship, acceptance, and later, in its refined form, the need for social relationship with individuals of the opposite sex. This is the great structure which eventually becomes consolidated and made meaningful and which well might characterize not only late adolescence, but also the rest of the person's life. As one traces back into a patient's childhood for the sources of failure, one sometimes finds a non-acceptance of one's role as male or female for some reason or other. Along with it there are signs of unbearable resentment, hatred, and feelings of rejection by one or both parents. These reactions and the denial of essential features of the person's own being expose the individual to insecurity. He is torn by repeated conflict, as well as by repeated failures in his interpersonal relations. Should a desolate child withdraw into the fortress of defiant loneliness and pretend that he is self-sufficient and that no one can hurt him and that he "doesn't care" and "things do not matter," it will be difficult to get him to expose himself again to the possibility of rebuffs and frustration. He might, in fact, work out powerful compensation and learn to manipulate people as he learned to master himself in the things necessary for his survival. Physical deprivation alone produces some frustration, but it is not the most important thing. It is only when the child senses that the deprivation is a threat to his personality that he is emotionally distressed and lonely.

A child may be led to conform to the requirements of his environment through fear of loneliness, but if he has the proper love and closeness to his parents he will later take over their principles and standards by himself and on his own. But if the child is browbeaten in a precarious family situation, he remains secretly rebellious. He incorporates moral values only under pressure and then one day he may suddenly overthrow this imposed regime rebelliously, indignant about values which are foreign to him. One of the essential elements of maturity is the ability to establish a good relationship and positive ties to the worthwhile people and things in one's environment. Those who are unable to accomplish this remain tense, anxious, unhappy, and lonely. The unloved child is a lonely child, and he will grow into a lonely adult. If hatred enters the picture, this will be the well-spring of loneliness and, because of it, the individual will be unable to build a bridge to his fellow men. Hatred is a sterile, useless, pathetic, and wasteful reaction and its intrusion will prevent a person from loving his family or his fellows and from making meaningful contact with them.

If a child's inferiority, due to circumstances which isolate him from others or make him ashamed, becomes a problem, this will be a punishing experience. The person who carries a dread inferiority within him fights a constant battle. He has to use up so much of his energy in battling himself that he cannot give himself to others. Occupied as he is with criticism of himself, he cannot tolerate correction or criticism from the outside. His own cup is already full to overflowing and he can't stand any more of it. Hence the explosion which is sometimes seen following some small incident—no one expected it.

Thus the child and adolescent brings his personality, already fairly formed, into adult life with him. What happens now depends upon the people he meets and the circumstances he encounters. If the circumstances are propitious, he will grow and mature emotionally, if he can give of himself in his various relationships. If they are not, he may have trouble and may even isolate himself from the group.

Now, what about the ordinary, garden variety of loneliness that is close to home? We probably should spend a lot of time upon the reactions of the basically lonely people whom one encounters in office or shop, but if we remember the essentials we have just mentioned we can fill in the details for ourselves. Just as each person is different, so too is each occupation; so we may draw our own conclusions. There are the chronically angry, the chronically belligerent, and the bitter who have isolated themselves psychologically from their fellow men. Something has happened somewhere along the line and they consistently feel that they are not getting a square deal.

The bores, the egoists, and the hypochondriacs can be more of a problem. They are defending themselves against inferiority and loneliness and they sometimes nest in the hair of their fellow workers. Lacking insight and sensitivity, they fail to see that they are their own most serious problem. They want new jobs in new places, not recognizing that their problems are built in and a change simply means that they will appear again in the new location, someone else will be blamed, and it will be time to move again.

Of all of the difficult persons we encounter, perhaps the extreme egoist is the most difficult to get on with, for he is hiding his fears and his loneliness under a multitude of disguises. He feels alone and afraid and, to compensate for these feelings, he turns all of his attention upon himself. No one must be permitted to know of his fears or his inferiority feelings. He fails to realize that in our present culture the opinions of no one can be absolute, but he is under pressure to be infallible. To obviate all chances of detection, he controls situations and conversations. His is a continuous push to aggrandize himself and make up for his inner insecurity. Some of these distressed folks will tie people to them by an insistent, persistent generosity and on the surface they will help people. You will always be able to tell those who are their beneficiaries, however; you can detect them by their haunted look.

The background reasons for the reactions of these individuals, as well as those of the super-sensitive persons in the home, factory, or office who are continually taking offense, and those of the suspicious who are forever on the alert so that no one puts anything over on them, the quarrelsome, the bores, and the other problem children, all would become plain to us if only we knew of the elements which contributed to their loneliness and their efforts to avoid it.

There are various subtle ways of trying to insure against feeling lonely; some of them are destructive. As one girl says: "Mother controlled the family and kept them close to her by her sweetness and her readily available heart attacks." Another was held close to home by mother's indigestion as soon as she showed signs of getting away. Almost miraculously she recovered as soon as the daughter's plans were cancelled. Psychiatrists speak sometimes of a separation anxiety which is really a fear of loneliness or of failure. It is legitimate and it appears when one has been in a specified, protected atmosphere for some time and must make a break from it for a new situation.

Some forms of alcoholism are escapes from loneliness, and in this illness a man even hides his true feelings from himself. Once well established in alcoholism as an escape and a refuge from insecurity, inferiority, guilt, or loneliness, however, the individual does not give it up easily. He conceals it, denies it, nurtures it, and gets cross at those who suggest he is a problem drinker. Incidentally, one of the reasons why Alcoholics Anonymous is able to help these individuals when other efforts fail lies in the fact that they recognize the sufferer's intense loneliness and they make efforts to socialize him and return him to the group. Compulsive overeating is another way of avoiding feelings of loneliness; it wreaks havoc with some patients and their families, although not to the degree that alcohol does. These individuals are functioning on an infantile level, and while overeating they are also getting back at some significant member of the family in this concealed fashion.

We certainly should not dwell too long on the unfortunate aspects of feelings of loneliness, however, for to be alone can be a blessed and useful experience, provided of course it is not tinged with any form of self-pity. Many artists are devoted servants of their loneliness; they are liberated by their creative work. Many times men have been driven to creative efforts by physical illness. Thomas Wolfe remarked that, "if man is to know the triumphant labor of creation, he must resign himself to long periods of loneliness." This holds true not only in art, but in all creative endeavors.

Many business and professional men suffer feelings of anxiety and loneliness because of their failure to get out in front. In this culture many contestants feel that they must place first, whatever the handicap, and that if they do not, they are complete failures. This attitude can ruin good men, particularly if they become at all envious or bitter. Wood says: "Happily for the solidarity of modern society, the threat of isolation does not always fall upon the envious, who would destroy what they cannot have, or upon the weak, who cannot face difficulties." Sometimes, as Bacon noted, "it lights upon an individual who honorably accepts the challenge laid down to him." And Emerson said: "A man's defects are made useful to him and he draws strength from his weakness and, like the wounded oyster, mends his shell with pearl." It is obvious that there are a large number of healthy, compensatory mechanisms open to everyone who refrains from pitying himself and feeling so alone.

It is said that the conquest of loneliness can be accomplished by all who are willing to find and destroy two foes and obstacles which are at the bottom of the trouble: they are inordinate self-love and hostility. Both make it impossible to communicate properly with people in the environment and render one unable to see or feel a real relationship with others. In examining himself when feeling terribly alone, Admiral Byrd said with rare insight: "The most likely explanation of the trouble lies within myself. Manifestly, if I can harmonize the various things within me that may be in conflict and fit myself more smoothly in the environment, I shall be at peace." This is the essence of this presentation; it would be a wonderful thing if more of us could believe this simple statement [or—subscribe to this simple truth:] "The most likely explanation of the trouble lies within myself."

Then there was one more thing which the same man thought and entered in his diary as he contemplated almost certain death after 43 days of isolation and loneliness. "At the end only two things matter to a man," he wrote, "regardless of who he is, and they are the affection and understanding of his family. Anything and everything else he creates are insubstantial. They are given over to the mercy of the winds and tides of prejudice, but the family is an everlasting anchorage, a quiet harbor where a man's ship can be left to sway to the moorings of pride and loyalty." Some of us would add a spiritual belief to that, but otherwise would let it stand as it is.

None of this is intended to encourage a lack of drive that might hold back our progress. It is simply to say that a man should carefully survey the situation in which he finds himself, decide where his various paths might lead him, and what his choice will cost him, and then make up his mind as to which way he will go. Ambition kept in bounds is consistent with a normal family life and a reasonable, happy existence, and all of this fits in with a reasonable, dedicated work pattern.

As to isolation—if I were given to composing slogans I would emphasize one, namely: *"Keep your lines of communication open."* Communication is the tie line that binds us to others; it is a safeguard against misunderstanding and the accidental rupturing of relationships. Once that line is impeded, neglected, or broken off in anger, our chances of reaching agreement with others are materially lessened and misunderstanding or misinterpretation is inevitable. Think of it, perhaps, as we do of the red telephone in the White House, the so-called "hot line" to Moscow, itself a most unlikely *terminus ad quem.* It is kept open at all times for emergency communication and it represents protection against failure of understanding, the kind of misunderstanding that could set off a major conflict. I suggest that it is necessary for individuals also to keep a hot line open at all times with family, friends, and fellow workers, no matter how tense a situation may be or how great may seem the provocation to disrupt communications.

Communication is not a function that is confined to what we know as civilized human society; it is a function that is very evident in all living things. The human animal, of course, is capable of more advanced methods of communication; he can do more than utter sounds. And, perhaps, it is just this state of higher development that accounts for the difficulties that he gets into in his daily experience with others. Man's ability to use words, whether in speech or writing, can act as a barrier to understanding, hiding his true thoughts and feelings as often as it reveals them. Psychiatrists, by the way, are particularly aware of the use of this subterfuge, for frequently they interview people who use words to conceal their problems and their real thoughts.

One final word to those of us who would like to get away from it all and be alone. We should realize that it is hard to do that. People cover the world, including the Pacific Islands. The only chance for escape is into space. And yet no place in the universe is so hospitable to us as the planet earth with its thin layer of enveloping, nurturing air and its hordes of annoying, *necessary* people. In the poem "Birches," Robert Frost said, "Earth's the right place for love: I don't know where it's likely to go better"—recognizing that not only are we physiologically dependent on our surroundings and companions, we are also strongly attached to them psychologically. Dr. Phil Solomon of the Boston City Hospital tells us: "Recent experiments show that the presence of a stranger in the sensory deprivation tests causes less serious aberrations." And, he says, the presence of a close associate or a member of the family —a wife, for example—is even more salutary. If most of our troubles on earth are caused by people, most of our troubles in space will, apparently, be caused by the lack of them.

It behooves us, therefore, to get along with and to understand our family, our friends, and those with whom we work. None of us can dispense with people. None of us is proof against loneliness. Should we begin to think we are sufficient unto ourselves and consequently unassailable, we would do well to recall Lowell's dictum:

> Console yourself, dear man and brother, whatever you may be sure of, be sure at least of this: that you are dreadfully like other people. Human nature has a much greater genius for sameness than originality.

REFERENCE

1. *Emotions and Sensibility in Ages of Anxiety* by George Rosen, M.D. A Comparative Historical Review, American Journal of Psychiatry Vol. 124, No. 6, December 1967.

2

A. RUSSELL ANDERSON, M.D.

*It is with much personal satisfaction that I make this
contribution to the Festschrift in honor of Dr. Bartemeier
upon his 75th birthday. Hope for man, with an interest in
every aspect of the individual and communal life, represents both his basic philosophy and his wide sphere of
activities during a vigorous and productive life.*

Some Considerations of Psychoanalysis and Other Therapies

THE VERY TITLE of this volume, "Hope: Psychiatry's Commitment,"
with its various related chapters, immediately foreshadows the breadth of
scope necessary for any consideration of the particular remedial efforts appropriate to a particular instance. In an ever-changing world, which is in so
many respects different from that of thirty years ago, we must be careful
to assess and reassess what is good for the race and society, and what is
good for a given person as he tries to live within this larger setting.

We know that not infrequently certain remedies are sought by the
individual because they have become popular or fashionable and allegedly
will produce the desired effect by a hidden magic. Within this category we
might consider the faith healers, certain routines of exercise, physio-
therapy, dietary fashions, and numerous drugs, as well as the more
bizarre methods of treatment such as Wilhelm Reich's orgone box, or
even the fad of Couéism which was so popular around nineteen-twenty.
As unsound and illogical as such practices are, they may lead to transitory
or prolonged spans of life which seem to be paved with gold. So, we are
always faced with what man is seeking, what compromises he will accept
and to what degree the rational and logical are available or acceptable to
the individual or the group.

In this short paper, I shall confine myself to a consideration of some types of psychological treatment which are designed for the individual. My aims are to discuss:

(1) The main features of psychoanalysis with its special emphasis on the understanding of man's inner life;

(2) those therapies which are based on the premise that man's behavior is explainable primarily in terms of his physiology or the external milieu; and

(3) those therapies which may be viewed as gradations between the two extremes outlined in (1) and (2).

Throughout, I shall consider the factor of transference, which in psychoanalysis is a therapeutic tool of prime importance, but which also plays a varying role, both qualitatively and quantitatively, in these other therapies.

I shall not attempt to outline the history or development of psychoanalysis, but shall briefly delineate its essential goals and methods of operation. Psychoanalysis rests upon a solid foundation of clinical observation. This has led to a body of theoretical knowledge which endeavors to explain the psychic make-up of man. It gives due weight to the constitutional matrix and the genetic course of maturation and development as shaped by internal biological and psychic forces in combination with external experience. These factors will determine the particular psychological constellation of each individual which, in turn, will determine his interactions with the external world and their relationships to his own inner experience.

Psychoanalysis combines the scientific study of man and his development with a technique of therapy aimed at the modification of those psychological abnormalities, defects, and conflicts which have arisen during the individual's long period of life leading to maturity. Psychoanalysis is based upon an exploration of inner psychic life. Only parts of this inner life are apparent to the observer and, under usual circumstances, much of it is hidden from the individual, himself. To bring it into more extended awareness, we rely on the one hand on the patient's introspection, free associations, and dreams; and on the other hand, on the analyst's empathy, intuition, and background of scientific knowledge.

Ideally, the psychoanalytic situation enables this inner life to reveal itself in a way that is unencumbered by influences and distortions imposed by the analyst, whose only purpose is to help the patient gain awareness of the meaning of his past experiences and to bring these into relation with his present life. Man's earliest experiences are never really erased, but still exist in the unconscious and exert a continuing but changing influence not only on his intra-psychic conflicts but also on his modes of adaptation and adjustment.

What is essential to this psychoanalytic situation if it is to be one in which our observations are to achieve an optimal degree of validity? Since the object of investigation is something as four-dimensional and complex as man, our technique must be as precise as possible. From one angle, the analytic room may be likened to a laboratory where the object of study lies on a couch, unable to see the observer who sits in a chair behind him. But, as pointed out by Lewin and Stone,[11,16] from another angle this analogy breaks down. For the object of investigation is not a corpse to be dissected, but a living reacting human being who is driven by the need for help to seek, to trust, and to reveal himsel to another real person. It is in this context that a relationship develops in which the patient becomes strongly attached to the analyst and manifests continuing and varying attitudes toward him. These attitudes, often complex, seemingly irrational, and painful for the patient, are repetitions of relationships rooted in the past which are now experienced anew in connection with the analyst. And it is these attitudes which we subsume under the term, transference. Transference supplies us with one of our major sources of knowledge about the patient's relationships with the original love objects of his childhood and hence facilitates our understanding of the patterning and texture of his current object relationships. Nonetheless, it is also the source of much of the analyst's difficulty and of many of his mistakes as he tries to help the patient to become aware of its ideational and affective content, and to reconstruct the story it has to tell. I shall return to this problem a little later.

It may be said that psychoanalysis has a dual role in that it serves both a therapeutic and an investigative or research aim. It functions as a scientific discipline with a study of the individual psyche in a multi-dimensional approach which encompasses five factors: the dynamic, the economic, the genetic, the structural, and the adaptive. This method of examination of each psychic problem from five different vantages has been designated as the metapsychological approach. The dynamic factor was the earliest one to be defined and refers to the interaction of psychic forces. The economic factor is essentially a quantitative one and deals with psychic energies in terms of their distribution and balance. The genetic factor entails the knowledge gained through memory and reconstructions of the interaction between past significant events and inner phantasy life and the way in which this interaction has influenced the course of development and pathology. The structural approach, which is fundamental and basic to an understanding of psychic activity, defines and studies the three psychic structures whose nature and origin are different and which interact with each other in various ways: namely the Ego, Superego, and Id. The adaptive factor attempts to assess the various ways in which the psyche uses its resources and functions to adapt to the external world as well as to certain internal needs and problems.

Inasmuch as the structural approach is a prerequisite for the comprehension of inter-psychic conflict, it would seem fitting to elaborate on it in some detail. It is true that our sphere of study consists solely of psychic phenomena. The biological matrix from which, a priori, the psychic drives arise is an unknown entity although it may account for those seemingly innate differences in individual drive endowment. We divide these drive derivatives broadly into two categories: the libidinal and the aggressive. The Id is that psychic structure which is the site of the psychic drives.

In order to satisfy the needs arising from the drives or to control them and defer satisfaction, man must develop a complex psychic structure which we refer to as the Ego. To accomplish this purpose, the Ego must have a knowledge of the external world, of the body and its functions, and of the self and the needs which seek fulfillment. It possesses certain innate autonomous functions such as perception, memory, the ability to learn, control of motor functions, and varying degrees of ability to integrate and synthesize experience. It must gradually develop other important functions such as control of impulses, sense of time and space, differentiation of the internal and external world, and the development of object relationships, i.e., a meaningful relationship with another person. Certain internal mechanisms will be developed which will serve as defenses against inacceptable impulses. It will also develop particular character traits which are firmly structured and serve a defensive function as well as a source of satisfaction. In order to implement these many functions, the Ego possesses a store of energy which is neutral in nature and available for any purpose. What is more, the aggressive destructive drives of the Id may become in part neutralized and thus become a source of energy at the service of the Ego.[9] Much of the Ego, including its defenses, is unconscious.

As I have attempted to imply, the many functions of the Ego make it possible for the individual to become aware of his endogenous drives and affects and develop methods for their control and deployment. It also is responsible for a detailed knowledge of the external world. Yet, given these abilities, we are still confronted with the fact that we have not explained the presence of a certain part of the Ego which is well organized and essentially functions as a separate structure. It possesses a well-established code of ethics by which it judges the actions and even the impulses and phantasies of the person. It exerts a continual influence through its power to evoke guilt and self-punishment or bestow gratifying approval. This part of the Ego is called the Superego. It may be poorly developed or the Ego may find ways of avoiding its influence.

These basic psychic structures may have differing constitutional potentials for development which gradually evolve in an "average expectable environment."[8] If we have markedly abnormal components in the biological substratum, in the external environment, or in the psychic structures themselves, pathology generally will arise.

Psychoanalysis finds that the inner psychic life of the individual has a basic continuity and that an understanding of the present inner life and behavior of the individual entails a detailed study of the entire life experience in the external world and in particular the relationships to other people. At the same time, these experiences must be viewed in respect to the significance and particular interpretation they are given in the internal psychic life where phantasies are ever-present and distortions, omissions, or denials will play an important role in shaping the full autobiography of the individual. As a result, we are faced with the fact that the inner experience, as well as the external behavior, are dependent upon the proper development of the functions of the Ego with its deployment of the drives and energy in such ways as will lead to mature satisfaction and solution of internal conflicts. We could say that pathology always implies either certain Ego or Superego deficits or a state of conflict or imbalance between certain inner structures and drives. It would follow that in psychoanalysis our goal would include more than relief of some symptom or increased satisfaction in the individual's life. Its main endeavor would be to bring about actual changes within the structure of the psyche and a re-allocation of energies so that more mature object relationships would be possible. In the process, crippling defense or character traits would be relinquished and the individual would be capable of a freedom to fulfill his needs and be aware of his phantasies. He could then develop a degree of objectivity that would allow an assessment of other people on the basis of reality, and they would not be experienced on the basis of repetitions from the past.

Let me briefly mention certain important aspects of the biographical study. The work of Mahler,[12] Spitz,[15] and Greenacre,[7] has given us new insights into the first three years of life. The infant must gradually differentiate itself from the mother and pass through a symbiotic period of existence to a definite individuation as a separate person. Thus, external and internal become distinguishable on the basis of a child's ego development to the point where his self-representations and object representations achieve some degree of stability and constancy. Simultaneous with ego development, and continuing through life, is the constant problem of the drives, which undergo changes in accordance with the well-known and predetermined courses of libidinal phase development.

The mother is the first important object toward whom the child will develop a number of different and ambivalent attitudes which will be accompanied by strong affects. The father soon assumes importance as the other main pillar in the fulfillments and conflicts of life. In fact, the basic attitudes and conflicts are built around mother, father, and siblings, and reflect the specific details of these relationships.

I shall now return to a consideration of Transference. In the analytic situation, there will be increasing evidence of various reactions and attitudes toward the analyst which will appear directly or be evident in his associations and dreams. Many of these reactions to the analyst will be inappropriate, both in relation to their content and their affective intensity, so that they are readily identified as transference reactions. As previously implied, the transference manifestations provide one of the main sources of information which makes possible the reconstruction of early object relationships.

Transference, as a basic phenomenon determining man's behavior in his object relationships, was early recognized by Freud[1,2,3,4,5] and has been carefully studied and stressed in the development of psychoanalysis. In fact, the transference reactions recapitulate the important relationships of the individual from the time he emerged as a separate being with a separate internal structure and with the ability to cathect and relate to other people. The content of these early relationships with their specific reactions, attitudes, affects and conflicts, as well as the defensive processes which serve to conceal or distort them, are to a large extent unconscious even though they enter into, and to a great extent determine, the attitudes and reactions in various phases of the individual's life. To a greater or lesser degree, they will determine the choice of people who will become important to him, as well as the interaction and type of relationships that will ensue. They are responsible for his repetitive life experiences which show an uncanny similarity to one another and which he will tend to explain as due to chance or the external environment. In other words, the individual tends to repeat his early relationships to his parents, siblings, and other important people in his life with remarkable exactitude. At times, he may be aware that he is seeking another mother or father similar to his own and that his conflicts and aggressions are repetitions of what ensued in these early and primary relationships. For the most part, however, their origin is hidden from him.

Transference reactions occur in some measure in all of our meaningful relationships with other people. Their intensity and breadth will depend upon the extent to which the individual has become independent and separated himself psychologically from the early attachments to people, such as mother and father, who were essential to his development and who may still retain a continued importance in his unconscious life. It will also depend on the degree to which the individual has a well-established set of ego functions such as a sense of reality, an ability to be objective, and more mature ways of gratifying essential needs. Then he will be more able to meet and know other people on the basis of a real objective appraisal and determine what type of relationship is mutually possible.

As I have said, transference is an ever-present part of life although, for the most part, it is not perceived by the patient or the people around him unless it leads to noticeably inappropriate behavior. Since it plays such an important role in the psychoanalytic understanding of the patient and his treatment, the psychoanalytic situation is set up in such a way that regression will occur and transference toward the analyst encouraged to develop. We must be careful to provide a situation where the transference reactions are not appropriate to the analyst so that they can be differentiated as transference and related to the appropriate source. This in turn leads us to a consideration of the analyst himself, who may have unresolved transference problems which can alter or interfere with the psychoanalytic situation.

I wish to stress again that in psychoanalysis we assume a complete continuity in the life of each individual. As Kris[10] has pointed out, "the past emerges into the present," and the past and present are the two extremes or poles of a continuum in the changing biography. Current behavior has a history and definite set of determinants that can be unearthed and placed in proper juxtaposition by a careful study through the analytic process.

Since transference is a reflection of these earlier relationships, it is of special importance for two reasons. In relation to theory and our under-

616.89   H771p
C.1

standing of the individual, it can be an important source of information about his early relationships which are not available in his memories. In relation to therapy, it is of crucial importance because only through a reexperiencing of the past with insight and conviction can the individual become free of these early object relationships so that his new object relationships will be established upon the basis of his ability to perceive and maintain objectivity toward his current experience and observations.

While transference is almost always present and can be at least partially understood by the analyst, it does not follow that the patient can gain insight with convictions so that the transference can be seen as part of the past rather than experienced as current reality. In the psychotic and borderline patient, the repetitions of the past relationships are often experienced as the current reality and are not subject to any permanent change. For example, the analyst is experienced as though he were the real father or mother. Deficiencies in certain functions of the ego, such as the sense of reality, inability to form solid object relationships, and lack of essential controls, make psychoanalysis and working through of the transference impossible.

The development of psychoanalysis was dependent upon the discovery of a new process, namely, the psychoanalytic method which made it possible to study the internal psychic life of man. I would like to consider briefly other methods of understanding man's life and behavior which do not consider in detail or tend to negate the significance of the internal psychic life.

The physiological approach is well delineated in the book "The Conditioning Therapies" edited by Wolpe, Salter, and Reyna. The research work of Pavlov and Bechterev on the conditioned reflex in animals provides the basic theory for this approach. Dr. Wolpe[18] states that "These methods stem from the conception that neuroses are persistent maladaptive habits that have been conditioned. There is persuasive evidence, both experimental and clinical, that the great majority of neuroses are fundamentally conditioned autonomic responses. . . . Experimentally it is possible to condition an animal to respond with anxiety to any stimulus one pleases," so that "one can obtain an emotional habit that is utterly refractory to extermination in the ordinary way. In human neuroses, one can usually elicit a history of similar kinds of conditioning." These findings led to the framing of the reciprocal inhibition principle of psychotherapy.

Dr. Salter[14] writes as follows: "Psychological events are physiological events, and conditioning is the modification of tissue by experience. But since our knowledge of these changes is incomplete, we manufacture psychological hypotheses. We do not want psychology to be a science of sterile abstractions. . . . Maladjustment is malconditioning, and psychotherapy is reconditioning. The individual's problems are a result of his social experience and by changing his technique of social relationships, we change his personality. We are not especially concerned with giving the individual stratified knowledge of his past—called 'probing.' What concerns us is giving him reflex knowledge for the future—called 'habits.' "

Early life and the period of growth and maturation would have no influence other than their lasting effects upon the physiology of the body and the establishment of particular conditioned reflexes. The essence of object relationships would be the presence of appropriate reactions, responses, and affective experiences to another person. The concept of transference would not exist.

The purely sociological approach would consider the individual from the viewpoint of the influence of the social milieu within which he has developed and lived. It would study the culture and the group patterns which would be assumed to have shaped and structured the behavior of the person and the particular way in which individual psychic mechanisms would be employed. The individual's actions, verbal responses, and affects would be modes of behavior to be understood and evaluated in relation to his culture and its particular norms and values. Upon this basis, his degree of adjustment or pathology would be determined. It is a simple conception of man and his external world which was portrayed in many 19th century novels and biographies. As Erich Fromm[6] states, "Common to all these theories is the assumption that human nature has no dynamisms of its own and that psychological changes are to be understood in terms of the development of new 'habits' as an adaptation to new cultural patterns. These theories, though speaking of the psychological, at the same time reduce it to a shadow of cultural patterns."

This external and sociological viewpoint would lead to an approach in which the interests of mankind and society would be the prime consideration in the evaluation and treatment of each individual. A man would be judged by his actions, and life would revolve around simple and definite purposes which would be self-evident on the basis of a well-formed religious conviction, current social values or strong patriotic commitments. Little attention would be paid to deeper psychological motivations or their origins which would be deemed irrelevant. Man would be viewed as a specific part or cog in a larger over-all social group or institution where his role would be determined by the structure of society at that particular time and place. This could possibly lead to a stable culture such as the Egyptians enjoyed for two thousand years. It is well exemplified in successful military structures or certain religious communities where for centuries an unchanged social structure is maintained.

At the present time, this sociological frame of reference is relevant to certain controlled societies as exemplified by the communistic countries or those subject to a dictatorship. Even in the large industrial areas there are certain social groups where individual expression is a hindrance and cause of dissension. Within such a milieu, education and conditioning would be the acknowledged methods of psychotherapy. There would be a response to the group or the leaders based upon the repetitions of early attitudes to the father and mother with varying degrees of compliance or rebellion. The therapist, with his authoritative positions, would accomplish his purpose by a stern or benevolent attitude. Inner freedom to develop as an autonomous individual would be pathological for all but the leaders.

Most psychotherapy would not be determined by these points of view in which only the physiological or sociological factors would be of importance. Likewise, it would not follow the path of psychoanalysis, although recognizing the importance of man's psychic life and the fact that he is influenced and shaped by his early life and interaction with other people. The main emphasis would be placed upon psychotherapy as a goal itself, rather than upon the development of a procedure which is a vehicle for the complete study of man's internal life and at the same time may function as a method of therapy.

H. S. Sullivan[17] says:

> As psychobiology seeks to study the individual human being, and as cultural anthropology seeks to study the social heritage, so psychiatry seeks to study the biologically and culturally conditioned, but *sui generis*, interpersonal processes occurring in the interpersonal situations in which the observant psychiatrist does his work. . . . Personality is the relatively enduring pattern of recurrent interpersonal situations which characterize a human life.

Man is viewed as part of an interpersonal situation rather than as a separate entity and the importance of adequate inter-communication is stressed.

The innate, biologically determined structures, potential reactions and responses are shaped into definitive patterns or dynamisms as a result of the specific interpersonal experiences. While the importance of child-hood experience is acknowledged, it is in terms of the development of interpersonal patterns, so that there is no need for a detailed knowledge of the internal life and the autobiography of the particular individual. The individual is always viewed in terms of the actual present interaction with a specific person and the interplay of the two personalities. As a result, there would not be an emphasis on the understanding of transfer-ence which could not be isolated because of the lack of neutrality on the part of the therapist. Instead of a study of the internal psychic life of the individual, the emphasis is upon the interaction of the patient and therapist in a current situation where unhealthy patterns would be worked with as defective methods of interpersonal adjustment rather than as parts of the psychic structure which must be studied so that psychic changes can follow.

The central emphasis in most psychotherapy is based upon the social and interpersonal factors as they appear in the patient's life and in his contacts with the therapist. The particular aspect of man's development which would lead to specific problems within his unfolding life would be viewed differently by various schools of psychotherapy or individual therapists. Alfred Adler[13] placed the point of emphasis upon the feelings of inferiority in the child due to organic defects or environmental factors which would lead to competitive strivings for power to assuage this inferiority complex. The initial helplessness of the child would lead to a drive for superiority, power, and prestige. The therapeutic endeavors would be directed to a "common-sense current approach" with open encouragement by the therapist.

K. Horney[13] would emphasize the helplessness of the infant leading to a basic experience of anxiety, i.e., his sense of being isolated in an un-friendly world. Otto Rank [13] predicated his approach upon the trauma of birth and the need for the individual to develop the will to accomplish a separation and develop as an individual. There is the more recent existential approach where the point of emphasis is upon the confronta-tion of the individual with his basic current experience and its accom-panying anxiety and guilt so that he can come to terms with himself, the basic facts of existence, and the people with whom he lives.

I have tried to outline in a very brief way certain essential aspects of psychoanalysis and other psychotherapeutic approaches which exist and are possible with our current ways of thinking and perceiving man. We must confess that our success in therapy is limited but at the same time recognize that this should be expected in a rapidly changing world. Psychoanalysis, with its unique method of studying man's internal psychic life, has striven to apply this method in a carefully scientific way in order to acquire an exact body of knowledge and fact upon which to base its theories. I would say that this is the primary purpose of the analytic method, and its major contribution. Its secondary purpose is to develop a sound method of therapy. In relation to its use as a therapy, we must recognize the limitations of such a basic and scientifically orientated approach, and decide when the purpose of therapy will be better served by the introduction of parameters and compromises—in which case we speak of it as psychoanalytically oriented psychotherapy.

The conditioning therapies are based upon a truly scientific approach to the physiological functions of the body as developed in the work by Pavlov and Bechterev. On the other hand, these therapies exclude any real consideration of man's psychic life and interaction with other individuals so that they present a biased and limited view of man. This does not mean that the method employed may not have a limited usefulness in a pragmatic way, but it does follow that we justly question the basis of the therapeutic success that is claimed—that is, whether it proceeds from the therapeutic processes described or from other factors not recognized in the oversimplified theory and approach. Success *may* be due to suggestion or the ever-present influence of transference reactions toward the therapist and his pronouncements.

We might well ask two questions about every psychotherapeutic system: 1) To what degree does it arise from a nontherapeutically oriented but carefully scientific study of man, and 2) to what degree are its origin and goal directly motivated by a purely therapeutic orientation where scientific considerations are considered to be valuable but quite secondary to the practical and pragmatic problems of the individual. The latter approach (which characterizes many psychotherapeutic endeavors) has resulted in a body of accumulated clinical observations which can be relied upon to bring clinical improvement in many situations.

REFERENCES

1. Freud, S., (1905). "Fragments of an Analysis of a Case of Hysteria." C.P., 7, pp. 116-120.
2. ———— (1912). "The Dynamics of Transference." C.P. 12.
3. ———— (1914). "Remembering, Repeating, and Working Through." C.P., 12.
4. ———— (1915). "Observations on Transference-Love." C.P., 12.
5. ———— (1916-17). "Introductory Lectures on Psychoanalysis." C.P., 16, pp. 431-447.

6. Fromm, E., *Escape from Freedom.* p. 14. (New York: Farrar & Rinehart, 1941.)
7. Greenacre, P., (1960). "The Parent-Infant Relationship." Int. J. of Psychoanalysis.
8. Hartman, H., *Ego Psychology and the Problem of Adaptation.* p. 23 (New York: Int. Universities Press, 1959.)
9. ———— "Notes on the Theory of Sublimation." *Psychoanalytic Study of the Child.* Vol. 10. (New York: Int. Universities Press, 1956.)
10. Kris, E., "The Recovery of Childhood Memories in Psychoanalysis." p. 59. *Psychoanalytic Study of the Child.* (New York: Int. Universities Press, 1956.)
11. Lewin, B., "Counter-Transference in the Technique of Medical Practice." Psychosomatic Medicine. Vol. 8, pp. 195-200.
12. Mahler, M., *On Human Symbiosis and the Vicissitudes of Individuation.* pp. 7-31. (New York: Int. Universities Press, 1968.)
13. Monroe, R., *Schools of Psychoanalytic Thought.* (New York: Holt, Rinehart & Winston, Inc., 1955.) Adler, A., pp. 337-343. Horney, pp. 343-349. Rank, pp. 576-594.
14. Salter, A., "The Theory and Practice of Conditioned Reflex Therapy." *The Conditioning Therapies.* pp. 23-25. New York: Holt, Rinehart & Winston, Inc., 1965.)
15. Spitz, R., *The First Year of Life.* (New York: Int. Universities Press, 1965.)
16. Stone, L., *The Psychoanalytic Situation.* pp. 12-17. (New York: Int. Universities Press, 1961.)
17. Sullivan, H., *The Interpersonal Theory of Psychiatry.* pp. 20, 110-111. (New York: Norton & Co., 1953.)
18. Wolpe, J., "The Comparative Clinical Status of Conditioning Therapies and Psychoanalysis." *The Conditioning Therapies.* pp. 9-10. (New York: Holt, Rinehart & Winston, Inc., 1965.)

3

JOHN C. WHITEHORN, M.D.

To my good friend, Leo Bartemeier, to honor his many years of able service in the care of troubled people, and in appreciation of the fidelity and grace with which he has fulfilled those responsibilities—truly a mature person.

A Working Concept of Maturity of Personality

THE PSYCHIATRIST does his clinical work in a particularly personal mode. Like other physicians he is concerned with infectious diseases, toxins, metabolic disturbances, congenital anomalies, genetic handicaps, and other relatively impersonal factors or processes which hinder people in coping with life situations. But the psychiatrist has a particularly strong interest in the patient's personal experience of coping, and in the possibilities of helping the patient cope with life with greater effectiveness and with less distress. All physicians, concerned with the health and welfare of their patients, have an interest in restoring their patients' self-confidence and effectiveness, but it is the psychiatrist who has this concern as the central point of his professional task.

Psychiatric patients in general are not coping effectively with their personal life situations. In general, the disability and distress which bring the patient to a psychiatrist are manifestations of some ineffectiveness or disturbance in social functioning. The psychiatric patient, in attempting to cope with his life situation, is characteristically using an unsuitable pattern of reaction—often grossly unsuitable. It is somewhat

Reprinted with permission of the *American Journal of Psychiatry*, Vol. 119, pp. 197-202, 1962. Copyright © 1962, the American Psychiatric Association.

inaccurate to say "attempting to cope with his life situation," for the patient often is not really coping with life, but only posturing, that is, demonstrating a pattern or attitude which has little or no useful effect in his life situation, but in which he persists. The attentive study of the patient's pattern of reaction, considered in relation to his life situation and personal biography, will often reveal that his current non-useful pattern of behavior has much relevance for some earlier issue in his life, unresolved at that prior time. As a clinician, eager to gain a useful understanding of psychiatric patients and their problems, I have found much help in the concept of "unfinished business." Intensive study may reveal that the current life situation, as the patient has been experiencing it, contains for him this older issue, and in this sense his mode of reaction has some relevance. To an outsider's commonsense view, the patient's behavior or feelings appear quite inappropriate. His behavior is very likely to be misunderstood by those with whom he is reacting so that he fails to be constructively effective, except as he may gain from others some dependency, protection and care, by reason of his distress and disability. Even the psychiatric expert may have difficulty in understanding the issue, as the patient experiences it.

The repetitive, ineffectual pattern manifested by the psychiatric patient is usually at first observation a puzzling phenomenon. Seeking appropriate words to describe the patient's behavior, one may at times resort to terms like "childish," or "infantile," or "adolescent." I recall, for example, a middle-aged woman patient, in a morose and gloomy state, who forcefully told me, "I'm no baby. I know what I want, and I want what I want when I want it." This statement has always seemed to me a beautifully clear-cut expression of an infantile attitude.

Such clinical characterizations of a patient's attitudes as immature have seemed to me at times very apt. They deserve careful study and systematic formulation—a task which has engaged much of my interest for some years.

When, a few decades ago, I began to give serious attention to this problem, there was ready to hand Sigmund Freud's beautifully clear and simple formulation of levels of immaturity, set forth in terms of his theory of libidinal determinism. This was the theory of erogenous zones, and of the fixation of libidinal interest at the oral, the anal, or the genital phase of psycho-sexual development. But this Freudian formulation seemed to me much oversimplified, and often quite beside the point. For me the significance of words connoting a level of maturity is that they indicate a concern with attitudes about responsibility and authority, only tangentially related to the libidinal interest with which Freud was so strongly preoccupied. The practically useful meaning of *maturity* or *immaturity* is centered, as I see it, on the humanly inescapable problems of leadership, authority and responsibility—inescapable because man is a domestic and social animal. The domestic and social patterns of living, which constitute the human way of living, contain inherently the problem of leadership. Freud was not altogether wrong, I think, in relating infantile attitudes to the mouth and anus. Weaning and toilet training are among the earliest experiences involving authority and frustration by other human beings. "Unfinished business" in respect to these issues is often encountered in the psychiatrist's work. But the original Freudian formulations here were somewhat misleading in placing all motivational emphasis upon libidinal interests.

In formulating our conceptions of human nature, we of the late nineteenth and early twentieth centuries have been strongly influenced by the Darwinian revolution. Psychology has become a subdivision of biology —"Psychobiology" as Adolf Meyer called it. Mentation got a functional orientation; perception, cognition, affect and conation were freshly conceived as preparatory aspects of behavior. That was all to the good, in my opinion. But in the early post-Darwinian enthusiasm for biologizing human nature, excesses occurred. Instinct theories, for example, were pushed to disproportionate extremes. Freud based his formulations of personality development upon the sexual instinct, on the basis of certain clinical observations and inferences. Yet, instinct is but a fragment in the life of man. In regard to instinctive endowment man is far surpassed by many animal species. Each human being is born weak and helpless and survives only by the sufferance and sympathy of others, enduring a long period of helplessness and inadequacy, indeed an unending dependency. Human beings, we may truly say, never do become wholly mature and independent, in the sense in which we might describe some animals in their adult stage as mature and independent. Human beings achieve such a state as we usually call *maturity* only by developing a good working accommodation to the inescapable fact of their inevitable interdependence.

Let me recite just a few of the items illustrative of persisting human immaturity: The adult human remains childishly curious and distractible; he seeks playful activity, sometimes at great cost; he does not develop fully the specialized capacities which distinguish his more maturely developed anthropoid cousins and which enable them, biologically, to live more independent lives. In comparative analogies, man is a weakling baboon, an incompetent chimpanzee, an awkward monkey. He does not even grow an adequate coat of hair.

The Dutch anatomist Ludwig Bolk accumulated an impressive body of evidence that the human adult resembles in many anatomical details the foetal state of his anthropoid ancestors or cousins. Bolk's observations prompted a foetal theory of the origin of man, namely, that man is a creature of ape-like origin who couldn't reach maturity but was condemned, so to speak, by genetic mutations to suffer a suppression of his previously more adequate ape-like biological potentialities. According to this theory, the effects of suppressor genes have kept man—in some respects, and to some degree—in a permanently foetal or infantile condition, compared to his immediate predecessors and the other anthropoids who took a different line of genetic development.

I make use of this theory to suggest that there may be a very sound reason why, in the discussion of maturity and immaturity, we are often embarrassed by our inability to give a wholly satisfactory definition of what we mean by maturity. As I have said, maturity in human life is an ideal rather than an actuality—something toward which we struggle but which we do not quite reach. At any rate, maturity is never a gift which comes to one like a trust fund upon reaching a specified birthday. Whatever approximation to maturity one may possess has been attained by active behavior, rather than by passive waiting for the maturation of instinctive endowment.

At the level of responsible human performance, human behavior and its motivation can be more adequately understood in terms of attitudes rather than of instincts—attitudes developed through social experience in a milieu characterized not merely by censorious and authoritarian controls but also by gregarious and protective tendencies. Thus, attitudes, socially cultivated, have much greater significance for social-emotional value and for practical effectiveness in human living than any human instinctive endowment.

For the professional student of human behavior concerned to establish sound observational supports for his motivational inferences, the term "attitude" has a further value. It provides a more directly verifiable concept for working with actual human beings than is provided by the concept of instincts. Instinct concepts, when utilized for the understanding of human behavior, are rather remote abstractions from the observable realities of human beings in action; such abstractions have for some workers the attractiveness of apparent depth and ultimate verity. Attitude concepts give one a somewhat less gratifying feeling of grasping the ultimate, but give a compensating sense of observational reliability because attitudes are more directly discernible than instincts, while at the same time attitudinal characterizations leave open the possibility for those who are so disposed to make further inferential leaps toward instinct formulations, if and when justifiable.

CHARACTERIZATIONS OF IMMATURE ATTITUDES AND IMMATURE LEVELS OF PERSONALITY DEVELOPMENT

Having presented, sketchily, a biosocial frame of reference, I shall now go back to the clinical descriptive work and present briefly a four-stage scheme for characterizing immature levels of personality functioning, which I have designated for obvious reasons as the infantile level, the childish level, the early adolescent level, and the late adolescent level.

Infantile level. At the infantile level one expects from others a limitless amount of service and consideration, without feeling any reciprocal obligation.

Childish Level. At the childish level there has developed some sense of responsibility, the kind that is completely erased by a good excuse. The alibi habit is a characteristic manifestation of this stage. Great circumstantiality of speech is a useful clinical clue. Persons at the childish level expect complete reliability in others but only perfunctory effort, up to the excuse level, in themselves. They may expend more effort in framing acceptable excuses than might be required to get a job done. Obsessiveness as a substitute way of establishing merit is rather characteristic of this level. Praise or blame is the focus of attention.

Early Adolescent Level. At the early adolescent level, exhibitionism and prestige-seeking are the outstanding manifestations. There is a strong push to assert one's personal significance, and to sustain it by repetitive demonstrations. Badges and trophies have high value as demonstrable symbols of prestige. The striving for self-importance requires extra-familial supports and these are characteristically found in idealistic hero-worship and in gangs.

Late Adolescent Level. The late adolescent level is the stage of "-isms"—romanticism, idealism, or cynicism, for example. The sense of social responsibility has become more generalized in the form of loyalty to a cause, as well as to a hero or a gang. The tendency to excess is still present, as in early adolescence, but it is doctrinaire excess rather than strenuous physical excess. The pseudo-sophisticated "line" of talk, the "wisecrack" and the sophomoric savant are easily recognizable manifestations. Sexual interests are expressed in pairing off and in courtship behavior, but success in this field, or the anticipation of success, may have the emotional quality of a conquest rather than of mutual devotion.

CAUTION

Now I should add a few works of caution in the use of these schematic propositions. First, they are highly schematic. Secondly, I have found by experience that young physicians, learning to study their patients from this point of view, tend to slip into the use of these terms as epithets, in effect accusing the patients of being infantile, or childish, or adolescent. The real purpose of these concepts is not to place blame, but to help one appreciate the patient's attitudes, for the better understanding of his distress or disability. The physician can be aided to get a more constructive value from these characterizations of immaturity by considering them in relation to human emotional needs.

THREE EMOTIONAL NEEDS

I have found it helpful, therefore, to relate the levels of immaturity to three emotional needs. 1. The need for affection; 2. The need for personal security; and 3. The need for personal significance. I have characterized them as *needs* because it appears to me that a person has to have some satisfaction in these three respects in order to develop and maintain the social assurance required for effective participation with others. The three form a series having relatively different degrees of importance at different stages of personality development. All three needs exist at all stages but the emphasis is different at different stages.

The Need for Affection. The predominant emotional need in infancy is the need for affection. Affection assures protection, care and nourishment; but affection means more. It fosters enthusiastic mutual responsiveness and attitudes of eager expectation in the most elementary social situation of parent and child. Affection provides some assurance of favoritism at a time of great dependency when some special favoritism is greatly needed. In some persons the infantile pattern of dependency upon affectionate favoritism persists far beyond infancy. One may say that such a person has clung to infantile values, or has been fixated at such levels through extreme attachment, but it is my impression that the principal reason for such an extreme block in development lies in the failure of the home to provide the sense of personal security needed to negotiate the next step.

The Need for Personal Security. In order to participate with comfort in the competitive life among other children, or even to endure without extreme distress the uncertainty aroused by parental absence, little children need to gain from their experiences a reasonable expectation that the universe is dependable. If mother has to leave, mother does come back; food is forthcoming at suitable intervals, and so is affectionate attention.

Later, the custom of sharing goodies, and the custom of taking turns, inculcate a faith that fair play characterizes the operations of the youngster's universe. This faith is supported and strengthened by the interventions of parental figures supporting principles of fair play. Without the faith built on such experiences one feels very much in danger, not only from aggressive attacks, but from one's own tendencies to aggression, which might elicit overwhelming retaliation.

Lack of support or lack of firmness in parental figures endangers this security; frequent and unpredictable conflicts between parents wreck it; favoritism and overprotectiveness from parents inhibit its development. The reasonable expectation of fair play is one of the conditions necessary for a person's eager exploration and adventure in the give-and-take of social living—not a guarantee of absolute justice, but just a reasonable expectation of fair play. Fair play is a good bargain for all concerned, and most youngsters appear to perceive that it involves obligations to adhere to fair practices oneself.

The psychiatrist not infrequently encounters patients whose faith in fair play or whose sense of security has gained so little validation from experience that they had had to rely throughout life upon favoritism in the infantile pattern. Lacking the sense of security that comes from a faith in fair play, some infantile personalities live life timidly and with great circumspection. Other infantile personalities, with careless abandon, dare foolish risks and impulsive adventures, apparently as means to gain repeated manifestations of the protector's favoritism and power. I have seen such examples in which it appeared that the protector took a childish delight in the extreme expression of favoritism and indulgence, and I have been tempted to label this partnership *infantilism à deux.*

The childhood phase of personality growth, with the emphasis upon the development of personal security, covers a good many years and a large experience of role-enactment, whereby the boundaries of social tolerance or social approval may be fairly widely explored.

The Need for Personal Significance. The widest extravagances in testing the limits of social tolerance are likely to appear in adolescence. In the usual course of events in our culture, one feels in adolescence an increased need to assert one's personal significance, sometimes very brashly, against authority figures such as parents, sometimes in exhibitionistic physical exploits, and often in late adolescence in a rather exaggerated radicalism or excessive reactive conservatism.

We are also familiar in our culture, perhaps more so than in other cultures, with the grown-up, middle-aged adolescent—grasping at opportunities for self-display, insatiable in the pursuit of badges of distinction, chasing after sexual exploits or other types of mastery, dramatizing attitudes of impudence or contempt of propriety.

In psychiatric case material one can find abundant evidence that difficulties of adjustment and psychopathological states often involve motivations based upon extreme needs to assert personal significance. The self-assertive behavior prompted by such needs may be quite annoying. As a clinician and a therapist, I do wish, however, to put in some good words for these adolescent motivations. Behavior thereby motivated may be exasperating, but the patients who manifest it do get well, pretty regularly. Such motivations may prove very useful at certain stages of psychotherapeutic strategy.

Toward a Mature Personality

Up to this point we have been concerned mostly with immaturity. Now we should consider maturity. Complete maturity is an ideal, only approximated in reality. In what we call the mature personality a manageable flexibility of social attitudes has been achieved. This is manifested in a variety of role behaviors, developed through life experiences which have served to fulfill emotional needs reasonably well.

The mature individual has not graduated to a stage in which he no longer has these needs; rather he has attained flexibility in accepting and acting out the roles which satisfy these emotional needs. In developing his personal accommodation to the basic condition of human life —interdependence—he has had gratifying experiences of leadership and of loyalty, of domination and of submission.

To get along with other people who are in varying stages of maturity a person needs to maintain the capacity for playful good humor. He can, on appropriate occasions, quit being soberly grown-up and enter into adolescent and childish activities with spontaneity and gusto. He can share with lively sympathy in the emotional values pertaining to those less mature levels of social development. He can not only enter into immature emotional contexts, but he can come out of them again, as occasion requires, and resume more responsible roles, also with good humor and with some measure of playful enthusiasm. Indeed, it might be said that the mature person, in order to maintain the emotional attitudes required by the fact of persisting interdependence and to handle the friction generated by such interdependence, has to retain and exercise some propensities for childishly playful curiosity and amusement.

Clinical Usefulness of These Concepts

I would find myself much handicapped in my professional work without some appreciation of the human being's need for affection, for personal security, and for personal significance, and without some means of recognizing levels of immaturity which characterize persons who have suffered critical deprivation of these needs. I would lack understanding of many patients whose anxieties and frustrations are not readily appreciated when viewed from an adult, commonsense point of view, but whose problems become understandable when one appreciates the immaturity of their personal development and the extent to which their sense of well-being is dependent upon the preservation of social contexts suited to immature levels. In such a frame of reference one can also understand better a person's temporary regression to earlier levels of immaturity in the face of frustrating and intolerable life situations.

How Much Free Choice?

Having spoken now at some length about the environmental deprivations which may seriously limit the development of mature attitudes, I should now try to balance the discussion by some reference to a person's role in his own development. It happens that I am not one of those who believe in complete, 100 per cent, determinism. To a small extent, but to a significant extent, human beings, as I see them, seem able to exercise some degree of choice in behavior.

According to the foetal theory of the origin of the human species, suppressive genetic mutations made man enduringly immature, as compared to the chimpanzee, and prevented him from developing the fully specialized repertoire of his Simian cousins. We may be handicapped by such deficiencies, but we have gained a degree of freedom in modifying our behavior. We have gained some chance of escape from the coercive force of instinctive patterns of life, and we have developed patterns of domestication and socialization which permit a certain degree of freedom of personal preference or choice.

It is indeed one of the significant achievements of civilization to have gained for so many an enlargement of their individual freedom of choice of behavior. The rules required by the social nature of human living are not too highly restrictive. Some leeway exists so that individuals may give acceptable expression to their temperamental differences, and thus participate with gratification and enthusiasm within the broad bounds required by their mutual interdependence.

Unfortunately, many people feel, unnecessarily, that they are oppressed or deprived, and fail therefore to develop their opportunities and employ their capacities. This is particularly true of the psychiatrist's patients. The basic psychotherapeutic task can be distinguished from merely comforting manoeuvres, or merely supportive, or corrective, or interpretative techniques. The basic psychotherapeutic task consists essentially in awakening a person to the more enthusiastic and spontaneous exploration of his available degrees of freedom, and in eliciting hopeful and constructive efforts along lines of his interest and competence. The potentialities thus evoked encourage the patient to cope more effectively with his life situation and may even lead to greater maturity and achievement than he enjoyed previous to his illness. It is one of the greatest gratifications to the psychiatrist when he is able to evoke in an immature patient the faith and enthusiasm and effort by which he achieves a more advanced level of personal growth.

4

BERNARD H. HALL, M.D.

Carl Sandburg, in describing the incomparable Abraham Lincoln, stated, "Not often in the story of mankind does a man arrive on earth who is both steel and velvet, who is as hard as rock and soft as drifting fog, who holds in his heart and mind the paradox of terrible storm and speech unspeakable and perfect."

Dr. Leo Bartemeier has these same extraordinary qualities. For indeed, he is both steel and velvet, hard as rock, and soft as drifting fog. How proud I am to have him as a friend!

When the Menninger School of Psychiatry was started in 1946, Dr. Karl and Dr. Will Menninger asked some of their closest friends to come to Topeka periodically to teach and supervise those of us in the School's first class. Dr. Leo Bartemeier used to come for a weekend once a month and I have had the unusual experience of presenting cases to him on Sunday mornings! His gentle, but firm deftness as a superior clinician and teacher had the residents fighting for time with him. By this selfless weekend contribution to the new Menninger School of Psychiatry, he enabled it to become the outstanding center of psychiatric education that it is.

I have learned a great deal from Doctor Bartemeier, but as with all great teachers, it is hard to point to just what skill or insight I can now trace back to him. Thinking about this, however, it occurred to me that I did learn, early in my career, an extremely important lesson from him. I am indebted to him for learning that a psychiatric clinician must always lead with empathy.

I do not think he ever told me this in so many words. It was a lesson learned by watching him work with patients and with staff, and by my wish to be like him. For it was from the very qualities of this man, being both steel and

41

velvet, hard as rock and soft as drifting fog, that I learned the singular importance of empathy to the psychiatric clinician.

Psychiatrist or Attorney for the Prosecution?

A BASIC TENET that we hold about the psychology of man is that all behavior has a cause and is significant in light of the patient's life story and psychic functioning. In addition, the behavior is economical in the sense that it is the best that the patient can do under the circumstances. This formulation about human behavior, which comes to us from Sigmund Freud, introduced a reason for the scientific belief in hope for the mentally ill. This formulation means that if we can develop our clinical skills and capacities and understanding, the behavior of any patient can be understood in light of that individual's individuality. Thereby there is reason to believe that the patient can be helped, not only to understand himself better, but to cope better and to function more autonomously.

I have little patience with colleagues who conduct an interview with a patient or a colleague with the stated objective "of making the patient anxious." What I learned from Dr. Leo Bartemeier was that this is a foolish way to try to be helpful to a suffering human being. We have to accept the patient as he is. We have to let the patient be sick and manifest his illness to us if we are going to be of help to him. Therefore, I become equally perturbed with any colleague who describes a patient as lacking in motivation, or a patient who is testing him. If the patient is lacking in motivation, that is a manifestation of his illness and that is the aspect of his illness to start treating immediately. And, if the clinician feels that a patient is "testing" him, I am convinced it is the colleague's reaction to the patient's illness that we are talking about and not the illness itself.

It is obvious that the stance of the clinician is to offer himself as a sympathetic and understanding listener against whom the patient can reflect his difficulties. I believe that the office in which the clinician works is extremely important. The distinguished architect, Mr. Bertrand Goldberg, once told me that he thought the psychiatrist's office should be more like a sculptor's studio than a mere office.

I always surprise psychiatric residents when I talk about the psychiatrist's office. It is my conviction that the most important thing about the psychiatrist's office is that the *psychiatrist* is comfortable in it. When I reflect that I spend one-third of my life in my office, I think I have every right to have it the way I want it. My conviction is that if the psychiatrist is comfortable in the surroundings in which he works, this will greatly facilitate the patient's comfort and the psychiatrist's ability to be helpful. In contrast to many, I think of the office as a personal area, and it should reflect the personality of the psychiatrist. Too much emphasis has been placed on austerity as a rule for psychiatrists' offices. Such offices leave me cold and I think such offices leave many *patients* cold. My own office is filled with books, old pharmacy bottles, favorite psychiatric historical items, and pictures of President Lincoln, John Hunter, and a print of El Greco's "Luke The Physician."

The extraordinary thing about one's office is how patients apprehend it differently as individuals and differently at various points in time in the course of their treatment. Often the patient's perception of the office is a commentary to his struggles, the nature of his current transference feelings, and the state of the recovery process.

One has some unanticipated experiences about what the patient "sees" in the office. I treated a rather hysterical girl for two years and she sat in the chair where a favorite photograph of the Ponte Vecchio was in full view. She never mentioned the picture. On one occasion I interrupted her treatment for a month's vacation. Her curiosity about where I was going was extreme. After my vacation and when I resumed seeing her, I was amazed at what happened. She came in, sat in the same chair as always, looked around her, and said, pointing to the Florentine picture, actually seeing it for the first time, "Now I know where you went on vacation. You went to Italy!" A picture of President Lincoln in my office often draws comments and I was very touched when toward the end of treatment a patient noticed the picture and said, "How appropriate for a psychiatrist to have a picture of President Lincoln in his office—psychiatrists also free slaves."

I once had the experience of having to use the office of a colleague who was on vacation while my office was being redecorated. I was uncomfortable in not being in my own usual chair. I was distracted by the paintings on the walls in my colleague's office—paintings which I would not have in my office at all. This was a miserable two weeks for me and for my long-term patients, and I am convinced that the quality of my clinical work was not the same during that time.

The office should have comfortable chairs and the patient should be allowed to choose where he sits. I prefer to sit below the level of where the patient is sitting, so that my six feet do not tower over him. I want nothing between us such as a desk. I feel, at the time of the first appointment, that the patient is a kind of guest in my home and I treat him exactly as I would a new guest in my private home. I see that he is comfortably seated, that he has an ash tray, is not blinded by the sunlight and, if he has traveled a long distance for the appointment, I may even offer him a cup of coffee. It is in this climate, after visiting briefly with the patient about general things, that I then ask him how he happened to seek out a psychiatrist at this time.

A psychiatrist, if he is comfortable in his office surroundings, will find it easier to be empathic to his patient's suffering. He will be less likely, in my opinion, to act like a prosecuting attorney with the patient. The attorney for the prosecution in his effort to elicit information and to prosecute the case very often cannot rely on an approach of empathy and may have to turn to rather rugged interviewing techniques in which he may even be forced to try to trap the subject in his testimony. Unfortunately, some psychiatrists follow a similar approach in trying to elicit information from a patient. I suppose most of us, until we learn the power of empathy in our work with patients, resort to more of a prosecuting attorney approach. Such an approach often has as its objective to "break the patient down" and elicit from him, with verbal coercion, "a confession of guilt."

My good friend and attorney, Mr. Gerald Goodell, reiterated my belief that the goals of the prosecuting attorney are different. The prosecuting attorney has as his goal to obtain a verdict of guilty, so that the person can be punished in keeping with the law. Mr. Goodell pointed out to me, however, that there is a definite trend in legal education to borrow the more empathic interviewing techniques from psychiatrists, as a departure from the traditional prosecuting attorney approach.

The psychiatric clinician approach and the prosecuting attorney approach may be contrasted by the way the question is phrased and by the feeling with which it is expressed. A psychiatrist can start with the assumption that the patient is going to resist giving an accurate history of his own sexual life and decide to outsmart the patient and "get the truth" by tricking him. If one has the confidence of the patient, then the patient is more likely to give his sexual history as he perceives it to be. A great part of the success in helping the patient discuss his sexual life candidly is to create a climate in which the patient can feel that this is an accepted part of his being; that he is with a physician; and that, with the veil of privileged communication, he can talk openly.

The prosecuting attorney's "patient" also has the problem that he knows very well that if he can withhold certain information he will not incriminate himself. He knows he will come off better by withholding or distorting "the facts." A psychiatrist's task is an easier one in that he tries to convey to his patient that the patient has everything to gain by telling the psychiatrist about himself as he sees himself, and that he will only cheat himself of the chance to get well by consciously withholding or consciously distorting facts about himself.

The situation becomes much more complicated when the patient is being seen at the request of a court or a medical department of a large industry. Very often when this occurs, the patient cannot let himself be a patient and, indeed, may not even feel that he *is* a patient. He may feel that he is there by coercion. He knows full well that if he starts acting like a patient and telling what is really wrong and what really happened, he may lose his job or incriminate himself legally.

We can easily fall into a countertransference trap when seeing an adolescent who is very often a reluctant patient. It is so easy, under such circumstances, to begin to act like a parent toward an uncooperative, resistive, "unmotivated" adolescent. Actually, adolescents take to talking about themselves relatively easily if they sense your concern about their struggles and if the clinician wonders out loud with him about how a young person could find himself in such a complicated situation. Certainly, the prosecuting attorney approach will only further alienate such patients, and their often silent and troubled relationship with one or both of their parents is immediately re-created with the psychiatrist.

So often, the adolescent complains that he is sick and tired of people lecturing to him about what he ought to do. Success in working with him is entirely dependent on empathizing with that very feeling the patient has, and then raising the question as to why he thinks this situation has come about. If his curiosity about what has happened to him can be aroused, maybe it will be possible to point out gently that what he seems to be saying is that in his stumbling efforts to grow up and find himself, he has provoked a situation with his parents and others that is only stunting his psychological growth and defeating his achievement of the very autonomy he so sorely desires.

Another error that can occur in the absence of proper empathic work on the part of the psychiatrist is that one can end up behaving like the attorney for the prosecution, telling the patient what the psychiatrist thinks the patient is feeling. Indeed, there are certain patients whose feelings become isolated and are not available to them and the psychiatrist may wish to say, "I wonder if you are not feeling such and such now." But in these therapeutic instances, one uses this approach to set a model by which the patient comes to know and recognize his feelings on his own.

The young psychiatrist is often frightened away from using a more empathic approach to his patients out of fear of over-identifying with the patient. One of the first dictums we learn when we enter psychiatry is, "It is a cardinal sin to over-identify with the patient." We grow up as clinicians living in horror that we will be judged as "over-identifying" with the patient or, as it is sometimes put, "over-involved with the patient." I hope I never have to supervise another young psychiatrist who does not get over-involved or over-identified with his patients. My thesis is that, at the beginning of a clinician's career, a certain amount of over-involvement is necessary for the eventual development of the empathic clinician who has learned to moderate his feelings and concerns for a patient in the patient's best interests.

Dr. Robert P. Knight used to teach us that our task was to step into the patient's life and feel exactly what the patient was feeling and then to be able to step back out, to help the patient reflect and come to an understanding of what he was experiencing, and why. Through experience, and particularly through able supervision, the young clinician begins to lose his fear of being branded as being over-identified with his patient, and he begins to develop the empathic skills necessary to do clinical work. Those clinicians who consistently keep an emotional abyss between themselves and their patients, who cannot over-identify with their patients in their early days in psychiatry, fail to develop empathic skills and, instead, lean more heavily on the tactics of the prosecuting attorney.

The young psychiatrist is often confused about empathy. He may well think that empathy will be perceived by the patient as approval of his behavior. In fact, the psychiatrist's apparent acceptance of his patient's behavior often provokes criticism from others. The psychiatrist is thus perceived as being without moral convictions, endorsing sexual licentiousness, and encouraging the rampant expression of aggression.

To fall into the trap of being approving or disapproving of the patient's behavior renders the psychiatrist ineffectual as a helper. Practically never does the patient come seeking approval or disapproval of his behavior.

More often than not, he comes so disapproving of himself that he is haunted with guilt feelings and depression. Most psychiatric patients have high ethical and moral standards for themselves. Their failure to live up to these standards, their stumbling efforts to do what they consider right, are commonly the source of their own suffering.

For a patient to be confronted by a judgmental attitude on the part of the psychiatrist may only compound the patient's difficulties. The patient may take such judgments and use them only to further harass himself. The psychiatrist in such a situation behaves toward the patient as the patient behaves toward himself and that is not what the patient is seeking help for.

If, on the other hand, the patient experiences the psychiatrist as nonjudgmental, as a person who seems to understand that human beings do a lot of stumbling in their attempts to cope with life, then the patient can, with the psychiatrist's help, begin a meaningful pursuit of understanding himself and thereby change the behavior that is objectionable to him.

Thus, empathy is nonjudgmental—it neither approves nor disapproves. It seeks momentary acceptance of things as they are, and becomes an instrument by which the patient can change and grow psychologically. Empathy is soft as fog, but it is also as strong as steel. Empathy is a manifestation of *concern* for one's fellow human beings. It is gentle and kind. But because it is concern, it is tough, durable, and powerful.

A priest-patient of mine once said, "You are undoubtedly the roughest, toughest confessor I have ever had." When I asked him what he meant, he said, "Well I can go to confession, tell what I have done wrong, receive absolution and a penance and the whole thing is forgotten. You never let me forget for a moment that I have a problem." I asked him if he really wanted me to let him forget about his problem which was bringing him so much misery and unhappiness.

An extremely important aspect of psychiatric practice, perhaps nearly equal to the importance of clinical acumen and clinical skills, is the constant monitoring of our own countertransference propensities. Countertransference, when it is not dealt with, can easily trip us from the emphatic approach to the approach of a prosecuting attorney. Freud taught us so clearly that our reactions to our patients can reveal feelings, attitudes, and expectations that are as inappropriate or unrealistic to the physician-patient relationship as are the patient's own transference feelings toward the physician.

It has always been striking to me that long before Freud the author or authors of the Hippocratic Oath required the vow: "Into whatever house I enter, I will enter to help the sick, and I will abstain from all intentional wrong-doing and harm. . . ." It is as if The Oath accepts that physicians, being only human, have to be on guard so that the patient is not exploited to gratify the physician's own psychological needs, expectations, attitudes, and hopes.

Our wish to be helpful as physicians costs us emotionally. And it is often hard for us, as physicians, to accept that we are only human and that there are limits to what we can do. Medical school days were a rude introduction for all of us to the limitations of our science. Each one of us recalls our first experience with a patient who died. Mine was a charming woman dying of leukemia, whose life we were able to prolong for a time with blood transfusions. She was able to leave the hospital long enough to attend her son's high-school graduation. A few weeks later she died, and I mourned her death. Our wish to help can be so great that it is personally painful when we cannot help.

It is easy for us to fall prey to our own needs which are unrelated to what is best for the patient. We have all caught ourselves infantilizing a patient whose suffering provokes emotions in us that momentarily blind our objectivity. And have not we all within time of quick recall had to act adroitly to check our feelings of annoyance and irritation with the patient who has not gratified us by getting well?

After all is said and done, physicians have the task of exercising their best judgment, and of doing their best to understand their sick and troubled patients, to help where they can to aid those forces in man's nature that strive toward health and happiness in life. The truth of the aphorism of Hippocrates, as Doctor Bartemeier has lived it for fifty years as a physician, has stood for centuries to remind us about our calling:

"Life is short, and the Art long; the occasion fleeting; experience fallacious, and judgment difficult. The physician must not only be prepared to do what is right himself, but also to make the patient, the attendants, and the externals cooperate."

5

CARLOS ALBERTO SEGUIN, M.D.

In the daily practice of psychotherapy, technique is, for many, the most important tool. Technique for them must be learned and painfully and faithfully applied if success is to follow.

There are other psychotherapists, however, for whom technique is a harness and who, along the years, create their own, which is nothing else but the sincere use of their authentic personalities. To me the latter are the true ones.

One of these true psychotherapists, engaging himself frankly and totally in his work, giving of his rich, warm and humane personality to his patients, is Leo Bartemeier, whose virtues reflect themselves in his successes as a psychiatrist. It is for that reason that I feel the following reflections are the best tribute I can make to him when we commemorate a moment in his fruitful life.

Beyond Instinct, Deeper than Libido

The "Psychotherapeutic Eros"

To speak about psychotherapy is to speak about human values. In the midst of the impersonal, automated practices of today, psychotherapy represents the truly human aspect of medicine. It is based upon interpersonal communication. It can be rightly understood only if the real essence of all human relationships is seen as directly related to affectivity. Psychotherapy is basically an emotional process. As such it is able to modify, deeply and fundamentally, the world of the patient just as any emotion changes profoundly the world of the moved.

But what kind of affect is the one that typifies the psychotherapeutic relationship? I have studied this topic elsewhere (Seguin 1963; 1965a,

49

b, c) and, avoiding repetitious details, I would like to point out, now, the main features of my position:

1. Psychotherapy is a particular kind of interpersonal relationship.
2. Its essence is the affective contact between therapist and patient.
3. Such affective contact cannot be anything else but love—a very special, differentiated and distinct form of love which I have identified with a new name: "the psychotherapeutic Eros."

The psychotherapeutic Eros—the love the therapist has for his patient—is a unique kind of love, distinct from all the others. It is different from the love a father feels for his son, a friend for his friend, a teacher for his pupil, a pastor for his follower. It is different, of course, from the lover's love. The psychotherapeutic Eros has special characteristics, both negative and positive. Among the former are freedom from a) authority or any tendency to possession; b) identification; c) dogma; d) imposition of values, rules or knowledge; and e) sexual attraction. On the positive side are: a) love for the patient or, rather, for the person of the patient (not a form of "humanitarian" love that the physician must feel towards the sick as sick, but an authentic movement towards the unique individual who is before him); b) indestructibility—a characteristic neatly distinguishing the psychotherapeutic Eros from any other kind of love;* c) duality of creation—the "psychotherapeutic experience" whose characteristics I have already studied in previous writings (Seguin, 1963; 1965a, b, c). The latter is an experience that partakes, on the one hand, of what happens when in love and, on the other, of what is lived in artistic creation or scientific discovery.

---

* The lover will cease to be a lover if his feelings are not returned, if his partner is unfaithful or if he finds indifference or scorn; a friend will not last long if he discovers that he has "nothing in common," nothing to share, with his supposed friend. A father will feel estranged (although his love will not disappear totally) if his son shows rebellion, opposition or any negative attitude; and a teacher will disavow a disciple who is no longer able to join him in the search for the road of excellence. The pastor, perhaps, may be more faithful—in that he will not lose hope even though his sheep may stray from the fold. Almost no one else but the psychotherapist, however, will continue to love in spite of everything. The patient may exhibit the complete gamut of negative feelings—he may be aggressive, hostile, intriguing, deceiving, mendacious, rebellious, incredulous or bellicose—and yet the psychotherapist will not cease to love him. On the contrary, perhaps all these feelings will augment his love, serving, as they generally do, to demonstrate precisely how much that love is needed.

"Conditioned" and "Unconditioned" Love

I shall try now to go deeper into the analysis of the psychotherapeutic relationship to uncover its rationale, meaning, value, and effects. At the very outset we ask ourselves: "How does the psychotherapeutic Eros act? What is the reason for its effectiveness?"

Allow me to attempt to answer these questions by offering a hypothesis which may serve as a framework for a comprehensive theory of neurosis.

Everybody accepts today the role that the mother-child relationship plays in the formation and deformation of personality, and the decisive influence it has during the first years of the infant's life. The mother's attitude is, therefore, of the outmost importance and should be closely studied.

Other than those rare cases in which there is a definite rejection of the child, maternal feelings may be classified in two categories. We shall call one of them "conditioned" and the other "unconditioned" love.

The mother whose love is "conditioned" will profess to love her child dearly and will try to show it, but she will always set conditions for that love to exist: "I love you, if you obey," "I love you, if you are a good boy," "I love you if you don't bother me too much." Even "I love you, if you are intelligent, or if you are pretty, or if you are like me." In sum: "I love you, if. . . ."

Where an "unconditioned" love exists, the mother will love her child with no ifs whatsoever. She will love him as he is, with his defects and his difficulties. She will love him, if we may say it, in spite of everything.

Obviously, the first one is not a true love, since love setting conditions hardly merits even the name of love. However, it is very difficult, if not impossible, to find a mother loving with a totally unconditioned love. It would not be pertinent to enter now into the consideration of the reasons for this phenomenon, rooted in the psychology and the pathology of the family, of society, and of culture. I would rather emphasize the importance the mother's love has in the shaping of a child's personality and hence in his later fate as a grown man.

Let us imagine now a mother offering a totally unconditioned love. We can understand, then, how her child will be in the best position to develop his finest possibilities and to grow up to become a conscientious and a responsible adult.

At this point, however, it may be necessary to clarify some points. To love unconditionally does not mean, of course, not to educate or correct. The mother who really loves her child loves him as he is but she will do everything necessary to bring about the maturation of the best that is in him and will work unremittingly to provide him with the proper environment for his growth.

It may be useful to recall Scheler's observation on the nature of love. He says:

> Every "you should be such and such" taken in a manner of speaking as a "condition" of love destroys its fundamental essence. . . . Love itself is what allows that, with perfect continuity, and in the course of the movement, there emerges in each case the highest value in the object, as if flowered "of itself" from the loved object himself, without any activity or direction on the part of the lover, not even a "desire." (Scheler, 1957).

To love unconditionally does not mean either to spoil or to pamper the child. We know only too well that indulgence and too much permissiveness are, instead of signs of love, spurious compensations, appearing in the most conditioned kind of love.

As a contrast to the cases of unconditioned love, let us imagine now what happens (and it happens daily) to children submitted to a conditioned love. The child has to fulfill one or several conditions if he wants to keep his mother's love. Because he cannot risk losing it, he behaves, or tries to behave, in such a way as to deserve it. He will be obedient, he will be "good," he will be clean, he will be everything he is able to be except "himself." Eventually, when he is not able to comply with his mother's conditions, he will resort to another mechanism: rebellion.

Always to be "as mamma wants" is for a child never to be himself. It is to constantly wear a mask; it is to thwart one's own spontaneous and free development. To make a child be "the way Mom wants him to" is to constrain his personality within rigid and narrow molds, imposing upon him neurotically artificial values.

Such a child will get so used to living with his mask on that he will never dare to show his real face. A moment will come, sooner or later, when the mask will eat his face up. Should he, then, want to tear the mask away, he will not be able to do it without pulling off his own skin with it and the child will become a neurotic. Indeed, if the mask is resistant enough and if personal conditions are adverse enough, he will become a psychotic. When the demands of the "I love you, if . . ." are impossible to meet ("I love you, if you are intelligent"; "I love you, if you are pretty"; "I love you, if you are better than the kid next door"), the child may resort to blind and systematic opposition to all values accepted by the mother, or, in other words, psychopathy.

The conditionally loved child grows up seeking the approval of others through claudications, renunciations and pretenses. As time goes by he will alienate himself more and more from his authentic self and sink deeper and deeper into falsehood until the moment when he is no longer able to stand the comedy. That man, then, suffering and in pain, will come to us for help.

I have elsewhere (Seguin, 1965a) qualified the psychotherapeutic Eros as an unselfish, undemanding, we-centered kind of love. It is the tender, on the part of the therapist, of a gift—the freedom to be—without conditions. Possessing that freedom at last, the patient is able to face and accept those parts of himself that he—with or without reason—learned so painfully to reject.

We can now understand the relationship between the pathogenetic theory of neurosis just outlined and the psychotherapeutic Eros. The neurotic, who never knew what it was to be loved "for himself," who never found any "condition-free" relationship (because he had not met it, or because he did not know how to live with it as a consequence of the threats and frustrations throughout his life), finds himself, for the first time, in front of a man, the therapist, who loves him with no conditions whatsoever.

It is, indeed, a totally new experience and, therefore, a disconcerting one. All the neurotic's life has prepared him to hide and escape, to disguise and deny. He cannot believe, he cannot trust, he cannot be sincere and, should he dare to, he will expect rejection, the loss of the "maternal love." Many a time he will, unconsciously, provoke rejection because he needs to confirm his fears and his distrust. In his relationship with the therapist all that will change. For the first time, he will experience a process of interrelation.

The Last Resistance

Since Freud, resistance has been thoroughly studied by the psychoanalysts. We all know that the patient will use every possible contrivance to prevent the therapist from reaching the innermost recesses of his mind, and that he will try—quite illogically—to end in failure every attempt to change his personality traits. When psychoanalysis was a very young science, the initial efforts made by the analyst to probe into the patient's instinctive past were met with his rejection. We see today that just the opposite is happening; shortly, after an initial period of disorientation—when such a period exists at all, given today's wide dissemination of psychoanalytic theories—the patient accepts willingly, and I would say merrily, all the explorations of the history of his libido. Soon afterwards, he not only handles analytic terminology as well as his doctor, but brings to his analyst dreams and associations which constitute suitable material for elaborate interpretations.

An experienced psychoanalyst should know how to deal with this intellectual defense, and also how to prevent the patient from "playing with dreams and symbols." Yet every day we see patients psychoanalysed by capable and reputable analysts, patients who are walking treatises on libido theory, but who still "nurse" their symptoms or revert to them now and then. We have met, furthermore, learned psychoanalysts who recognize themselves as not being free from neurotic residues in spite of their well conducted didactic analysis and their repeated "reviews" conducted by respectful and experienced colleagues.

I have asked myself over and over: Are we not, perhaps, in front of a much subtler form of resistance? Could it not be that all the sexual and libidinal phantasmagoria is but a protective screen, an extreme defense, behind which the deepest, most authentic, really true human aspect of the patient hides?

I shall try to make myself clearer. For Freud and his contemporaries, just to discover and be able to discuss libidinal problems was a real accomplishment. Sexuality was then so hidden, so denied, so covered-up, that to have brought it to light seemed a phenomenal achievement. The exposure of the unconscious—through a limelight focussed upon sexuality—gave the early analysts the belief that all resistances had been shattered and the most profound knowledge of human psychology was at hand. The alluring fascination of these perspectives prevented everybody from thinking that, behind the magnificent décor, beyond the polymorphic screen, there might be hidden more profound and perhaps more transcendent phenomena. Psychoanalysis, fighting as it had to on every front (against society, culture, religion, and against its patients themselves) let itself be deceived by that astoundingly effective mechanism of resistance—the patient's libidinal history—without realizing that it might be only that: another resistance. The patient traditionally plays with interpretations useful for putting the analyst off and preventing him from going deeper. He covers his spoor with endless discussion about his instinctive evolution. Through clever interpretations, carefully interwoven at every level, he shuts himself and his doctor out of where all that is really human lies and where he himself dare not look.

But what is there, beyond the instinctive level, that must be so jealously protected from analytic approach? I believe that in the answer given to this question lies the key to the future of a really human-centered psychotherapy.

Beyond Instinct . . .

Beyond instinct stands Being; deeper than libido exists Love. If we are able to overcome the last resistance, the screen of the patient's sexual history, we shall reach the very nucleus of the human being, that which makes him what he is. Once the vicissitudes of the libido have been conquered, we confront the essence of human feeling: love. And the neurotic shies away from the confrontation, for he is ill-prepared for love—much less for a bare encounter with another human being, or with his unmasked self.

A confrontation with Being and Love must be a confrontation without masks, without subterfuges. It is a bare-faced, flat-footed, and terribly risky encounter for the neurotic who, all his life, has been forced to disguise himself lest he lose his mother's love and, with it, the chance to survive. Furthermore, the renunciation of masks brings the neurotic face to face with his own freedom and personality. No longer can he take refuge in pretenses and excuses. He must love, not as a puppet manipulated by his mother's conditions, but as a flesh-and-blood man.

Having been subjected to "conditioned" love, he himself does not know at first how to love differently. He conditions *his love*—a fact which has led him to a series of unauthentic liaisons loaded with selfishness and far from the fidelity to being which love implies. The abandonment of his masks places before him the possibility—even the necessity—of really loving, and that fact frightens him. Thus he dallies for a while, exploring his libidinal past, analyzing the sexual symbolism of his dreams and thoughts, and inventing ingenious interpretations of his actions at the instinctive level.

Psychoanalysts have been wrapped up for too many years in the libidinal network of their patients. They have been drawn into the interesting game of deciphering the mystery of symbols and the adventures of instinctive evolution, thus permitting their patients to avoid the probing beyond their instincts and deeper than their libidoes.

These observations are not, of course, the product of theoretical speculations. On the contrary, they are the outcome of daily experience and the study of the patients' records. Moreover, any sensitive psychotherapist, who is not too limited by the rigidity of his own technique, will find them to be true in his practice. He will see, then, how, after a short time, every patient will readily attribute to himself any libidinal fixation or any known or unknown complex, but also how, should the therapist try to lead the patient to be himself and to love, the analyst will meet the utmost resistance—sometimes even flight. If the therapist knows how to help his patient through this stage, if he assists him to renounce, once and for all, his masks, then he will have contributed to the recovery of a human being.

To free a fellow-being to love is an accomplishment unattainable through technique alone. If we want to achieve such a feat, we must be able to offer love ourselves—the psychotherapeutic Eros that will allow the patient to reconstruct his existence in an environment without "conditions." Then only can the psychotherapeutic circle complete itself—with love begetting love; sincerity, honesty; compassion, humaneness; and understanding, maturity.

REFERENCES

Sartre, J. P. (1948): The Emotions. Outline of a Theory, Philosophical Library, New York, N. Y.
Scheler, M. (1957): Esencia y Formas de la Simpatia. Edit. Lozada, Buenos Aires.
Seguin, C. A. (1963): Amor y Psicoterapia, Editorial Paidos, Buenos Aires.
Seguin, C. A. (1965a): Love and Psychotherapy. Libra Publishers, New York, N. Y.
Seguin, C. A. (1965b): Der Artz und sein Patient. Hans Huber, Bern und Stuttgart.
Seguin, C. A. (1965c): El abrirse, el amor y el permitir en psicoterapia. Sem. med. (B. Aires), 127, 725.

Part I

Section Two

SOME SPECIFIC PROBLEMS
IN PRACTICE

Specific problems in the clinical practice of psychiatry
are legion. Although it is necessary to think in categories,
what is of primary and specific interest to the clinician is
the particular human being before him.

In this section four clinicians consider areas of concern
which have emerged from their interaction with patients.
By means of an historical survey, Doctor Martin outlines the
psychotherapies of marital partners. Doctor Solomon, in a
case study, explores the psychic implications of the concept of existence. Doctor Rome speaks about the causes
and complexities of malingering, while Doctor Rosen reflects
on the psychotic aspect of suicide.

6

PETER A. MARTIN, M.D.

As I look back, it is easy for me to trace the connections between my psychiatric and psychoanalytic training with Leo Bartemeier and the development of my interest and research in the treatment of marriage partners.

A dictum which we all have been taught is that the psychiatrist and the psychoanalyst vis-à-vis the patient stand for reality. If there are two people in a room in a psychotherapeutic situation, one of them should know what reality is—preferably the therapist. As Freud in his writings about our therapeutic endeavors said "There where id was shall ego be; there where the unconscious was shall consciousness be. Consciousness is the candle which brings an area of light to the darkness of the unconscious. Like the people of Holland, both as therapists and as individuals who practice what we preach, we try to reclaim from the sea (the unconscious) as much land (the conscious) as possible. . . . the property of being conscious or not is in the last resort our one beacon light in the darkness of depth psychology."

In watching Dr. Bartemeier interview patients and in his supervision of our psychotherapy, I and my fellow residents at the Pontiac State Hospital and at the Haven Sanitarium, as well as my fellow students at the Detroit Psychoanalytic Institute where he was our supervising analyst, were aware that here was a man who was without peer in knowing what the reality was and in asking the insightful questions which would bring further clarification to areas of confusion. He knew how to ask what seemed to us to be a million questions about such things as the eating habits, sleeping habits, and bowel habits of the patient and once such material had been gathered there would emerge a sharply focused picture of the patient's character. The fascinating part was that the sharply focused knowledge of external reality brought out in bold relief this underlying inner psychic reality. The outer and

*inner realities were head and tail of the same coin. A
light from the conscious was turned on to see the darkness
of the unconscious.*

An Historical Survey of the
Psychotherapy of Marriage Partners

PERHAPS FIFTY PER CENT of all patients who seek psychotherapeutic
treatment do so because of marital difficulties.[2] Of the other fifty per
cent, perhaps one-half recognize, during the course of analysis, the existence of serious marital problems. These figures are not surprising when
one considers the intimate nature of marriage. Surpassing in intensity
even the mother-infant bond, it naturally conduces to the development
and expression of disturbed interpersonal relationships.*

Grotjahn[3] defines the "marriage neurosis" as the transfer and projection of unresolved, unconscious conflicts from the past of both partners
into the present—that is, of conflicts generated in the parental families
and perpetuated in the marriage situation. He also says that the mother-
child symbiosis is the prototype of the later family, that it is the basis of
the child's conscious and unconscious. This prototype thus lies underneath
later family relationships, be it that of the child to his father, brother,
sister or that of a grown-up to a husband or wife.

This definition of "marriage neurosis" might be amplified to include
the concept that it is also the basis of an implicit contract, consciously
or unconsciously agreed upon before marriage. The contract may later be
breached if one of the partners changes or finds himself or herself unable
or unwilling to maintain the original terms. Unless the second partner
accepts the new codiciliary terms, marital disharmony, accompanied by
symptom formation in the decompensating partner, is apt to occur.

An example of a breach of an implicit-but-unstated contract (which
was based on the marriage neurosis) and its disturbing consequences was

---

* It is significant that in a survey of the married in treatment improvement in therapy was more frequently found among those patients who did
not report a marital problem as a major reason for entering treatment than
among those patients who did.[2]

the disharmony in a marriage, between a confused, non-thinking, rule-following man and a dynamic, vivacious, career-oriented woman. The implicit contract was that *she* could continue to pursue her personal interests without interference from *him*. *She* was to be allowed both marriage and a career, and *he* was to show gratitude and count himself fortunate to have gotten her. This man, weak to the point of at times seeming to lack an ego, prized his wife as an alter ego, and she was eager to accept the role he imposed upon her, since she believed it would be an assurance of no demands to change her usual way of life after marriage.

The status quo was maintained for several years until the husband developed severe panic reactions (repudiating his part of the implicit contract) and thereupon entered analysis. The agreed-upon relationship had not met his expectations because the wife had continued her independent activities and was not at home enough to fulfill his demands. In his leech-like attachment to his wife, the patient had become oppressive.

During analysis he recounted this dream: "A man is swimming in shallow water—an odd, ludicrous figure. He is crawling around, not really swimming but going through the motions." In another dream sequence, he saw himself in the kitchen, talking with his wife and her parents. The latter were supporting their daughter's determination to remain involved in her career and other activities outside the home. The wife declared that she was going to continue to do whatever she wanted to do. The husband left the kitchen and went upstairs, pouting, whereupon his wife followed him, saying, "This is the only way I can make the marriage work. This is the only way I have a chance. If I stay home with you and the children, I will wither and dry up and become sick myself." As he awakened from this dream, the patient thought, "No wonder she feels the way she does. I have been too gloomy, oppressive, self-centered, and unaware of her needs."

The breach of implicit contract and the original marriage neurosis become very clear through these dreams. Some of the patient's unconscious fantasies (which became conscious during his analysis) were ones in which some strong, successful man fell in love with the wife and, because of this attachment, helped the couple to achieve success—professional, financial, and social. The patient's unconscious was tuned to his wife's unconscious, as was hers to his. She was involved in extramarital activities with powerful, aggressive men. He unconsciously realized and consciously denied these involvements. This material became a resistance to the analysis.

Whenever the patient, through his analytic work, became more adequate, his wife would work to undermine his new strength and reestablish the old equilibrium. She was particularly destructive in their sexual relationship. When he had built himself up to being especially virile in a sexual experience, bringing both himself and her to full orgasm, she responded typically. Instead of rewarding him with the admiration and awe he desired, she flipped him over so that she was on top and—working furiously—had six tremendous orgasms of her own. (Throughout the recital of this story, one could almost hear the wife's strident, exultant soprano—"Anything you can do, I can do—*better!*") The patient subsequently became crestfallen and depressed—exactly as his wife wanted him.

She was vehemently opposed to any alteration of the original agreement. The unverbalized contract, ratified by the husband's acquiescence to the wife's demands, had stipulated that the man should become an extension of the woman, furnishing her with the penis she did not have. The wife's desire for a penis and a masculine role were unresolved conflicts with her mother, the husband's passiveness and desire for an alter ego were unresolved conflicts from his mother-child symbiosis. Any improvement on the husband's part was, to the wife, a breach of the unwritten clause that required him to be submissive and her dominant.

Now what is the treatment of such a marriage? A successful analysis of the husband might eventuate in either the loss of his wife or the necessity for her to undergo treatment in order to be able to cope with her husband's newly fortified position of adult adequacy. Over the years, marriage therapists have repeatedly been confronted with such dilemmas and have diligently sought the most expedient techniques for resolving them. What follows is an effort to trace the history of marriage therapy and the efforts of its practitioners to make viable relationships out of moribund ones. I shall not try to evaluate the various trends in the field but only to show their many diversifications and directions.

THE CLASSICAL APPROACH—PSYCHOANALYSIS

In the classical approach to marriage therapy, the therapist takes into psychoanalysis the mate who has designated himself or herself the patient—and never sees the spouse. The reluctance to see the spouse arises out of the analyst's fear that such communication will endanger the trust and confidence the patient reposes in him. The very essence of psychoanalysis is an intense dyadic relationship between patient and therapist. It also involves free association, interpretation, transference, resistance, and unconscious mental activity. The patient freely associates; the analyst interprets. Because the *transference neurosis* is the cornerstone of psychoanalysis, every possible effort must be made to keep it free from contaminants, such as the distrust and jealousy that might result from the analyst's being available to the spouse. A sound, therapeutic alliance established between the conflict-free portion of the patient's ego and the analyst contributes greatly to the success of the analysis, as does the resolution of transference-countertransference deadlocks.

In the classical psychoanalytical approach, change in the marital relationship is a goal incidental to change in the individual's psycho-dynamics. Yet, because improvement in the mental health of one partner is often positively correlated with improvement in the well-being of the other, a successful analysis may result in an improved marriage relationship.[2] One frequent outcome of analysis is the ability of the patient to move toward the resolution of his marital problems—more often to improve than to dissolve his marriage.

In order to resolve his marriage problems through classical psychoanalysis, however, the patient must have enough basic strengths to allow for structural changes in his ego, regardless of whether the partner changes psychodynamically. If the patient has the necessary ego-strength, one of four outcomes may be expected:

1. *A one-way change with improved relationship.* The analysand, having psychodynamically separated and individuated, becomes capable of functioning successfully in the marriage, even though the mate fails to cooperate in fulfilling previous dependency needs.

2. *A two-way change with improved relationship.* The change in the analysand brings about a positive change in the responses of the mate and, consequently, a new and successful relationship.

3. *A two-way change with deteriorated relationship.* In about seven per cent of the cases, the mate responds to the patient's improvement by developing serious psychological disturbances of his or her own. The improvement of the patient causes a shift in pathological equilibrium with a resultant decompensation in the untreated mate—either necessitating treatment, contributing to a divorce, or creating new burdens for the successfully treated partner.

4. *A one-way change with deteriorated relationship.* The change in the analysand, without accompanying change in the mate, leads to an "impossible situation" with resultant divorce, instigated by one or the other of the marriage partners.

If the patient has not adequate ego strength and the analysis is unsuccessful, one of at least three outcomes may be predicted:

1. *An unchanged, though still unsatisfactory, relationship.* The marriage may continue as before, disturbing and frustrating to one or both partners.

2. *Divorce instigated by the patient.* The former analysand may instigate divorce in an effort to attribute his lack of change and his personal difficulties to the marriage.
3. *Divorce instigated by the mate.* The untreated mate, having waited in hope of a change and now despairing of one, may instigate divorce or legal separation.

PSYCHOTHERAPEUTIC APPROACHES OTHER THAN PSYCHOANALYSIS

In an effort to achieve effective therapeutic changes in the marriage neurosis and marriage contract where success had not resulted from classical psychoanalysis, several analysts pioneered in finding new combinations of treatments. We begin our historical survey of the literature illustrating changing attitudes toward treatment of marriage partners with a review of the work of a psychoanalyst, Dr. Clarence P. Oberndorf.

Clarence P. Oberndorf (1934). Consecutive and Concurrent Dyadic Psychotherapy

In 1934 Dr. Oberndorf, following his treatment of a couple with folie à deux, made observations on the role that the marriage relationship played in symptom formation. His patients, a husband and wife, had held similar paranoid symptoms and had, far from venting their neuroses on each other, directed them against the world. The equilibrium of their relationship was maintained by their having a common enemy—reality. Subsequently, Dr. Oberndorf treated five married couples in consecutive dyads[4]—that is, first one mate and then the other (Figure 1). Eventually he evolved the technique of seeing the two partners of a disturbed marriage concurrently, although not together at the same time, and conducting the analyses as if the patients were strangers to each other. In so doing, he broke with the classical psychoanalytical tradition of never seeing the patient's spouse.

Bela Mittelmann (1948). Concurrent Dyadic Psychotherapy

More than a decade later, Bela Mittelmann also treated mates simultaneously but in separate analytic sessions.[5,6] Yet his innovation and contribution to marriage therapy went beyond Oberndorf's in that they stressed more forcefully the significance of the mates' inter-relationship through psychotherapy and the advantages to the analyst of this therapy-generated relationship (Figure 2). The technique enabled Mittelmann to observe both the healthy and the neurotic interactions between mates, as

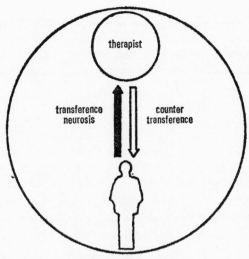

at completion of psychotherapy #1

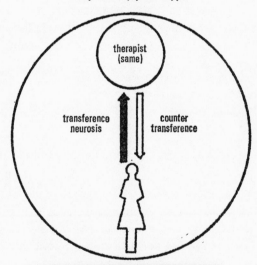

CONSECUTIVE DYADIC PSYCHOTHERAPY
(separate and consecutive sessions)

OBERNDORF (1934)
(based on psychoanalytic model)

Figure 1

well as to pick up trends in each far more rapidly than he could have were only one person reporting to him.[7] Mittelmann, like Oberndorf, noted that the neuroses of husband and wife complement each other and that there is a dovetailing of conflictual and defensive patterns.

Peter A. Martin and H. Waldo Bird (1952). A Collaborative Dyadic Approach (The Stereoscopic Technique)

At the Pontiac State Hospital and the Haven Sanitarium, Dr. H. Waldo Bird and I, under the supervision of Dr. Leo Bartemeier, began to evolve yet another technique because we saw that, in a particular group of patients, the classical psychoanalytic technique was not feasible. Some of our patients were so resentful of their mates, so disturbed, and so defensive that we were often dissatisfied with the results of the psychotherapeutic hour and yearned for more knowledge of what was going on in the hours away from therapy. Thus we devised a plan whereby we saw the marriage partners of each other's patients and then compared notes.[8]

The stereoscopic technique serves a purpose similar to that of the optical instrument for which it was named; it gives greater depth to the therapist's understanding of the patient by presenting two different views, which, when fused, produce an added dimension. The technique differs from Mittelmann's and Oberndorf's in that each partner is seen by a different psychiatrist and that these analysts regularly review together the reconstructed versions of important events in the lives of the marriage partner (Figure 3).

The collaborative, or stereoscopic, approach has the advantage of allowing for an immediate recognition of distortions of reality in the productions of the patients and, consequently, for understanding the instinctual impulses being warded off in each mate, as well as characteristic ego defenses. In patients lacking the ego strength necessary for dyadic psychoanalytic therapy, it was found that the neurotic symptom, conflict, or regression was fixed not only in the patient's personality, but also in the powerful emotional forces tying him or her to the marriage partner. For example, neurotic symptoms or regression to a psychosis might be the choice of one marriage partner in preference to separation from, or murder of, the "normal" mate. By comparing the productions of the mates, the psychiatrists could understand their complementary neuroses— that is, the forces which both drew the partners together and pulled them apart.

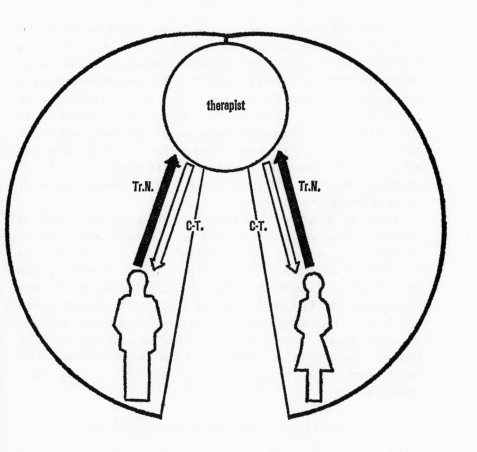

CONCURRENT DYADIC PSYCHOTHERAPY
(separate but concurrent sessions)

MITTELMANN (1948
based on psychoanalytic model)

Figure 2

Furthermore—and as Grotjahn notes[3]—the skillful use of insights developed by psychiatrists working together helps in the analysis of a resistance which censored information. This resistance may not necessarily be anchored in the neurosis of the patient; it may actually be anchored in the relationship between the marriage partners, and have become an important part of the "marriage neuroses." In evolving our technique, Dr. Bird and I tried at all times to remain aware of the importance of distinguishing between a resistance rooted in the patient (sometimes so subtle than its interpsychic implications almost went overlooked) and an intractable marital reality situation interfering with the therapeutic action of the analysis.

The study of the current relationships between the spouses and the transference neuroses in the individual therapies made possible the reconstruction of even the earliest symbiotic and separation phases of infant-mother relationships. In this respect, the therapeutic approach in the individual therapies was psychoanalytically modeled. But two new relationships—that between the psychiatrists and that between the patient and the mate's psychiatrist—were added and used for diagnostic and interpretative purposes. Through the dyadic relationship between therapists, moreover, the countertransference reactions of the psychiatrists to the patients were more accurately discerned and dissolved for greater therapeutic effectiveness.

Alexander Thomas (1956). Simultaneous Dyadic Therapy

More than two decades after Oberndorf's innovation, Alexander Thomas wrote a paper illustrating the shift in emphasis taking place in marriage therapy during the 50's.[9] He reported favorable results with simultaneous analytic psychotherapy modified by the use of the interpersonal relationship between marital partners (instead of the relationship with the therapist) as the prime focus for the delineation of the neurotic patterns and the impetus to change. This modification was made possible by the therapist's accurate knowledge of the interplay between husband and wife through his contact with both. Therapeutic attention was thereby shifted from the patient-therapist relationship to the family relationship. By 1954, this shift was so widely condoned and accepted that, whereas formerly a psychiatrist could not afford to consider the patient's family, now he could not afford to neglect it.[10]

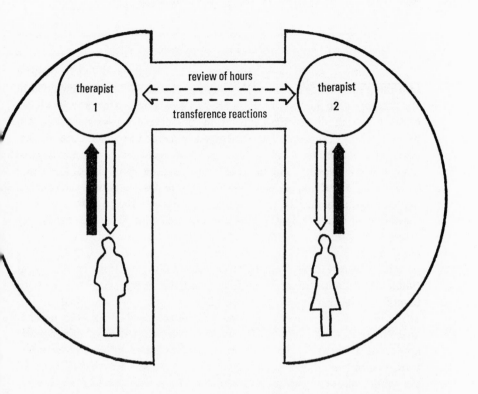

COLLABORATIVE (DYADIC) APPROACH
(the stereoscopic technique)

MARTIN and BIRD (1952)
(based on psychoanalytic model)

Figure 3

Don D. Jackson, Virginia Satir, Andrew S. Watson (1959)
Conjoint Marital Therapy, Triadic Therapy

Conjoint marital therapy brought even larger issues of family therapy into the picture since children, if present in the marriage, were included in the therapy. Don Jackson is considered to be its originator, and its theoretical approach differs markedly from the classical psychoanalytic approach. It has been defined as a therapeutic method in which both marital partners are seen together by the same therapist or co-therapists (one male and one female) and in which the signaling symptom or condition is viewed by the therapist as a comment on the dysfunction of the couple's interactional system.[11] In conjoint marital therapy, the patient is seen by the therapist as a family-surrounded individual with real problems originating in the present. This view—in addition to the idea that the patient is enmeshed in a fixed scheme of behavior where each family member is expected to behave in a mutually acceptable fashion—results in an operational approach based on the postulate that the interpersonal relationships involve two levels of communication allowing for double-bind relationships (Figure 4). Herein lie the fundamental differences between the psychoanalytic intrapsychic approach and the interpersonal psychotherapeutic approach. There is no development of transference neuroses, no countertransference resolutions. It is based on the here-and-now but because of the unfortunate early death of its founder, this therapy does not have a well developed theoretical foundation.

It is obvious, of course, that a therapist can see both marriage partners at the same time using the psychoanalytic emphasis on transference and resistance. This therapy would be called conjoint and triadic. The emphasis under such circumstances would be on the transference analysis and not on the interactional analysis of the therapist—as in the treatment devised by Greene.

Bernard L. Greene, Alfred Solomon, Noel Lustig (1960)
The Combined Approach

The combined approach makes use of individual, concurrent and conjoint sessions when, in the opinion of the therapist, both triadic and dyadic transactions are necessary either for successful treatment of the marital transaction or for successful treatment of one of the partners. The approach is very flexible and lends itself to the styles of various therapists and to the personalities and situations of various married couples.[12] The approach is based on the transactional concept of the nature of marital

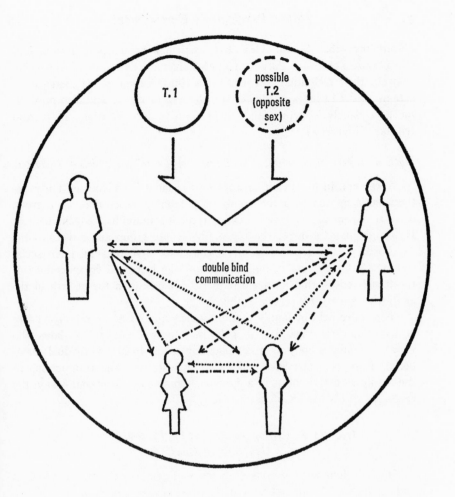

CONJOINT MARITAL THERAPY (FAMILY)

DON JACKSON (1959)

(not based on psychoanalytic model but on interpersonal therapeutic approach)

Figure 4

disharmony—that is, the idea that particular homeostatic transactions characterize a marriage. Although another shift away from classical psychoanalysis, their technique still involves a consideration of transference reactions (constituting a *triangular* transference neurosis) and also provides for psychoanalytic depth study of projective identifications in marital tensions (Figure 5).

Nathan Ackerman (1950). The Family Approach to Marital Disorders

Ackerman, in his definitive work on the family,[13] advocates a psychotherapeutic approach to the family as a family, rather than as a group of related persons, each of whom is receiving individual psychotherapy. He contemplates a direct therapy of the family group and advocates the psychoanalytic interpretation of unconscious dynamics in their social context. Although cumbersome because of the increased complications of the transferences, this approach pays rich dividends in the growth in the analyst's capacity for reality testing.

The entire field of family therapy is new and changing rapidly. There is a tendency for therapists to polarize into two groups: 1) those who view the family merely as a complicating factor in any individual member's intrapsychic struggles and 2) those who view the transactions of the family as determining, in a dynamic—sometimes beneficent—way, the responses and attitudes of its members.

Georges R. Reding, et al. (1964). Treatment of the Couple by a Couple

In their four-way sessions with married couples, Georges R. Reding and co-workers[14,15] at first viewed their therapy as a combination of two individual treatments. In their 1967 publication, however, they emphasize the relationship between the patient-couple and the therapist-couple, rather than the individual relationships of the four participants and the impact of the patient-couple's communications upon the relationship between the two therapists. They now pay specific attention to the current thoughts and affective reactions of the therapists towards each other, making extensive use of transference and countertransference interpretations from couple to couple during the four-way sessions. Their combination of transference and countertransference concepts with psychodrama, mediating between interpretation and verbalization, limits the intensity of the transference neurosis which the patient couple can develop with the therapist couple. Such limitation is in keeping with the treatment goals

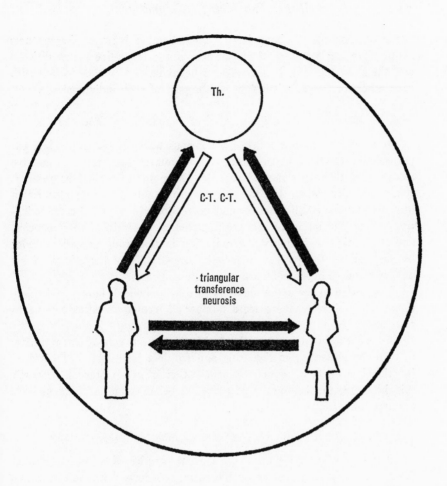

CONJOINT AND COMBINED (TRIADIC) THERAPY

GREENE, et. al. (1960)

(psychoanalytic and transactional)

Figure 5

—the opening up of channels of communication between the partners rather than the fostering of maturation of the respective personalities— and the substitution of better ways of behaving and communicating with each other for deeper self-insight on the part of each individual.

Martin Blinder (1960). Married Couple Group Therapy

Most of the papers published by various workers describing their experience in treating married couples in groups have shown a positive response to the experiment, but a few have indicated serious reservations.[16] Blinder claims that the therapy group obtains for its members a healthier marital equilibrium through correction of perceptual communicative errors, alleviation of reciprocal anxieties, analysis of discrepancies, and facilitation of intimacy. Participation in the group process, Blinder believes, allows the patient to examine constructively the effects of his behavior and to experiment with alternate responses.

In addition to the many methods used in individual, family and traditional group therapy, there are a number of techniques either unique to married-couple group therapy or of special importance in such therapy. Blinder believes that persistently positive interpretation of intent serves to turn the patient from defensive and fruitless justification of his dysfunctional goals to constructive participation in group process. Through this, he is free to examine the effects of his behavior and experiment with alternatives.

S. R. Slavson (1965). Coordinated Family Group Therapy

Slavson,[17] who believes that the current practice of working with the family as a unit may do irrevocable harm, has devised a modified group therapy. It is based on the observation that the capacity for tolerance in one particular member is frequently overtaxed to the point where his resistances become intensified and his hostility overt. In coordinated family group therapy Slavson employs the following practices:

1. The adolescents are placed in like-sex groups.
2. The fathers and mothers are seen in separate groups, arranged according to the age and gender of the children.
3. Seriously disturbed parents, whose distortions would interfere with the progress of the groups, receive individual psychotherapy, in addition to that obtained at their regular meetings.

Each of the three groups is presided over by a different therapist—a practice which prevents the involvement of a staff member with both a

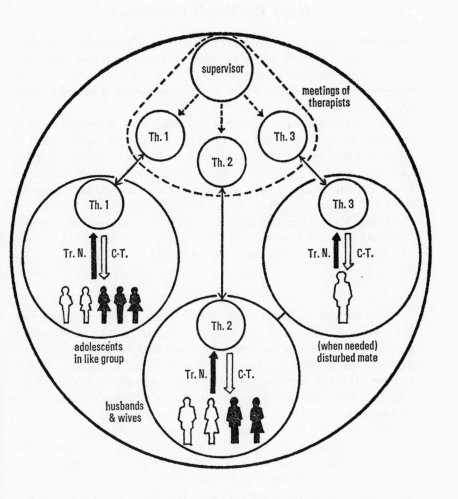

COORDINATED FAMILY GROUP THERAPY

SLAVSON (1965)

(psychoanalytic origin)

Figure 6

parent and a child at the same time (Figure 6). This separation of function prevents distortions of the therapist, decreases resistance, and avoids confusion in the transference. It also prevents the abrasive effect on vulnerable members of the family that Slavson sees as a hazard of many types of group therapy.

The coordinating process involves an extensive set of protocols kept by the three therapists and used as the basis for the regularly scheduled integration conferences. In these conferences, critically conflicting situations and damaging acts usually manifest themselves in the communications of one or more of the family members, and this material alerts the appropriate therapists to take steps to correct or diminish pathology as it appears in the group. Slavson sees the sharing of the same supervisor by the three therapists as an aid to control. He also recommends this method as a way of achieving flexibility and individuation in treatment.

SUMMARY

It is clear that the literature on marriage therapy and marriage neurosis is originally predominantly psychoanalytic in nature. As such, the therapeutic emphasis was on the development and analysis of the transference neurosis. The classical psychoanalytic approach, the concurrent, the consecutive, the collaborative and combined approaches maintained this emphasis. The main change in direction took place when therapists began to de-emphasize and even avoid the transference neurosis. The focus first moved from the patient-therapist transferences to the transferences between the marriage partners, and, finally, to something entirely new. This "something new" was the effort to establish constructive relationships between the partners in the family setting through their experiences in the therapeutic situation without emphasis on the deeper understanding of transference reactions within the individual patient. Such an approach implies that a change in the marital relationship produces some alteration of the personality of the individuals involved.

Another approach illustrating the trend from classical psychoanalysis was Roy Grinker's transactional model for psychotherapy.[18] Grinker describes avoidance of the development of a transference neurosis but recognizes that he is still dealing with transference phenomena, which he views as communications between the therapist and patient tacitly recognizing the fact that the present is colored by the past.

It is possible that these changes in emphasis will in time recede and allow emphasis on the transference neurosis to surge to the front again.

But I do not think so. I think there will continue to be experimentation and inventions to meet the necessities of our changing social order and changing patterns of marriage and family living. In the medical schools at which I teach, the residents show an avid interest in learning the various techniques of treating marriage partners, families, and groups. If they are given such training, they will undoubtedly use and promulgate the new techniques—and probably introduce further innovations.

In order to achieve flexibility and specificity in his approach, a psychiatrist must be versatile. Ideally he will suit the psychotherapeutic approach to the specific couple. However, I cannot overemphasize the importance of the following observation: there is no magic power in any single technique; every technique has both advantages and disadvantages. There are many ways to "skin a cat," many practicable ways to accomplish the same job. What is important is the skill, training and experience of the individual using the technique. This determines its degree of efficacy. The practitioner of a particular technique is more important than the technique itself. Also, the interpersonal relationship inherent in all forms of psychotherapy makes the personality structure of the therapist, his ability to inspire trust and confidence in his patient, his sensitivity, his flexibility, and his capacity for empathy fully as important as his skill as a psychotherapist.[19]

It was my experience with the stereoscopic technique that psychoanalytic training made me more capable in the use of the new approach. Conversely, my experience with the stereoscopic technique made me more capable in treating a disturbed marital partner in psychoanalysis. Psychoanalytically-trained therapists can use the new techniques more successfully than therapists *not* trained in psychoanalysis. The history of marriage therapy clearly points to psychoanalysis as the genesis of the recent trends. It is also clear from the literature that many of the new techniques are not adaptable to patients with severe character disorders, borderline psychosis, and severe psychoneurosis. Hence young therapists should not resort to any of the recent techniques as substitutes for training in intensive psychotherapy. A thorough understanding of conventional technique, plus versatility and flexibility, is a mandate for the therapist who must handle today's varied and complex marriage problems.

REFERENCES

1. Freud, S. The Ego and the Id. *The Complete Psychological Works of Sigmund Freud.* Volume XIX. Hogarth Press, 1961.
2. Sager, C. J., et al. The Married in Treatment. Arch. Gen. Psychiat. 19: August, 1968. p. 206.
3. Grotjahn, Martin. *Psychoanalysis and the Family Neurosis.* W. W. Norton & Co., New York, 1960.
4. Oberndorf, Clarence P. "Psychoanalysis of Married Couples." International Journal of Psychoanalysis, 25 (1938) 453.
5. Mittelmann, Bela. "Complementary Neurotic Reactions in Intimate Relationships." Psychoanalytic Quart. (1944) 13:479-491.
6. ———— "The Concurrent Analysis of Married Couples." Psychoanalytic Quart. (1948) 17:182-197.
7. Sager, C. J. The Treatment of Married Couples. *American Handbook of Psychiatry.* S. Arieti, Ed. Basic Book, 1966. Volume III, p. 214.
8. Martin, Peter A. and Bird, H. Waldo. "An Approach to the Psychotherapy of Marriage Partners—The Stereoscopic Technique." Psychiatry, XVI:123-127 (1953).
9. Thomas, Alexander. "Simultaneous Psychotherapy with Marital Partners" Amer. J. Psychotherapy. X:716-727 (1956).
10. Grotjahn, M. "Analytic Family Therapy: A Survey of Trends in Research and Practice." *Individual and Family Dynamics.* Edited by J. Masserman. Grune & Stratton, Inc., 1959.
11. Satir, Virginia M., "Conjoint Family Therapy," in *The Psychotherapies of Marital Disharmony,* Edited by Bernard L. Greene, The Free Press, New York, 1965.
12. Greene, B. L., Broadhurst, B. P. and Lustig, N. "Treatment of Marital Disharmony." *The Psychotherapies of Marital Disharmony.* Edited by Bernard L. Greene, The Free Press, New York, 1965.
13. Ackerman, Nathan W. *The Psychodynamics of Family Life.* Basic Books, Inc., New York, 1958.
14. Reding, Georges R. and Ennis, Barbara. "Treatment of the Couple by a Couple." Brit. J. Med. Psychol. (1964), 37, 325.
15. Reding, Georges R., Charles, Lois A. and Hoffman, Michael B. "Treatment of the Couple by a Couple II." Brit. J. Med. Psychol. (1967), 44, 243.
16. Blinder, Martin G. and Kirschenbaum, Martin. Archives General Psychiatry 17, July 1967, 44.
17. Slavson, S. R. "Coordinated Family Therapy," International J. Group Psychother. April, 1965.
18. Grinker, Roy R. "A Transactional Model for Psychotherapy." Archives of General Psychiatry. 1:1959: 132.
19. Wolberg, Lewis R. "Is Psychoanalysis Dead?" Editorial in Medical Tribune, Nov. 28, 1968. 0. 15.

7

JOSEPH C. SOLOMON, M.D.

This chapter on the psychoanalytic view of existence is dedicated to Leo Bartemeier whose very existence has enriched the existence of many others.

Cogitor, Ergo Sum

WE ARE FAMILIAR with Descartes' philosophical concept "cogito ergo sum." This formulation suggests that one's existence is contingent upon the ability to think. Recent investigations have shown that "thinking" does not develop in a vacuum but is an outgrowth of stimulation and communication. It is the purpose of this presentation to clearly define the concept of "I am" as a manifestation of human existence and as the basic foundation for the formation of the ego. Stated differently, the concept postulates that the human infant becomes an entity when he develops the knowledge or awareness of his own existence. This can only be accomplished through the medium of an awareness of the mother who is similarly aware of him. I am therefore offering a revision of the Cartesian formula to read: "Cogitor ergo sum"—"I am thought about, therefore I am."

XENIA'S DREAM*

A patient reported a fascinating dream that started a whole chain reaction in my thinking. Never, either before or since, have I heard a report of a dream of a similar nature. Many colleagues, especially ones who have been making studies of patients' dreams, were consulted, but no one had ever heard of such a dream. Yet the dream would seem to have wide clinical implication.

---

* Much of the material of this presentation appeared in the author's paper, "Alice and the Red King," referenced in the bibliography.

Here is the dream:

> There is a giant lying on the grass. There is a big round circle above
> him indicating that he is dreaming (like in the comic strips). I'm in
> that dream just doing ordinary things. I get the idea that I exist only
> in his dream. It is important for him to stay asleep, because if he
> wakes up, I will disappear. This is a tremendous fear.

Even without having a clinical description of this patient, the astute
reader can draw many inferences from this dream. One suspects the patient has a very tenuous hold on reality, and that a plausible cause for
this was a serious problem with the patient's father. Furthermore, one
would suspect the anxiety expressed by the patient is related to primitive
urges for self-preservation and union with a parent.

The patient, Xenia T., was a 36-year-old single woman who entered
analysis because of severe anxiety over recurring thoughts of becoming
psychotic like her brother, who was a patient in a mental hospital. Her
father, a physician, urged her to get assistance because of her extreme
obesity, which could not be controlled because of her compulsive eating.
The patient was not seriously concerned about her weight, which probably exceeded 250 pounds, and she had no desire to change her eating
habits.

The patient's speech mannerisms were eccentric. She was very loqua-
cious and, moreover, spoke in a loud voice as if she were addressing a
huge audience. She gave the impression that she must continually make
her presence felt; yet, at the same time, she always considered herself
very insignificant. She was always surprised when others recognized her
or listened to what she had to say.

The patient considered herself a thoroughly dependent person, which
indeed she was, but she acted in a bossy, officiously managerial manner
whenever she had the opportunity. She was fearful of men and marriage.
She used her obesity as a foil for warding off romantic involvements. As
a child she had never wanted to be a girl. She played football with the
boys and avoided all feminine activities. This pattern persisted, one example being her exaggerated interest in spectator sports. Although her
homosexual inclinations were well-defined, she showed no tendency towards
overt homosexual behavior. Her disturbance in object relations probably
was derived from the fact that she saw very little of her physician-father.
Her mother was also a physician and was more aggressive and authoritarian than her father. Her mother had been responsible for the care and
punishment of the children. Although the patient knew many people, she

never allowed herself to be close to anyone, male or female. On the other hand, she was devoted to her two dogs. Although she was a peculiar person in many ways, she functioned to her own satisfaction until the age of twenty-five when her mother died. Shortly thereafter, her maternal grandparents died and her brother became psychotic. She watched him develop delusions of being Jesus Christ. Her fears of insanity then took hold, and her character traits and compulsive actions became intensified.

From her early childhood Xenia exhibited strong scoptophilic and exhibitionistic drives with the accompanying reverse polarities, namely, the inability to notice things about her and the fear of being noticed. She also struggled with the opposing motivations of omnipotence and helplessness. In an attempt to cope with her conflicts, she remained regressed to an early level of infantile thought processes. From an early age she centered her thinking around the idea that her very existence was contingent upon the maintenance of a masculine image. She accomplished this by incorporating some aspects of her father, which led her to eat like a man and talk like a man. An early memory of her father eating a poached egg on toast in four bites impressed her considerably.

Although the patient professed a great deal of hostility to, and fear of, her father, it was revealed in working through her Oedipal situation in the transference that her greatest libidinal gratification came from being at home while her father was asleep. Her loud talk and eating habits were related to the dinner table situation when her father was home. The wish fulfillment function of the recurrent dream can be understood from learning of the patient's enjoyment of her father's presence at home and the absence of his criticism when he was asleep, along with his tendency to leave her and ignore her when he was awake. The groundwork for her underlying fears of abandonment and oral preoccupations had been laid earlier when her mother, because of illness, left her for a period of nine months beginning when the patient was one and one-half years old.

When Xenia first reported the dream, she attached little signficance to it. As the analysis progressed there was occasion to refer to the dream many times both as an interpretation and as an association by the patient. Xenia gave some structure to the dream by stating that she sometimes does not feel real and might vanish as a dream vanishes when a person awakens.

ALICE AND THE RED KING

Whether it was by accident or by motivation from some unconscious forces set in motion by this patient's dream, the author picked up Lewis

Carroll's "Through the Looking Glass."[2] His attention was arrested by the following passage:

> . . . she checked herself in some alarm, at hearing something that sounded to her like the puffing of a large steam-engine in the wood near them, though she feared it was more likely to be a wild beast. "Are there any lions or tigers about here?" she asked timidly.

> "It's only the Red King snoring," said Tweedledee. "Come and look at him!" the brothers cried, and they took one of Alice's hands and led her up to where the King was sleeping.

> "Isn't he a *lovely* sight?" said Tweedledum. Alice couldn't say honestly that he was. He had a tall red night-cap on with a tassel, and he was lying crumpled up into a sort of untidy heap and snoring loud—"fit to snore his head off!" as Tweedledum remarked.

> "I'm afraid he'll catch cold with lying on the damp grass," said Alice, who was a very thoughtful little girl. "He's dreaming now," said Tweedledee: "and what do you think he's dreaming about?" Alice said, "Nobody can guess that." "Why, about *you!*" Tweedledee exclaimed, clapping his hands triumphantly. And if he left off dreaming about you, where do you suppose you'd be?" "Where I am now, of course," said Alice. "Not you!" Tweedledee retorted contemptuously. "You'd be nowhere. Why, you're only a sort of thing in his dream!"

> "If that there King was to wake," added Tweedledum, "you'd go out —bang!—just like a candle!" "I shouldn't!" Alice exclaimed indignantly. "Besides, if *I'm* only a sort of thing in his dream, what are *you*, I should like to know?" "Ditto," said Tweedledum. "Ditto, ditto!" cried Tweedledee.

> He shouted this so loud that Alice couldn't help saying "Hush! You'll be waking him, I'm afraid, if you make so much noise." "Well, it's no use *your* talking about waking him," said Tweedledum, "when you're only one of the things in his dream. You know very well you're not real."

> "I *am* real!" said Alice, and began to cry.

> "You won't make yourself a bit realler by crying," said Tweedledee, "there's nothing to cry about."

> "If I wasn't real," Alice said—half laughing through her tears, it all seemed so ridiculous—"I shouldn't be able to cry."

"I hope you don't suppose those are *real* tears?" Tweedledum interrupted in a tone of great contempt.

"I know they're talking nonsense" thought Alice to herself: "and it's foolish to cry about it." So she brushed away her tears and went on, as cheerfully as she could. . . .

Xenia was asked if she had read *Alice in Wonderland* or *Through the Looking Glass*. For a long time she steadfastly denied ever having read or heard anything of these books. Later she admitted she may have glanced at the *Alice* books but said that she never liked them. Rather, she indicated she associated the giant of her dream with Jack and the Beanstalk and Robin Hood and not with Alice. If she had heard the story of the Red King, she probably repressed it because of her need to deny her libidinal interest in her father. However, it is likely that Xenia's dream arose from purely intrinsic sources. We feel that we are obliged to conjecture that Lewis Carroll's fertile imagination and the patient's neurotic imagery must have originated from comparable sources.

It is surprising that the type of dream Xenia reported does not occur more frequently because it is so closely bound to the primitive concept of existence. The basic "need for attention," which is such a universal motivation in childhood, we believe actually to be a search for reassurance that one's image appears in the mind of an important person in the life of the individual.

It is interesting that the dream-fantasy of both Xenia and Alice represent the projected thoughts of a little girl into the mind of a powerful father-person, which could reveal much about the thought processes of Lewis Carroll. Greenacre's[3] study of the life of Carroll is helpful here.

Both Xenia and Lewis Carroll were strongly influenced by magical thinking. Carroll (actually Charles Dodgson) was a mathematician. This suggests that he used the precision and predictability of numbers to master his impulses and uncertainty. His other identity, that of the writer, permitted him to give vent to his sadistic and erotic impulses, albeit in a nonsensical whimsical fashion. Dodgson was a shy individual with strong ties to his mother. He both admired and feared his father, to whom he found it difficult to speak. When he spoke to his father, he stuttered badly. Xenia used loquacity as a defense, but at the same time, she never looked a person in the eye when she spoke. Carroll displaced his imageries on to Alice Liddell, who served as an object of identification and gratification. His interest in little girls was a displacement and denial of his libidinal ties to his mother. Likewise, Xenia also showed sexual interest in little boys and older people but fled from her contemporaries.

Carroll and my patient had poor relationships with their fathers. No behavior seemed to make any impression on their fathers, at least so each thought. As a defense against the fearsome qualities of his father, Carroll depicted his authoritative male figures as weak, emasculated men—e.g., they either blundered, or fell off their horses, or, in the case of the Red King, were asleep. His women, on the other hand, were strong and punitive. My patient, like Carroll, was never able to cope with masculine men. She had a few male friends who were obviously homosexual. With them she felt safe.

A characteristic of the Alice stories is the use of disappearance as a form of punishment. Greenacre considered the vanishing of the Cheshire Cat as a castration phenomenon. If this is plausible, Xenia's dream might also be looked upon from this point of view. In therapy, however, interpretations at this level were not too successful. It turned out that the extent of the anxiety experienced by Xenia, and perhaps by Carroll as well, was of a more archaic nature. It embodied the concept of nothingness, of non-existence, of death. Carroll reduced some of his fears by converting them into grotesque nonsense fantasy. My patient, too, defended herself by incorporating the masculinity of her father, and by making her presence felt through her large size, her loud voice and her overbearing manner.

Greenacre's study of the life of Lewis Carroll was helpful in understanding some of the thinking processes of my patient. Xenia's dream of appearing as the dream of a giant who would make her disappear on awakening was similar to Alice's fantasy of the dream of the Red King. Greenacre's statement that the Alice books "reproduce the spirit of the preverbal era" was thoroughly applicable in the treatment of Zenia.

Inasmuch as disappearance from the mind of a parent image leads to fear, we are obliged to assume that the presence in the mind of the pertinent parent leads to gratification or satisfaction. It is this very point which I should like to emphasize in this paper as constituting the phenomenon of existence. As such, it represents a phase of ego growth and is one which has its derivatives in an on-going ego function.

EXISTENCE AND CASTRATION

The castration phenomenon bears an important relationship to the fear of non-existence or death. Burton's[4] recent survey showed that a large majority of psychoanalysts believe that fear of death is secondary to castration anxiety. (He considers such "thanatophobia" a counter-transference phenomenon.) It is far more reasonable to feel that castration anxiety is partial death, i.e., mutilation, and is of a less archaic nature than death itself. In this respect we can utilize the concepts expressed in this presentation to understand some other symptoms of human behavior, particularly sexual exhibitionism. When the man exposes his penis to a strange woman, his greatest libidinal charge comes from his organ having been seen. This assures him that it is still there. This may also explain the absence of female genital exhibitionism and the prominence of female breast exhibitionism because it confirms the fact that something is there.

EXISTENCE AND THEOLOGY

The concept of existence being dependent upon the image in the mind of a parent figure is an ancient one. In the Hindu religion, particularly the Vedanta, the existence of man is predicated upon the dream of the deity. The dream of the Supreme creative power (Ishwara) controls the entire cosmos. Actually, it is not a sleeping dream but is described as an act of cosmic ideation. It is believed that man's existence is created by the thought processes of Ishwara and man's existence as such ends when the deity goes to sleep. The whole universe is created and destroyed in alternate cycles depending upon the successive thinking and non-thinking of the Supreme being.

The concept of the waking awareness on the part of the deity controlling the existence of man is the reverse of the existence being dependent upon the sleeping figures of the giant and the Red King. But the relationship of the psychic process of the parent figure and the phenomenon of existence is unmistakable.

The Greek philosopher, Philo,[5] whose concepts, like those of Plato and Aristotle, influenced later Christian philosophers, stated that God has a direct share in the rational and irrational processes of the soul:

> But neither has the mind the power to work—that is, to put forth its energies by way of sense perception—unless God sends the object of sense as rain upon it.

The concept that the existence of man is dependent upon God's awareness was propounded by St. Thomas Aquinas[6] in his Summa Theologica. He quoted the New Testament:

> "Upholding all things by the word of His power" (Heb. 1:3).

He stated that both reason and faith require us to say that creatures are kept in being by God. He quoted Augustine:

As the air becomes light by the presence of the sun, so is man illumined by the presence of God, and in his absence returns at once to darkness.

Maritain[7] expounds the Catholic point of view of existence by quoting St. Thomas and adds a few observations which have psychological and/or philosophical implications. He speaks of existence as a subjective phenomenon of perception with the added ingredient of "essences" or "natures" which are reflections of divine linkages.

The secular philosopher Bishop Berkeley[8] had much to say about existence. He reasoned that objects exist only because we perceive them. This led him to subscribe to the principle of *esse est percipi*—i.e., to exist is to be perceived by some mind. He went on to say that individual human existents exist in the mind of human persons as well as in the mind of a Supreme being. From this he believed that he had adduced the proof of the existence of God.

From the commentary by Gardner[9] in his *The Annotated Alice*, there is the suggestion that Carroll consciously used the concept of Alice and the Red King as a reflection of the Berkeleyan theme. Gardner also pointed out that the dream of the Red King has been the source of much discussion among philosophers, including Bertrand Russell.

EXISTENTIALISM AND PSYCHOANALYSIS

Before going further in the discussion of the metapsychology of human existence, let us examine some of the contributions of the existentialists on this subject.

The existentialists describe two elements in the formation of an existence—namely, the "natural" and the "ontological." The "natural" factors they define as the anatomical and physiological realities of the organism. The "ontological" factors, perhaps because they are more difficult to understand, they explain by resorting to older metaphysical ideas.

Ontology is defined as the science of being or reality. It is considered to be that branch of knowledge which investigates the nature, essential properties and relations of beings as such. In this connection, May[10] offers the statement that man must be understood in terms of those characteristics which make him human and without which he could not exist. Kirkegaard,[11] the father of existentialism, was a religious man who explained the concept of existence along purely theologic lines. Maritain also, it was pointed out, adhered to the notion that the desire for being and the anguish over not-being is resolved by faith in God. The "atheistic" existentialists—particularly Heidegger[12] and Sartre[13]—have a more difficult time explaining existence. In fact, they do not explain it at all. They say, "We exist because we exist."

Heidegger refers to the union of man with his environment as the phenomenon of "being-in-the-world." Sartre refers to two aspects of existence, "being-in-itself" and "being-for-itself" or "nothingness" as presumably synonymous with human consciousness. We find this concept quite incomprehensible. It may be Sartre's particular way of dividing the natural from the ontologic. Sartre says that man conquers his feelings of nothingness or non-existence by the use of the will, whereas the theologians turn to faith in a Supreme being.*

It seems clear that the concept of "being" versus "non-being" represents basically the operation of the survival or self-preservative instincts. Non-existence is the fundamental survival threat, the threat of disintegration of the self. In infancy and in neurotic persons it is the threatened loss of the primitive ego integrity. The disturbances in the state of being or existence, whether they emanate from the outer world or from within the individual, still do not explain the positive fact of awareness of existence itself. We are thus obliged to bring out in scientific terms the concept that can best be epitomized by the words "I am."

It is difficult to grasp any truly scientific aspect to the so-called ontologic factors. We hear such statements as "beyond all time," and "unmeasurable dimension." When pinned down for more exact definition, an ardent existentialist stated that *ontologic* is synonymous with *religious*. This, of course, brings us back to such concepts as "the soul" and "divine essences," which have been amply postulated by Jung.

Closely related to the subject at hand are the concepts of *ego* and *self*, which Jung delineates. He considers ego as being formed by the consciousness of environmental phenomena which make the child aware of his own body. Self, on the other hand, he equates with the "soul," which is a cosmic or mystical element in the psyche derived from a collective unconscious and manifesting itself in the dream, in religious ecstasy,

---

* Varying degrees of adherence to mystical, magical, or metaphysical ideas have been expressed by numerous thinkers on this subject. Authors not referred to in the text are many. For more extensive reading on this subject, the following names are offered: Nietzsche, Jaspers, Maral, Merleau-Ponty, Jeanson, Dondeyne, Luijpen, Minkowski, Reinhardt.

in rapture, or erotic entrancement. He could very well have applied his terms the other way around. That is, he could have said that the consciousness of the body is the self and the ego is the soul.

PSYCHODYNAMICS OF EXISTENCE

We shall next offer a few points that hopefully will help in understanding the concept of existence as a phenomenon of human development. Certainly, Freud did not emphasize existence as such, but his writings indicate cognizance of it in many ways.

The anxiety experienced by Xenia can very well be described as *existential anxiety*, the term introduced by Heidegger. A better term is *existence anxiety*. Xenia was worried that if her image were not present in her father's mind, she would no longer exist. Because this manifestation seems so closely bound to the basic self-preservative instincts, it appears likely to be an archaic form of thinking that may be quite universal in the growth processes of all human beings. By definition, *anxiety* is the experiencing of fear with no known or visible cause. It is the anticipation of an unconscious threat from the instincts, superego or object relationships.

Kirkegaard defined anxiety as a desire for what one dreads, and compared it to an alien power that lays hold of the individual.

In Xenia's case the anxiety she experienced had a life of its own, quite disconnected from her real life situation but one which clearly had its roots in her earlier life experiences. Nevertheless, the primary fear, that of her possible non-existence, continued in the form of an obsessive idea which permeated her whole life. The tenaciousness with which she held onto this idea and the associated compulsive behavior was to her self-preservative. For her to give them up would reactivate the original separation anxiety that she had experienced as an infant.

It will be remembered that, because of illness, her mother had had to leave the year-and-a-half-old Xenia for a period of nine months. Bowlby's studies on separation anxiety are very illuminating here. He describes three stages that the child experiences when he is separated from mother. They are (a) protest, (b) despair and (c) detachment. The phase of protest is one of either anger or fear. He refers to the fear as "primary anxiety." It might be better to call it "fear" because it is not derived from unconscious sources but from the actual threat that the child experiences when the mother-child union is disrupted. The phase of despair is the depressive phase where the child gives up hope of recalling the mother and nothing else can console him. The phase of "detachment" has been misnamed, because Bowlby describes it as one in which the child re-attaches himself to other persons or to substitute objects, such as his thumb, the security blanket, toys or pet animals. This is the phase of repair or restitution. The mother's importance dwindles.

All the phases of reaction to the original separation of mother and child which later can be manifested as fears of rejection and still later as fears of castration and social ostracism have their representations in the secondary perceptual thinking of the neurotic processes. These are discernible as varying degrees of (a) tension, (b) resignation and (c) accommodation. Each of these may set up imageries and sensations which act as subterranean sources of reality distortions for the afflicted individuals and produce the clinical syndrome of neurosis or character disturbances.

Let us now return to the imagery of the patient and the concept of existence anxiety. Hora states it very clearly:

> Existential anxiety stems from the need to have our existence confirmed by our fellow man. We are driven to reach out with our voices, and experience a connection through being heard by another power.

In short, what is meant by existence anxiety is built-in fear that has originated when the image of the self is not apprehended as existing in the mind of pertinent individuals or, we might add, when the object itself disappears.

With Xenia, the need to feel important to her father was motivated by her genital strivings to him. However, the form that this affinity took was based upon the original separation or existence anxiety that had been fixed in relation to her mother. Having failed to be perceived by mother, she turned to father. Her father never gave her any actual reason to feel important, either in a general sense or, in particular, to him. For that reason her Oedipal relationship was completely permeated with the theme of the concept of existence that had been established earlier and amplified by his mode of communication (or lack of it) to his daughter. It is noteworthy that Xenia repressed all of her sexual feelings. Even her masturbation was not considered by her to be sexual. This sexual repression may have had some relationship with the repression of actual memories of having read or heard the story of the Red King, though we recall she claimed she associated her sleeping giant with the sleeping giant in Jack and the Beanstalk.

Xenia's dream is reminiscent of Frenkel-Brunswick's description of her own analysis in which her analyst interpreted her behavior as resembling a "Cordelia motive." The analyst had suggested to her that she was displaying in her life the role of Cordelia, the youngest daughter of King Lear. To her answer that she had read most of Shakespeare's dramas but not King Lear, the analyst replied that Cordelia was the best and most generous daughter of King Lear, who nevertheless preferred his other two daughters because of their flattering attitude. At the time it was offered she refused the interpretation with considerable emotion but received it more favorably later on. Much later, after coming to this country, she discovered in looking through old notes that at the age of about fifteen she had copied the entire role of Cordelia. Thus, she must have been concerned at that age with the fate of Cordelia, with whom she had identified herself, later repressing not only this identification but also all other memory of the play. If Xenia had read the story of the dream of the Red King, it could easily have been repressed in the same manner as the Cordelia story wherein the Oedipal wishes were repressed and an identification with a fictitious character remains. With Xenia an archaic imagery of existence was retained in an act of regression. Although many features of Xenia's thinking were of a regressive nature there probably also existed a certain amount of undeveloped ego function because of the failure to have mastered her early needs to establish an independent autonomous existence. This leads us to the consideration of the concept of existence as a phase of ego integration and to the concomitant concept that when there is disruption of this process there is ego disintegration or disorganization. Let us turn our attention to infant development and some other behavioral phenomena.

During the infancy period the mother literally has the power of life and death over the baby. The parasitic position of the human infant makes it imperative that all of the innate instinctual functions be satisfied by the physical presence of the mother or mother surrogate. For the first six months the specificity of a particular mother does not seem to be vital. After that, it is necessary for the child to recognize and become fully aware of the existence of one particular mother. At the age of eight months, Spitz[14] has shown us, a strange mother is unacceptable and frightening. The appearance of such a non-mother is a reminder of the non-appearance of the real mother.

The knowledge of the existence of the mother is determined by the stimulation and gratification of the child's perceptual apparatus. Before being able visually to recognize its mother, the baby has appreciated her through her gratification of his need to suck, to obtain nourishment, to be warm, to smell, to be passively and rhythmically moved through space and to hear familiar sounds. The familiar sounds to which the infant first responds with a feeling of relaxation are the heart beats of the mother, according to researches by Salk.[15] Later this is replaced by mother's spoken voice and the familiar lullaby. A patient who could not bear to be alone was comforted to a degree by the sound of the radio, to which he listened incessantly. He was a hi-fi enthusiast. (We are surrounded by ubiquitous "canned" music, thus never "alone.") Bowlby[16] also emphasizes the infant's need to cling and his later need to follow.

There is a distinct connection between the feeling of existence on the part of the child and the appreciation of the existence of the mother. The emotional or perceptual experiences of the infant-mother union must occur before there is established the awareness of one's existence. In theologic terms, this emotion is recaptured in religious people by the Holy Presence. Sensually, it probably is the same as the oceanic feeling, the Nirvana principle and some forms of aesthetic experience. It is the epiphany of Joyce and Yeats, the manifestation of Divine power, or moment of Divine revelation, and "the moment in and out of time" of Eliot. It is likely also the Dharma of Yoga and the Satori of Zen Buddhism.

Silverberg[17] formulated the basic instinctive motivations of the infant as drives to see, touch and swallow the mother. The subsequent derivatives of these motivations are the wishes to *be* seen, to *be* touched and to *be* swallowed by the mother, which serve to close a harmonious circuit in a primitive conflict-free intercommunication system between mother and child. The knowledge of the satisfactory mutual coexistence of mother and self forms an early beginning of the ego.

The taking of the Sacrament does not have its full effect unless it is accompanied by the intense emotional experience which has been described as the equivalent of the infant-mother union. This emotional experience of the Eucharist is depicted as the spiritual union between Christ and the faithful. In the Catholic Church, particularly, the emotional experience of the Eucharist leads the individual to a state of grace within the framework of the Church. This is a special form of existence which places one in the position of being favored with God's mercy over and beyond justice. It is a supernatural gift bestowed upon man for his salvation.

The favor for being in a state of grace is that which is to be attained in Heaven. The ultimate reward is the beatific vision. This vision is the immediate sight of God in the glory of Heaven, as enjoyed by the blessed dead. In other words, there is an anticipation of a new level of existence, the perpetual one, that of immortality. If one observes and is observed by the immortal parent, then one attains immortality himself.

A devout Catholic patient demonstrated the theme of this presentation during one of her analytic sessions. She was a rather disturbed young woman who had had one acute schizophrenic break but who was making a fairly good adjustment at the beginning of her analysis. She was comfortably married and engaged in professional activities but was hampered by severe recurrent anxiety spells. These are her verbatim remarks:

> From the time I was in the sixth grade I became afraid of people. I felt inferior to everyone. I became studious and felt that I had to be perfect. I was a good girl in God's eyes. This held me together. I knew God loved me. He cared for everyone in a special way. Even if I were the only person in the world He would die for me. Because I was always in a state of grace He knew I existed. This kept me alive. If not for this I know I would have died. As long as I believe in God I knew that He would not turn away from me.

At a later session this patient became very distressed about the hereafter. She said that she was afraid of Heaven because one cannot be married there and she would miss her husband. Apparently, the live human relationship with her husband had become more important than the mystical one with the Deity, which at one time had been of supreme importance to her.

Melanie Klein[18] believes that the destructive impulses are primary motivations of the infant and that the loving mother acts merely to neutralize these forces, thereby imparting to the child the feeling of life. Separation from mother merely accentuates the aggressive impulses, which are presumably derived from the death instincts and are projected outwardly upon the mother. This gives rise to the phenomenon of persecutory anxiety.

Stokes[19] subscribes to this view along Kleinian lines but adds some interesting observations. He states that the sense of loss of the mother brings with it a "taste of death," since it is the first libidinal reaction to the pull of death. This involves the duality of life and death instincts, which has not been accepted by all analysts.

It is this "taste of death" that we can speak of as the fear of nonexistence. The primitive fear of death need not be predicated upon a death instinct, which rather suggests a wish for death. The innate fear of harm is exhibited by all animals, who fear the threats of known or unknown dangers. In the case of the infant, the death threat does not emerge from the actual threats from the outside but rather from the absence of the gratifying or neutralizing maternal image. As stated, Klein believes that the threat comes from the overwhelming aggressive impulses.

When there has been a minimum of threats or when the threats have been mastered by the organism, there are stored memories of gratification. It is the accumulation of stored memories of mastered experience that constitutes the ego. This implies that the ego develops as an acquired psychic function. There is no need to postulate any other device or mechanism which seems to give the ego the properties of a special organ. Nor is there any need to theorize along mystical or magical lines when there are adequate explanations along purely biological principles. Freud[20] spoke of the ego as a coherent organization of mental processes, also as the residue of abandoned objects. The second factor lends "qualities" or "character" to the ego. It is the collection of "internalized objects" or what we should prefer to call the *memory traces* of the images of the important people in the life of the growing individual which constructs the ego and, in earliest life, the first confirmations of the state of existence.

Developmental Factors

Let us examine a few more observable facts. Before the age of nine months, the human infant acts as though objects which he cannot see do not exist. Later he learns to look for hidden objects and awaits the appearance and disappearance of the mother. Actually, the alternation of appearance and disappearance can become pleasurable, as in the peek-a-boo game.

The toddler closes his eyes or hides his face and believes that he is invisible. If he does not see you, then he thinks you cannot see him.* From this ideation the association develops that if the image of the parent is thoroughly implanted upon his mind, the child senses that his image must be present in his mother's mind. When the child is certain that his image is present in his mother's mind, he can then share in her power.

The feeling of power derived from the mother at first comes from being actually in her presence. Dangers are dispelled when the child looks up from his crib and sees her reassuring countenance. It has been pointed out that this is the origin of prayer and the search for God high up in

---

* Variations of this theme occur in unstable people and some children who wish to combat fear by making themselves invisible. They close their eyes so the burglars will not see them, or, even more fantastic, they try to stop their thoughts and in this way to be invisible. Another derivative is the covering of the eyes at the masquerade ball in order to hide one's identity.

Heaven. Later, the child not only needs to see his mother, but he needs the constant reassurance that his presence registers upon her. Afterward, the process of incorporation or internalization of the knowledge that one exists as an image in a loving parent's mind gives the child a sense of his own importance. This does not become complete in any individual. The residual of the need to be in someone else's mind is the need for attention and the constant search for being important to somebody or to everybody. Exhibitionism and scoptophilia are both derived from this source. Stated differently, existence is related to noticing and being noticed.

Paranoid illness likewise may have its roots in existence anxiety. Defensively, the paranoic gives up the quest for love (which he perceives as hopeless anyway) for the quest for power. The paranoid person's sense of integrity must come from without; yet he sees others as disinterested. Freud commented that the paranoid patient interprets indifference as hate because it represents a failure to give wanted love. Paranoia is seen to be related to early infancy when the child perceives the mother passively as affecting him but not being affected by him, a perception that is realistically reinforced by the unresponsive parent. Not feeling noticed by the parent, important to her, or capable of having impact on her, the potentially paranoid child feels like nothing. Restitutive defenses of grandiosity and omnipotence ensue.

The concept of the wish to deny the existence of noxious or painful objects is seen in the negative hallucination. This is the basis for repression. Xenia did not want to look at conflictual areas in her life; therefore she did not see them and thus they did not exist. She denied her sexual feelings completely, especially for her father. Instead, she regressed to a level of merely existing in his mind. This was enough for her to survive. Consciously, she strove for a position of importance to her father but never expected to attain it. Hence, she felt unimportant and strove to compensate in many ways.

Sibling rivalry classically illustrates a child's sense of being threatened when his image is replaced by the image of the brother or sister. The Oedipal triangle illustrates his feeling jeopardized by a parent. We can adduce the fact that existence is an ego function from the quantitative degree of preoccupation that individuals have with this modality. The individual suffering from a schizophrenic process may be one whose ego is so poorly organized that he often displays an inability to appreciate his existence. Such a person in therapy may report that he (or she) only exists in the presence of the therapist. When he leaves the therapist, he feels he no longer exists.

At this point I should like to differentiate *existence* from *identity*. These two concepts can be subsumed under the headings "to be" versus "to be something." Existence as an ego function comprises survival as an autonomous unit. The child has mastered some of his early survival needs, largely gastro-intestinal, and can function to some extent as an entity with an ability to utilize his external world only when specific needs arise. The words of a confused, 19-year-old girl who was making progress in therapy are quoted verbatim:

> It is important that my image must exist within you, so that you can be within me. I am aware of your strength—then I can have it within me. Now I feel that I can have life, a life of my own. I can face all the past that has happened to me and handle anything that may come up in the future.

This statement clearly indicates the transition from existence to identity. It is the movement from "I am" to "This is who I am." Existence implies survival; identity implies a design or style of existence. The "who" is contingent first upon the clues in the communication system between mother and child, and later, between the father and the child.

Many elements of ego functioning in the establishment of Xenia's existence and identity were revealed in the course of her therapy. She demonstrated many infantile introjections, projections, and re-introjections, or *projective identifications*. Her mother, for example, was looked upon as a good understanding mother upon whom Xenia depended. The cruel, hostile, unfriendly mother image was repressed and incorporated into her own image of herself. Thus, she considered herself to be evil and unworthy. This allowed her to maintain the mother image as a loving figure whom she needed for the purpose of finding out what to do and how to act.

Xenia also projected a good image of herself into the mind of the father, as demonstrated by her dream. It also became evident that she re-introjected the male image of father into herself. This led her to acquiring his masculinity as a spurious identity. She also displaced and projected her hostility to her mother onto her father, fortifying her own fears of his actual power over her. Defensively, her helplessness was also projected outwardly, allowing her to feel powerful over other people. This form of tyranny over the others assumed to be helpless gave her a reason for her existence and created a form of temporary ego mastery.

The similarity of Xenia's defenses to those of the paranoid patient is obvious.

In the course of therapy it was necessary to point out to Xenia the various identification processes and their resulting conflicts as defensive maneuvers in her efforts to survive. She was able to relinquish these defenses only after she had established a state of existence in the therapeutic situation. For a portion of time, it was useful for the patient to sit up and face the analyst so that the actual presence of the therapist and her awareness of herself as a communicant confirmed her own existence as a person. Group therapy was a helpful adjunct.

The concept of existence as a person is still a far cry from the establishment of a true ego identity. An ego identity is essentially the integration of the self that has emerged in the various orbits of operation in which the individual lives, e.g., family, social situation, occupation, church, etc. Thus it is composed of such items as: sexual identity, family identity, racial identity, religious identity, occupational identity. Out of this synthesis there is established a sense of values, characteristic of the mature adult.[21]

FURTHER CONSIDERATIONS

It can be adduced from the foregoing discussion that a requisite condition for early ego formation, the inception of self-awareness is the feeling of being important to someone who is important to the self. Such a feeling, of course, should originate in the mother-infant union. In gastrointestinal terms, the language of the infant, the feeling of a self is attained by either devouring or being devoured by the object which nurtures.

Through the process of mutual internalization, the infant is able to overcome the natural threats of the outside world. At birth, he experiences a contest with death—suffering pain, suffocation, cold and possibly hunger. The contact with his mother (or her representatives) neutralizes the frustrating or frightening threats of the external world.

As the mother continues to reappear when needed, it becomes apparent to the child that he is known to her, just as she is to him. Their knowledge of each other establishes a dyadic relationship that is necessary for survival. As growth continues and autonomy develops, the triadic relationship, that including the father, becomes manifest. The intrusion into the dyadic system reactivates the original feelings of threat experienced at birth and taxes the growing organism into new areas to be mastered. The father generally becomes the symbol of authority, holding power of punishment and sway over life and death. This identification of father with punishment and mother with rescue is to some degree the same in both boys and girls. The coping mechanisms, however, are different. The boy reacts with hostility, the girl with seduction.

The residual of the need to feel important, like the wish to be the favorite or only child, exists in some degree in all people. In some it is the wish to retain the feeling of importance once held as a child; in others it is the wish to possess something that one has never had but wants. In any case, it is the motivating force that continually presses us on for new achievements. After the child attains his importance in the family, he seeks to be important to his peers and later to his mate and to the world.

Adolescence is the period when the individual attains a recognizable, identifiable self. Next comes the period when he gets ready to choose a mate. The ultimate goal, of course, is the establishment of an intimate and binding relationship with a partner of the opposite sex. Anything less than a state of true intimacy may result in pseudo intimacy—for example, homosexual relations. Pseudo intimacy, or false closeness, is a defensive maneuver to ward off loneliness, anxiety, depression or ego disintegration.

A true romantic and, later, a permanent conjugal relationship follow the general principles outlined in this presentation: *cogitor ergo sum.* It becomes "we think about each other; therefore we exist for each other."

REFERENCES

1. Solomon, J. C.: Alice and the Red King. The Psycho-Analytic View of Existence. Int. J. Psycho-Anal. 44:63, 1963.
2. Carroll, Lewis: Through the Looking Glass, and What Alice Found There. Macmillan, 1871.
3. Greenacre, Phyllis: Swift & Carroll—A Psychoanalytic Study of Two Lives. Int. Univ. Press, N. Y., 1955.
4. Burton, A.: Death as a Countertransference. Psychoanal. & Psychoanal. Rev. 49:3, 1962.
5. Philo by Wolfson, H. A.: Howard Univ. Press, 1947.
6. Aquinas, St. Thomas: Basic Writing of St. Thomas. Vol. 1. Pegis Anton (ed.) Random House, N. Y., 1945.
7. Maritain, J.: Existence and the Existent. Pantheon, N. Y., 1948.
8. Berkeley, G., Sampson, G.: The Works of George Berkeley D.D., Bishop of Cloyne, G. Bell & Sons, Lond., 1897.
9. Gardner, Martin: The Annotated Alice. Clarkson N. Potter, Inc., N. Y., 1960.
10. May, Rollo and others: Existence a New Dimension in Psychiatry. Basic Books, N. Y., 1958.

11. Kierkegaard, S.: Fear and Trembling (1844). Princeton Univ. Press, 1941.
12. Heidegger, H.: The Question of Being. Twayne, N. Y., 1958.
13. Sartre, J. P.: Being and Nothingness. Philosophical Library, N. Y., 1956.
14. Spitz, Renee: Psychogenic Diseases in Infancy. An Attempt at their Etiological Classification. Psychoanal. Study of the Child 6, 255, 1951.
15. Salk, L.: Newspaper story by T. F. James. "Sound of Love." Amer. Weekly, Aug. 21, 1960.
16. Bowlby, J.: Separation Anxiety. Int. J. of Psycho-Anal. 41:89, 1960.
17. Silverberg, Wm.: Childhood & Personal Destiny. Springer, N. Y., 1952.
18. Klein, Melanie: On the Development of Mental Functioning. Int. J. Psycho-Anal. 38:84, 1958.
19. Stokes, A.: A Game That Must Be Lost. Int. J. Psycho-Anal. 41, 170, 1960.
20. Freud, S.: Beyond the Pleasure Principle. Complete Psychological Works of Sigmund Freud. Vol. 18. Hogarth Press, London, 1953.
21. Solomon, J. C.: A Synthesis of Human Behavior, An Integration of Thought Processes and Ego Growth. Grune & Stratton, N. Y., 1954.

8

HOWARD P. ROME, M.D.

In his quiet way, Leo Bartemeier with dignity and enormous patience has counseled the troubled, been a guide to the perplexed and a teacher par excellence. We who are his friends do ourselves honor by this tribute to him.

Malingering as Crypto-Suicide

THE PROBLEM OF MALINGERING is a heterogeneous one. The cause and complex nature of the deception and of the symbolic transformation that serves as a disguise of the underlying motive have been the subjects of inquiries since Biblical times. King David, sore afraid of Achish, King of Gath, feigned madness and escaped to the cave of Adullan. Rachel secreted the idols that her father Laban held in great esteem. When he searched for them, she remained seated in his presence, saying: "Let it not displease my lord that I cannot rise up before thee, for the custom of women is upon me." (Be it noted that Rachel had concealed the missing idols beneath the camel seat on which she sat. Had she risen before her father, as was the custom, their whereabouts would have been disclosed.) And Suetonius tells of a Roman knight who, to secure exemption from military service for his two young sons, amputated their thumbs and was subsequently stripped of his property (as were his sons of their inheritance) by the emperor Octavius Augustus.[1]

The clinical manifestations of malingering are protean. Traditionally they have been classified according to their more or less superficial characteristics rather than their latent motivations. However, once this frame of reference has been perceived, one outstanding characteristic is transparently evident: it is a variant of the generic theme of identity and its derivative attributes. A loss of self, a loss of ability, a loss of responsibility, or total self-destruction are myriad alternatives either overtly or in one

99

of their crypto-forms. Death negates self completely. In the case of the impostor, the loss of self takes the form of assuming the identity of another.[2,3] Like suicide and imposture, malingering is an attempt to cancel out the self—specifically through loss of ability or responsibility. In the extended sense of the term, then, all instances of malingering are instances of crypto-suicide—that is, of hidden, self-destructive actions.

Because the problem has social origins as well as psychological roots, one must, in studying it, include not only an analysis of intrapsychic dynamics but also an exploration of the milieu from which these behavioral expressions derive. The milieu determines the psycho-economics— that is, the specie of exchange in which the barter of interaction takes place. Generally speaking, affect and affective exchange use the media of more or less subtle non-verbal communication. Because, in our culture, signs and symptoms are a more highly valued currency than verbal symbols, body-language and body-behavior are more persuasive than words. They can express eloquently a plea for help or make a bid for alms. They can even elicit from a casual passer-by that prized virtue in Western culture—charity! And in recent times, there has been a partial acceptance of the ultimate gesture—suicide—as an anguished plea for succor.

Unfortunately, not everyone in a culture holds the same beliefs. Consequently, unconcealed suicide is still often considered a stigma on the individual as well as his family. In the event of a successful attempt there are sometimes penalties levied on the suicide's legatees, and in the event of an unsuccessful try, there are frequently penalties levied on the individual himself. It is probably this attitude toward actual suicide that conduces to what I have termed crypto-suicide—a less than overt, but nonetheless self-destructive gesture.

Crypto-suicide is a masked attempt to conceal not only the overt act of self-destruction but also the latent effects that, despite desperation, impel its disguise through a symbolic transformation of true motives. One can recognize crypto-suicides among alcoholics who freely admit that they intend to drink themselves to death; among habitual drug users; among the accident-prone; among those who repeatedly use hallucinogens (to "blow" their minds, as they significantly state it),—and, of course, among malingerers.

As long ago as 1870 an editorial writer in the *British Medical Journal* called attention to the self-destructive nature of malingering:

> The investigation of feigned diseases has hitherto been restricted too exclusively to those in which some known object is desired by the

malingerer. . . . It is well known that there are malingerers who assume their maladies without any ostensible object in sight and to the destruction, apparently, of their social happiness. It is this phase of the subject which we should like especially to see carefully and clinically studied.[4]

The author goes on to recognize in the transparency of the ruse the implicit plea for help:

> We may note that in many cases the clumsiness of the artifice and the ease with which it is allowed to be detected are characteristic of the disease.

And in 1872 William Roberts reported observing:

> . . . A number of very remarkable instances of simulated disease where the motive to deceit is altogether inscrutable or is so greatly out of proportion to the inconvenience and pain and danger of the condition simulated as to suggest an alteration of mind approaching, if not actually reaching, the confines of insanity.[5]

This author continues with a case report of a 14-year old boy whose mother complained that he had "vomited tubes for two months" and then produced "a piece of glistening membranous tube *three miles long* and as thick as the thumb which had been vomited by the boy, as she alleged, as they were coming in the train."

> I found the boy was her youngest child (she was a widow) and evidently a pet of herself and of his two grown-up brothers.
>
> His mother and brothers likewise continued, in spite of the clearest demonstration, quite unshaken in their belief in the genuineness of the symptoms. . . . No conceivable motive could be assigned for this imposition. The boy bore an unblemished character for truthfulness, and of the bona fides of his mother and brothers it was impossible to entertain a doubt.[5]

Malingerers who perpetrate fictitious lesions have to be distinguished from other patients not only by the unaccountable perversity of their behavior but also by the demonstrated malignancy of their affliction. Ticknor in 1834 described a classical instance of this, saying:

> Miss Lucy Parsons . . . (who demonstrated) . . . an extraordinary example of the amount of disease the system can sustain when nature is playing her wildest freaks . . . has sustained a character

for genuine piety and [has] lived with her two maiden sisters who
have had the sole care of her for more than 20 years . . . and there
can be no reason why she and her sisters would wish to deceive.[6]

And Hector Gavin, in 1835, related a case where

. . . a man simulating paralysis of the arm allowed the amputating
knife to be placed beneath it, and would have submitted to the operation. He was detected by being thrown into a river (being a good
swimmer) where he was obliged to strike out with both arms to
save his life. . . .[7]

From such data as these and others concerning patients diagnosed as
having Munchausen's syndrome, several observations may be made.[8,9,10,11]
The parataxic distortions of reality that characterize the patients' perceptions of themselves and of others are clearly of psychotic proportions.
The malingerers' remarkable tolerance for pain is bewildering to clinicians,
as is the indefatigable persistence of persons administering punishment
to themselves. There is also a singular absence of such affects as guilt
and depression, that has led observers of malingerers to compare their
emotional response to *la belle indifférence* of the hysteric at one time,
and the equally convincing instance of the guiltlessness of the paranoid at
another. The malingerer's acting-out may be interpreted as another mode
of psychological defense, even though its characteristic expressions are
somewhat different from the usual neurotic and psychotic reaction types.

An undifferentiated ego lies at the base of repeated self-injury. It lacks
the capacity to select stimuli which lead to consummatory acts in the
present; hence it dooms the malingerer to an appetitive behavior which
searches in random, self-defeating, stereotyped fashion for a satisfaction
that is not there. The blocks of consummatory behavior have been set
by the malingerer's life experience and the patient lacks the adaptive
facility to be other than compulsive.

The paradoxical part of the malingering game[12] is that it is truly a
plea for help—but a plea based on a symbolic confusion that is the tragic
result of a failure in communication. While it is evident that the person
is, in one sense, quite conscious of his acts—indeed, he even executes
them with a cunning which implies careful premeditation—it is also clear
that in a more important sense, he acts as if he were divorced from the
knowledge of what he is doing.

There is, however, another dimension to be considered: that while
this behavior is necessary to the equilibrium of the malingerer, it is not

self-sufficient. To yield satisfaction, malingering must be abetted by collusion of a very specific nature. The consciously expressed willingness of others to be involved is of less importance than their traditional symbolic value as care-taking persons. The true test of the collusive care-taker is his response to the proffered disability.

A typical sequence of the patient's testing and the care-taker's reaction follows this pattern: if a minimal lesion fails to provoke the desired response, the malingerer intensifies his effort without a realistic appreciation of the caricature he is portraying. There is rarely satiety in the interchange. In fact, the more outrageous the lesion· the greater the reaction. And the reaction· usually constituted of equal parts of revulsion and compassion· may be manipulatively escalated until the care-taker approximates the expectations of the patient. In a rare instance, a measure of unalloyed contact may be made, and the pretender will truly expose his wounds and speak feelingly of his wretched state, his dependence, his need to grovel and debase himself to justify his bare, unshriven existence.

In general, it appears that the primary site of psychopathology, as it were, is in the area of the interpersonal relations between the patient and a parent with whom his identification has been hostile. There are data that prove that the patient experienced repeated brutality which resulted in actual physical injury. In a somewhat belated and contrite recognition of this, the parent often attempts to assuage his guilt by behavior that serves to over-determine the entire experience. The consequence of this pattern is not only the distortion of the love-hate relationship but also chaos in the entire repertoire of symbolic values. Pain and physical suffering become the prime legal specie in such a sado-masochistic power struggle.[13] The facade of deceit is just a part of the learned economy—an acceptable opening gambit which ostensibly disavows hostile feelings, at the same time that it provides an acted-out penance for them. It is in this way that the malingerer euchres the world of the attention, solicitude, and physical devotion that he seeks.[3]

The doctor, however, is generally less easily bilked than the collusive care-taker.

In 1835 Hector Gavin delivered a prize essay "On the Feigned and Factitious Diseases of Soldiers and Seamen, on the Means Used to Simulate or Produce Them, and on the Best Modes of Discovering Imposters." In it he pointed out that it was "the duty of medical officers to protect the public service from imposition of this kind"[7] and illustrated his essay with ways and means of revealing impostures.

Glowing coals and hot sealing wax put on the hand or forehead of the imposter will draw from him expressions of pain. Individuals have been roused from a feigned paroxysm by dropping into the eye a few drops of alcohol . . . the Indians recommend a little of the expressed juice of a pod of Cayenne pepper to be put into the eye. . . . Blowing Scotch snuff up the nostrils is said to be an effectual means of rousing suppressed sensations. . . .

In so prescribing Gavin was probably giving vent to the spleen felt by the majority of physicians before and since his time.

Just as the milieu accounts for the problem of crypto-suicide, so does it generate the typical physician's response to it. The medical profession is traditionally one of the pillars of organized society. Hence its members claim a nobility that carries with it status privilege and the companion weight of responsibility for the maintenance of the Establishment, whose canonical code is basic to the social ethic.

The physician is a legatee of attitudes toward malingering that were established in the Middle Ages about the time that Western Culture began to subscribe to the Copernican theory of the universe, in place of the Ptolemaic. With the realization that his earth was not the center of the universe, man developed a compensating sense of the importance of himself as the dominant creature on his own planet, however subordinate that orb is in the total galactic structure.

For the first time in Western history, status became important to even the common man. A striving upward, an awareness of the possibility of social mobility, provoked personal ambition and enterprise, in addition to the condemnation and shunning of the lowly, the diseased, and the destitute. This opprobrium also stemmed, no doubt, from the knowledge that many vagrants sought to escape from the poverty rife in England and on the continent by securing admission to hospitals, where they eked out a livelihood by pretending to be chronically sick or crippled.

During the Reformation, the condemnatory attitude toward the malingerer was reinforced by the Puritan ethic. The central issue of Puritan philosophy was an ascetic approach to all social conduct and obligations. The rising middle class was motivated by a morality that stressed responsibility and was, therefore, hostile to sloth, that it construed as both fruitless and frivolous conduct.* As Weber puts it the spirit of

---

* Thus the Danish *skule* (to scowl, to keep aloof) entered Middle English as *skulk* (to play the truant from work, to lurk on the periphery of the active, industrious world).

capitalism had its roots in "the religious valuation of restless· continuous, systematic work in a worldly calling."[14]

Physicians, ever the pursuivants of authoritative society, are diametrically opposed to everything that manifest malingering stands for. Furthermore, physicians are generally, as Gavin observed, uncomfortable when confronted with behavior that seems "without any ulterior object." They are confounded by persons who "seem to experience an unaccountable gratification in deceiving their officers, comrades, and surgeons." When faced with evidence attesting malingering, most physicians react with the affect, as Gavin points out, that reflects the hostility inherent in the act of deception itself. This appears despite the fact that the hostile challenge is proffered in the form of signs and symptoms marshaled for doctors in general—not just for a particular physician singled out as target.

What is the explanation of the usually hostile response to malingering? One of the more obvious answers to this question is that the role of patient carries with it certain built-in expectations. When these are blasted by the discovery of feigned symptoms, the resulting drama creates discord—and not infrequently this discord is supercharged with anger, indignation, and resentment (on the part of the physician, as well as the patient) at being duped and tricked.

Parsons defines "being sick" as "a biological state which suggests remedial measures requiring exemptions from obligations, conditional legitimation· and *motivation to accept therapeutic help*."[15] Parsons also points out that the physician-patient interaction could not operate without a relation of "trust" that is expressed ideologically in the medical doctrine that a patient must be able to have "confidence" in his physician. In turn the physician tacitly asks and expects a voluntarily assumed sacrifice. It is incumbent upon the patient to strive actively for recovery by cooperating with the physician. Thus, the traditional physician-patient relationship rests upon the expectation of these fiducial commitments.

When he discovers that he is dealing with a malingerer· the physician often attempts to stabilize his shaken professional role by undertaking a relentless exposure of the patient's duplicity. Thus he acts to retrieve control of what he perceives as an unbalanced situation in which he has *been* controlled. Sometimes the physician's self-image is sufficiently threatened to provoke a loss of "neutrality" and a mobilization of countertransference affects.

In the past, the dominant affect, anger, has even taken such cruel and aggressive forms as those described by Gavin, who tells, for example, of "a woman 30 years of age, who had sustained the proof of fire (and who bore the cicatrices of three considerable burns which a surgeon had made to discover if there was fraud) without wincing; but who afterwards being put in prison for murder, avowed the simulation. . . ."[7]

In summary then, the malingerer is committing an act of crypto-suicide. This is a special instance of psychopathology characterized by distortions of affect, ideation and behavior which in some aspects of an identity-crisis assume psychotic proportions. The clinical difficulties that are encountered in the recognition of the malingerer reflect his early life experience with authority figures. This syndrome appears to be a consequence of a hostile identification with a sadistic parent whose behavior vis-à-vis the patient during the formative years has fostered this skewed pattern of self and object relations. The factitious lesion epitomizes this sado-masochistic interplay. Finally, the history of the medical care of the malingerer recapitulates on a broad cultural level the intrafamilial conflicts that make the malingerer, like the tragic King Lear, a man "more sinned against than sinner."

REFERENCES

1. Bassett, Jones, A. and Llewellyn, J. L.: *Malingering or the Simulation of Disease.* P. Blakiston's Son & Co., Phila., 1917.
2. Crichton, Robert: The Great Imposter, Random House, N. Y., 1959.
3. Grinker, R. Jr.: "Imposture as a Form of Mastery." *Arch. Gen. Psych.* 5:449-452, 1961.
4. Editorial Comment: "Motiveless Malingerers." *Brit. M. J.* 1:15, 1870.
5. Roberts, W.: "Cases of Motiveless Simulation of Disease." *British M. J.* 1:306-307, 1872.
6. Ticknor, C.: "Case in Which Sand Was Voided by the Mouth, Rectum, Urethra, Nose, Ear, Side and Umbilicus and Attended by Various Other Anomalous Symptoms." *Amer. J. Med. Sci.* 14:91-95, 1834.
7. Gavin, Hector: *On the Feigned and Factitious Diseases of Soldiers and Seamen.* University Press—Edinburgh, 1838.
8. Spiro, H. R.: "Chronic Factitious Illness: Munchausen's Syndrome." *Arch. Gen. Psych.* 18:569-579, 1968.
9. Ireland, P., Sapira, J. D. and Templeton, B.: "Munchausen's Syndrome." *Am. J. Med.* 43:579-592, 1967.
10. Asher, R.: Munchausen's Syndrome." *Lancet* 1:339, 1951.
11. Bursten, B.: "On Munchausen's Syndrome." *Arch. Gen. Psychiat.* 13: 261-268, 1965.
12. Simmel, E.: "The Doctor-Game, Illness and the Profession of Medicine." *Int. J. Psychoanal.* 7:370-384, 1926.
13. Brenner, C.: "The Masochistic Character: Genesis and Treatment." *J. Amer. Psychoanal. Assn.* 7:197-226, 1959.
14. Weber, M.: *On Protestantism and Capitalism in "Theories of Society"* Vol. II, p. 1262. Edited by T. Parsons, E. Shils, K. D. Naegle, and J. E. Pitts. Free Press of Glencoe, 1961.
15. Parsons, T.: *Social Structure and Personality.* The Free Press of Glencoe. 1964. pp. 274-277.

9

JOHN N. ROSEN, M.D.

Over the years, Doctor Bartemeier and I have discussed a number of psychiatric problems, ranging in scope from the diagnosis and treatment of a particular patient to the ways and means by which treatment could be improved and extended to the thousands of individuals whose needs are not adequately met. Of all the problems that we have discussed from time to time, I can think of none more urgent, or more basic to our mutual interests, than the problem of suicide. Doctor Bartemeier has expressed his views on this topic from time to time, and I have expressed my views, at least briefly, on previous occasions.* Now I would like to take this occasion to offer some further reflections on the problem of suicide.

Some Reflections on the Problem of Suicide[1]

A GREAT DEAL has been written about this problem, and much of the literature deals with it in isolation from the context in which it arises, namely, the unconscious motivation of an individual who is psychotic. For instance, in his paper on the complexity of motivations to suicide attempts Stengel has said: "Attempted suicide is a non-fatal act of self damage carried out with the conscious intention of self-destruction."[2] And he has said· further, "this is the only definition about which clinicians can be expected to agree." Speaking as a clinician myself, I certainly do not agree with this definition, especially with its emphasis on the *conscious* intention of self-destruction. I would say such an intention is seldom if ever to be found in the motivation of suicidal individuals.

---

* For instance, see John N. Rosen, *Direct Psychoanalytic Psychiatry.* New York: Grune & Stratton, 1962.

Another recent paper suggests that self-destructive motives are often present, and that, accordingly, suicide occurs when there is a loss of control over these motives.[3] This seems to be saying that a given individual will kill himself unless he is continuously prevented (by his own internal controls) from doing so. In my own clinical experience, I do not find any evidence to support such a notion.

Many other publications have helped to create the impression that conscious self-destruction is a real human motive and a frequent cause of death. If we had only this literature to guide us, we would be led to believe that suicide occurs when an individual decides that his best course of action is to kill himself, and that such a decision is essentially rational and conscious, whether it is reached abruptly (as in the stereotyped case of the investor who has suddenly lost a fortune in the stock market) or gradually (as in the stereotyped case of the bereaved person who has for months been brooding over the loss of a loved one). It follows from this line of thinking that, if only we had somebody standing by (preferably on the spot, otherwise on the telephone line from a "suicide prevention" service), he could intervene in the decision-making process and perhaps talk the suicidal person out of it.

In my view, this line of thought misleads us, and it misrepresents the suicidal person's state of mind. Seen from a distance, his actions may appear to be deliberate, rational, and conscious. For instance, he tidies up the papers on his desk, writes his secretary a check for next week's salary, composes a note to his family, takes off his shoes, raises the window of his office, climbs out onto the ledge, checks to see what obstructions might arrest his descent, and then launches himself outward at an angle calculated to clear them as he plunges toward the sidewalk below. So it appears from a distance.

However, as it is seen from the vantage point of a clinician who really knows such persons and their circumstances, suicidal behavior does not occur in the manner just described. Essentially it is psychotic behavior, like acting in a dream, and it occurs when the individual literally doesn't know what he is doing. For instance, in one case which I will present later on in more detail, a woman who jumped from a window and survived, said later: "Momma told me to come to her and all the people [pedestrians on the sidewalk?] who were there, and when I got there she was not there, nobody was there." There was no question, in this case, of a deliberate, rational, and conscious decision to commit suicide. Had the woman not survived then her death would have occurred as an acting-in of her psychotic fantasy. We do hear, in her explanatory statement, one of the clues to an understanding of suicide which I shall present further on. But it is evident to me that, in this case, the individual did not consciously know what she was doing. In other cases, I have known individuals who survived suicide attempts to express shock and terror when they eventually realized (consciously) what they had almost done. And in every case, as far as my clinical experience goes, the individual is invariably dreaming, psychotic, before and after (if he survives) the suicidal act.

So I would say that every suicide, as far as I know, occurs in the context of a psychosis, more specifically in the depressed phase of manic-depressive psychosis. Every suicidal individual is psychotic. Although it can be viewed and often is viewed out of context, as a special problem for which special measures are required, in my view the act of suicide is only one of the various ways in which the turbulent psychodynamics of the psychotic individual may be expressed. Other ways include homicide, smashing of inanimate objects in the environment, hallucinations of widespread destruction (*Welt untergang!*), and so on.

Of course there may be exceptions to my general statement that suicide occurs in the context of the depressed phase of manic-depressive psychosis. For instance, I know of cases in which self-destruction has been accidental. A person has planned to make a suicidal gesture, perhaps to upset his family or to gain attention, and something has gone wrong—he has slipped from the window-sill on which he meant to stay, or he has miscalculated a "safe" overdose of sleeping pills, or the gun really was loaded after all. Even in these cases, however, where we could regard the death itself as accidental, the individual must be psychotic or nearly psychotic to use the threat of suicide as a means of interpersonal communication. Normal people find other means of communicating or, more likely, they do not become involved in such a "sick" interpersonal situation in the first place.

Again, there may be exceptions in other cultures or other historical periods where suicide is part of an explicit code of ethics, so that it is actually expected to occur under certain circumstances. An aristocrat has disgraced the memory of his ancestors, a leader has involved his people in humiliation and defeat, a husband has been dishonored by the actions of his wife. Frankly, I do not know enough about such other cultures or other historical periods to comment on them, or even to venture any suggestions about the mental health of their people. My views are based on my clinical experience in this culture and this historical period, in which social codes of ethics are implicitly or explicitly opposed to suicide, but in which, nevertheless, suicide occurs with considerable frequency.

As I understand the suicidal individual, it is not the ethical codes of his society as a whole which influence him. Rather, it is the dictates of his own superego· whose perverse influence can be expressed in the statement: "Be still, be quiet, be dead." While the superego reflects social values to some extent, it is largely an embodiment of the early maternal environment in which the individual was born and spent his childhood.[4] In a word, the superego embodies "mother," and if its maternal influence is malevolent and deadly, then the individual's ego will feel an urgent need to comply with the wishes of "mother" by destroying himself. Hence I have developed the concept of suicide as "infanticide by proxy" even when it occurs in adulthood or old age. Anything to please mother.

In order to clarify my views on suicide I will now present some of the clinical material from approximately 30 years of experience in dealing with suicidal individuals.

First, a case in which self-destruction might have resulted *accidentally* from the actions of an individual who was emotionally disturbed, but not overtly psychotic, at the time. The following episode occurred in a well-known New England resort during World War II. A young man, from a highly regarded Bostonian family, was picked up by the police for attempting to induce several Coast Guardsmen, who were stationed there and had been drinking, into some homosexual practices. This occurred on a Saturday night, and instead of being jailed, he was released to appear in court the following Monday morning. He brooded over his plight and the disgrace of exposure, and felt he could not face it. There is a tower in this town resembling somewhat the Washington Monument, in which one can climb stairs to the top, and on top there are four observation windows that are open. There is a ledge about six feet below the level of these windows; it is about two feet wide and it goes around all four sides of the monument. Below it is a sheer drop of several hundred feet to the sidewalk. Early Sunday morning· a crowd gathered below to see on this ledge a young man in shirt sleeves, his arms outstretched, leaning against the wall of the monument and screaming for help. The police entered the building and rescued him by raising him up to the window through which he had climbed and pulled him in. I talked to this young man, heard his story, and between his sobs and regrets· he kept repeating, "I wish I could have done it." One can easily see that he might have lost his balance, become dizzy, and crashed to the ground below. He certainly could not have survived this fall, and he certainly would have been listed as a suicide.

When self-destruction is not accidental, as it would have been in the case just described, we often find that the suicidal individual has been acting as though he or she were dreaming, and that the individual's conscious experience may have nothing to do with death.

I have already mentioned the woman who jumped from a window, fortunately not killing herself. Prior to this episode, she had become increasingly depressed, and when she was brought to me, she presented the clinical picture of a manic depressive-depressed psychotic, in a state of considerable agitation, who could hardly sit still and had been sleepless for several weeks. Her productions characteristically related to her "worthlessness" and what an "evil" person she thought herself to be. With intense feeling, she said on a number of occasions that she should not be allowed to live. As a precaution, two assistant therapists were assigned to her case twenty-four hours a day. They slept in the same room with her, in a third-floor apartment in New York City, and between her bed and the two windows in the room. Shortly thereafter one night, she managed to get to the window by leaping over their beds· and she jumped! She was taken to a hospital and I immediately rushed to its intensive care unit, where I found her in shock with multiple fractures, some compounded, and considerable bleeding. When she saw me, she kept whimpering repetitiously, "Momma told me to come to her and all the people who were there, and when I got there she was not there, nobody was there."

In this case, where the patient survived, she actually heard her mother calling to her to come, to hurry, that the people were waiting; and she felt that she was obeying her mother and hurrying to get to her. Had she died, this would have been the kind of suicide that I consider genuine, rather than accidental. The patient had no conscious intention of destroying herself.* Unconsciously, she was obeying her mother who said, "Come, jump out of the window." Such is the mechanism of infanticide by proxy.

Here is another case in which the patient clearly did not consciously know what he was doing when he tried to kill himself. This was a young man whose wife and child had left him six weeks prior to his being brought to me for treatment. He had been seen in his home town by a psychiatrist who had referred him to me because he was sitting day and night at his desk with a revolver in his hand, beset with ideas of self-destruction. He

---

* Moreover, she seemed to feel no pain from her various injuries. I have wondered if this could be an instance of "hysterical anesthesia."

also presented the classical picture of psychotic depression. Two strong, young assistant therapists were assigned to his case, and they lived with him on the ground floor of a hotel in New York City; they brought him to my office daily for the therapeutic interviews. One morning, I had the impression that the patient was more than ordinarily involved with his unconscious mind, perhaps because he seemed so dreamy and hard to reach. I told the two assistants to be especially careful not to leave him alone, and they heeded the warning. At that time my office was at 83rd Street and Park Avenue, and after the treatment session they walked downtown toward their hotel. As they reached the hotel, the patient said that he had to go to the men's room, which was below the street level in the hotel, and they went with him. There is a door that covers half the toilet cubicle, leaving a space about a foot above the floor and about two and a half feet on top. This door can be locked. The assistants stood outside the cubicle waiting for the patient when suddenly a gush of blood appeared on the floor below the door. Assistant "P" leaped over the top of the door and landed on the patient, who had a razor in his hand and was slashing at his throat. He got the patient out of the cubicle while the other assistant called me at my office, and I got there within minutes. The patient was considerably exanguinated. He was struggling to free his hand from Assistant "P's" grip, screaming that "it" was stuck in his throat and that he had to pull 'it" out. This he tried to do all the way to the hospital. He had a deep wound in his neck, it was still oozing blood, and we rushed him to the emergency room. The surgical resident proceeded to disinfect and suture the wound. It was almost a miracle that the razor cut only down to the carotid sheath and did not sever either the carotid artery or the jugular vein.

Subsequently, the patient became paranoic with a fixed delusional system. He felt persecuted and he maintained that somebody was after him. He talked of disappearing to a distant island. There, surrounded by the sea, he would be a beachcomber, and there he would be safe.

Based on my experience with such cases, it is my opinion that the only condition under which genuine suicide can be carried out is in the depressed phase of manic depressive psychosis. Having become psychotic, the individual is no longer protected by the defenses of a (pre-psychotic) neurosis. But he is not (yet) sick enough to achieve self-protection and self-defense through a schizophrenic reorganization of the inner and outer environment as occurs in paranoia or hebephrenia (frequently, the manic-depressive depressed psychotic, in the course of time, will regress further to either the paranoid or hebephrenic state). It is this in-between condition, in which the individual is no longer protected by neurotic defenses and not yet protected sufficiently by psychotic defenses, that true suicide is most likely to occur.

Further, I think it is important to understand that suicide is seldom, if ever, imagined to be a destruction of the self. Sometimes the individual imagines that it is "something in him" which has the ego imprisoned and tortured. Hence the individual is attempting to destroy this part of himself (the superego) in order to free himself from it. When I refer to "parts of the self," I am speaking of mental functions which are integrated and united in the normal individual, but which are disintegrated and disunited in the psychotic individual. It may be no exaggeration to say that, in the psychotic individual, the ego and superego have always been more or less in conflict. A patient once described it by saying, "This is the Third World War."

However, even with a long history of psychological conflict between an ego and a superego which have always been disunited and disintegrated to some extent, it seems to me that suicide of the non-accidental variety does not occur *prior* to the onset of a psychosis. Then, with the schizophrenic-like split, unconscious functioning takes over; and under these circumstances, true suicide can be achieved. Until such time as the dreamy condition develops, no man has the courage to step off the Empire State Building to make sure that his destruction will be sufficiently violent. But once he has entered the dreamy condition, he is no longer restrained by normal judgment or fear.

I cite the case of a young man who had made several suicide attempts before I undertook his treatment. One day, in the company of his assistant therapists, he was walking along Central Park West in New York City. He had hardly spoken a word all day. Suddenly he dashed away from the assistant therapists, and started to climb the fire escape of a tall building. He rushed up the stairs, stopping at about the 6th floor and looking over the railing. I can only conjecture that it did not seem high enough to him yet to smash the superego adequately. He continued on, stopping at every other floor or so and peering over the railing again, until, on the 14th floor, he leaped to the ground below. We will never know what he was thinking. But it is interesting to consider that, although his judgment with respect to the basic problem may have been faulty, nevertheless his judgment with respect to some of the details may still have been sound. Instead of jumping from the fire escape on the second floor of the building, he climbed high enough to make sure that he would be smashed when he hit the sidewalk or street. But no psychotic tries to walk through a wall instead of a doorway, and similarly no psychotic tries to smash himself by jumping from a chair or table when tall buildings and skyscrapers are readily available.

In some of our discussions prior to the writing of this paper, we recognized the great ambiguity of suicidal actions, and we debated whether suicide represents a smashing of the ego by the superego (this would be infanticide by proxy) or whether it sometimes represents a smashing of the intolerable superego by the ego (even though this looked like "suicide," it would really be a kind of homicidal act and could be designated "parenticide by proxy"). Perhaps both elements are present in any act of suicide, with a predominance of infanticidal motivation in some and parenticidal in others. In every-day life, parents are occasionally murdered by their child, and, more often, a child is murdered by one of its parents. Either way, the act itself is likely to be quite brutal, and violent, even though its perpetrator may be as close to "dreaming" as the truly suicidal individual. For instance, we know of one case involving a woman who threw both of her infant children out of a hotel window into the courtyard below. Having done so, she went downstairs to the desk clerk and told him matter-of-factly, "You'll find my two babies outside." She was quite psychotic and her two babies outside were quite dead.

It is our responsibility to understand, if we can, the thoughts and actions of suicidal individuals. Their own explanations of what they are doing make little sense on a conscious level, but can only be understood with the help of their own associations (if they survive) on an unconscious level of meaning. For instance, a boy who jumped out of the window and killed himself left a note which said, "Goodbye forever 'til I see you in Heaven, Mother. . . ." Had the note stopped there, it might have seemed thoughtful and rational, indicative of conscious understanding on the part of the individual, and, incidentally, very much in opposition to our concept of infanticide by proxy. However, the boy's note went on to say: "I must do this because Father split the marble and cut both of my eyes." In order to gain insight about his irrational thoughts, it would have been necessary (had the suicide attempt been unsuccessful) to get the boy's associations to "marble," "eyes," and so on. As it is, the note leaves us with no more than a tantalizing glimpse of the bizarre world which this unfortunate young man perceived.

Another example of the psychotic irrationality that we encounter when suicidal individuals try to explain their actions occurred in the case of a man who had inherited one of the greatest fortunes in the country. At his death he left his wife and children in excess of one hundred million dollars in trust, together with other valuable property. However, his suicidal note protested that he could not face the prospect of seeing his children starve, since bad investments had "impoverished" him to the point of destitution. We know that the man had, in fact, lost a few hundred thousand dollars in a "bad investment" that he had made shortly before his suicide, but he had also made many good investments, so that his immense wealth was not really diminished by what he had lost. Yet *he* felt impoverished. I can only conjecture that his ego might have been impoverished of libido—that is, exhausted from its life-long struggle with a superego which was ultimately intolerable.

I hope that these reflections, gathered from my years of experience with suicidal individuals, will help other psychotherapists to understand better the problem of suicide as they encounter it in their experience. I have emphasized the irrational, psychotic aspect of suicide and have given little attention in this paper to other aspects of suicide, such as its moral implications or its emotional impact on those who survive the suicidal individual. Both of these aspects are of interest to Dr. Bartemeier, as well as to me, and I hope to include them in a more comprehensive paper on suicide, a project for the future.

Perhaps the present paper should close with this thought: If it is true, as I believe it to be true, that the suicidal individual does not consciously know what he is doing, then clearly it becomes our responsibility to save and maintain him, until such time as he does know what he is doing. In a special sense, then, the problem of suicide seems to make us our brother's keeper, and it is that note of responsibility and compassion which we find throughout Dr. Bartemeier's work, and for which we love and honor him now.

REFERENCES

1. I wish to express my gratitude to James W. Cochrane, Arthur L. H. Rubin, and Charles T. Sullivan for working with me on this paper.
2. Erwin Stengel, "The Complexity of Motivation to Suicide Attempts," *The Journal of Mental Science*, 1960, *106* (445), p. 1388.
3. T. L. Dorpat, "Loss of Control Over Suicidal Impulses," *Bulletin of Suicidology*, December 1968, pp. 26-30.
4. John N. Rosen, *The Concept of Early Maternal Environment in Direct Psychoanalysis*, Doylestown, Pa.: The Doylestown Foundation, 1963.

Part II

PSYCHIATRY'S COMMITMENT IN THE LABORATORY

He who does not hope for the unexpected will not find it.

—HERACLITUS

The search for the unexpected has intrigued men in every field of endeavor. This search leads men apart from the crowd—not for the sake of solitude, but because they travel uncharted courses in quest of new or deeper understanding. If validation of their hypotheses were the only reward of research, research would be a far less attractive venture. It is the attendant serendipity which rewards the labor. And hope motivates the search.

In this part of *Hope—Psychiatry's Commitment,* we have four examples of exploration of human behavior. As Dr. Anderson pointed out in Part One of this volume, psychoanalysis serves an investigative or research aim, as well as a therapeutic role. Although Dr. Levy does not use the psychoanalytic method in his research of "Maternal Feelings Toward the Newborn," he does use psychoanalytic theory. Doctor Brosin and his co-authors used film recording to study human behavior. Dr. Elkes encourages psychiatrist, psychologist, mathematician and communications engineer to cooperate in the development of new symbolic systems for the study of behavior. And Doctor Masserman considers human behavior in the light of man's Ur-objectives.

10

JOEL ELKES, M.D.

> *Dr. Leo Bartemeier and the author have often discussed*
> *the issues presented in this paper. It is included in this*
> *volume as a mark of the author's profound esteem and ad-*
> *miration for Dr. Bartemeier.*

Language and Observation in Psychiatry

IF THE ACCURATE description of behavior be essential to research in psychiatry, language must provide the weights and measures in this field. Yet where does "Behavior" end and "Language" begin? Is "verbal behavior" a model of "other" behavior? How accurate are such models in clinical investigation? And what of the relation of language to the non-verbal, subjective experience, so central to the business of psychiatry? I would like to raise some issues concerning the function of language in psychiatry, to give some instances of devices in current use, if only to point out the pains which go into their making, and the constraints under which they operate. A thorough exploration of the limits of language is presented in Susanne K. Langer's writings (1942, 1957); and the problem of communication and validation of subjective clinical data has been examined by Henry K. Beecher (1959a)

There can be little dispute of the attributes of language. Language is "our most faithful and indispensable picture of human experience" (Langer, 1942, p 76), a heuristic symbolic instrument shaping modes of observation and interpretation, and interpenetrating deeply with

* This chapter is an abridged version of a paper originally delivered as a Harvey Lecture in 1962 to a predominately non-psychiatric audience. Reprinted by permission of Academic Press, Inc.

experience. Phonemes and morphemes condense meaning into words, and the relation between word-symbols is regulated by rules of syntax and grammar. Such rules—rules of astonishing logic and economy—go, as Whorf showed (1956), into the fabric of even the most primitive language. They make for the smooth use of language as an instrument of social adaptation and communication. They order the relation of the fact-symbols to each other, and to the world which they represent. To serve such adaptive functions, the rules imposed by syntax must be strictly followed, and the symbols presented in a certain order. It is evident that "Tom followed Harry" does not mean the same as "Tom follow Harry" or "Harry followed Tom." Conventional logic imposes a linear, sequential quality, which has come to be known as "discursiveness" (Langer, 1942, p. 77), and it is in this sense that the laws of reasoning and logic are sometimes known as "the laws of discursive thought" (Langer, 1942, p. 77).

There is, however, another quality in words implicit in the one just discussed. For, while carrying certain meanings in one context, words carry a totally different meaning in another; and even standing alone they may—as anyone who has traced the origin of a word in a dictionary—carry an accretion of different meanings in a sort of strange algebra and calculus of their own. This economy, this logic, this dependence on context are characteristic even of the most primitive language (Whorf, 1956). Words are thus not mere labels, cards, stacked for reference in one of Broca's areas; they are states, sets, depending on relation, and context; they carry multiple meaning. Carnap in "The Logical Syntax of Language" (1937), has examined the capacity for expression of any given linguistic system. What is remarkable in that analysis is how little our ordinary means of communication measures up to the standard of meaning which a serious philosophy of language, and hence a logic of discursive thought, demands.

It would thus seem that there are large areas in communication and in self-communication (i.e., the symbol making not exteriorized in overt behavior) which are not represented by ordinary language. For whereas grammar and speech are essentially sequential, linear, and discursive, the characteristic of these other subjective states is the multiple simultaneous presentation of internalized objects and relations. The form of the "unspeakable" is as different from the "speakable" as the structure of a dream, or even a daydream, is from the structure of deliberate action. In such symbolic forms totality is apprehended simultaneously at different levels; mutually occlusive elements coexist; time is of no consequence;

and serial ordering in time (that backbone of causal reasoning) gives way to simultaneously perceived relationships. The philosophy of language tends to dismiss this type of presentational activity as falling into the sphere of subjective experience, emotion, and feeling. As Russell (1927) put it: "Our confidence in language is due to the fact that it shares . . . the structure of the physical world. Perhaps that is why we know so much physics and so little of anything else."

I would submit that we know so little of that large "anything else" because, all too often, we have tried to force discursive language and method on phenomena for which they were inappropriate. Nor is a relegation of such matters to the mystique of intuition at all helpful. There is nothing mystical, for example, about recent developments in sensory physiology. Here the data suggest a unique capacity of the brain to build up a central representational system through the juxtaposition of simultaneously coded transforms of multiple sensory inputs, modulated and gated by an interplay between central and peripheral, specific and nonspecific systems (Livingston, 1958). Sense experience is thus a fundamental way of creating form; and a mind working with meaning must have organs that supply it with forms (Langer, 1942· p. 84).

I would now like to consider some empirical approaches to the problem of measurement in clinical psychiatry with special reference to the effects of drugs on human behavior. These various approaches have been ably reviewed (Uhr and Miller, 1960).

SUBJECTIVE AND OBJECTIVE OBSERVATION IN THE SINGLE SUBJECT

Take pain. Like other subjective experience, pain can manifest in motor behavior; however, it need not. It is a sensation difficult to define operationally; one "known to us by experience, and described by illustration" (Lewis, 1942). There are other puzzling features about pain. In the single individual it can be estimated by a variety of experimental procedures, registering the so-called pain threshold (Beecher, 1959a, p. 92). Yet a careful review of the field leads Beecher to the surprising conclusion that "some 15 groups of investigators have utterly failed to demonstrate any effectiveness of morphine on experimental pain threshold" (1959b).

This sounds odd, in view of the patent usefulness of the drug in the clinical situation, a usefulness which is confirmed when the drug is tried in a carefully controlled clinical setting. Here there is remarkable agreement between data from Lasagna and Beecher's laboratory (Beecher,

1956b, pp. 104-105; Lasagna and Beecher, 1954) and from the group of Houde and Wallenstein (1953) concerning the effectiveness of 10 mg. morphine in pain of different origin (postoperative vis-à-vis metastatic cancer), and agreement concerning the reproducibility of data in successive experiments extending over three years by different groups of investigators in the same laboratory (Beecher, 1959b, pp. 104-105). In reviewing the effect of morphia on wound pain (Beecher, 1959a, p. 164), Beecher explains how attitudes toward a wound determine the need for the drug. Thus, soldiers, to whom a wound can be the symbol of survival (rather than evidence of injury), require less morphine than civilian postoperative patients, to whom (despite far less tissue damage), the operation may signify severe disability. The subjective reaction to the injury, the "psychic processing" (Beecher 1959a, p. 158) in a total behavior situation, modifies not only the original sensation, but evidently its reaction to pharmacological intervention. Mood and attitude are thus all pervasive; and the measurement of change of mood is an all pervasive problem in psychiatry.

There are a number of scales to quantify mood. Anxiety and depression, being common symptoms, have been particularly studied in this respect. Taylor (1953) and Cattell (1960) have developed instruments for the measurement of anxiety; Cattell isolated a "universal index" and a number of more discrete factors. A number of scales have been elaborated for estimating depression (Grinker et al., 1961; Hamilton, 1960). Such scales, although still in the process of trial, appear to be reliable (Hamburg et al., 1958), there being good agreement among raters, and also between subjective self-assessment and objective observation.

Another method, founded on the work of Nowlis and Nowlis (1956) has been developed by Clyde (1960). It makes use of a list of adjectives describing various mood states in simple, nontechnical terms, found empirically to be least ambiguous. Each term is printed on an IBM punch card; the subject is asked to sort these cards into four piles to describe the degree to which they describe his feelings, ranging from "not at all" to "extremely." Patients like this card sorting task, and prefer it to a check list. After being sorted, the cards are fed directly into an electronic computer, for scoring and analysis. Specific categories of mood and behavior (such as "friendly," "aggressive," etc.) can be arrived at according to the grouping of words which describe them. Above all, subjective self-ratings can be compared with observer's ratings. By having a central clearing house for the cross validation of this and other scales, confidence levels for various instruments can be determined and clinical reaction forms (as manifested by clustering of items) agreed upon.

These scales have a further advantage. Being self-administered, they make possible the careful study of fluctuation over time in a single case, and particularly of diurnal variation and variation on successive days. These variations can be quite marked, and can vitiate baseline readings (Knight, 1963). It is also possible to use these scales to gauge interaction between personality structure and the effect of a particular medication. Pain, anxiety, anger, and depression, all common enough clinical symptoms, can at present be approached in quantitative terms.

It is much more difficult to quantify other symptoms, such as the disorders of perception or of cognitive function manifested, for example, in the states induced by the psycho-dysleptic ("psychosomimetic") drugs. For here, as we saw, the flux, the speed, the intensity, the variety, the strangeness, the multiplicity of phenomena strain language and instruments built with ordinary language. Silence can be more eloquent than words, and the small guttural noise can carry the quintessence of meaning. The experience can be projected in a drawing, or in a poetical condensation. It can also be item-analyzed, in a self-rating questionnaire. Some 47 items have been listed by Abramson, Jarvik et al. (1955); some 300 in a card sort test used by Ditman (1960). Yet here a difficulty arises. Answering a questionnaire requires attention; attention breaks continuity; the very act of attending, or of speaking, may alter the phenomena; the answers, even if they are informative, are only partial answers; and the more trained the subject and observer, the more familiar with the inner space which he is exploring, the more informative the answers. Such item analysis, however, has great merit. It gives rank or order and pattern to individual responses and maps the distribution of symptoms over time. A shorthand can be devised to describe various categories and their fluctuation over time, and such categorization can be reinforced by retrospective self-description and the playing back of tape-recorded responses. The symptoms can also be related to striking alteration in the sense of time, noted in these states (Boardman et al., 1957). One other advantage of this longitudinal approach is that symptom intensity can be correlated with metabolic findings. Thus, in our laboratory Dr. Szara has attempted to correlate symptom intensity produced by diethyltryptamine, a powerful dysleptic, with the pattern of excretion of its metabolite, 6-hydroxydiethyltryptamine. There are some (admittedly slender) indications of a possible correlation between symptom intensity and the excretion of 6-OH-diethyltryptamine in man (Szara and Rockland, 1962).

What is the objective counterpart to this kind of subjective observation in the single subject? The sensory or social isolation experiments demand such observation (Solomon et al., 1961). There, the throat microphone, the periscope, the closed-circuit television camera are useful technical devices. However, we may briefly note one situation in which the behavioral output of an isolated individual is continuously monitored in a controlled situation. This approach is based upon Skinner's (1938) classical studies. It allows a piece of behavior to "operate" upon the environment in the light of past occurrence, so as to "obtain" a "reward" or "avoid" "punishment." The behavior thus determines the consequences of behavior. The "reward" and "punishment" can be presented at regular ("fixed") or irregular ("variable") intervals, altering the levels of expectancy. Moreover the reward can be actual (Lindsley and Skinner, 1954) (candy, visual displays) or symbolic (points, won or lost, as in a game). Dr. Weiner, in our laboratory, favors the latter course; he is also exploring the relatively unknown area of the influence of "cost" in human operant behavior (Weiner, 1962). By suitable automatic programming, the "cost" of each response intended to procure a reward can be altered (i.e., the apparatus set so as to ensure that points are *lost* every time the subject seeks his reward); the economy with which a subject uses resources at his disposal can thus be assessed. The task is essentially a vigilance task—the detection of a light on a frosted glass panel, for which the subject is allowed to look by pressing a lever. Gain of points is signified by a bell. The responses are recorded on a cumulative recorder. The behavior under "cost" and "no cost" conditions is strikingly different; and already individual differences between subjects in terms of handling "cost" and "no cost" contingencies are apparent. This approach may, in time, give one an insight into the way individuals of different personality structure, (or, for that matter, psychopathology), handle the very rapid transitional states (i.e., changes in anticipatory set) which some of the procedures demand. They also may teach one something of the individual variation in the experience of time; of the individual meaning of "gain," "loss," "reward," and "punishment." It has been of great interest and encouragement to Dr. Weiner, Dr. Waldrop, and their colleagues that patients respond to "symbolic" incentives more readily than to actual minor material rewards; and that performance remains remarkably stable in certain contingencies. With the equipment now available at the Behavioral and Clinical Studies Center of Saint Elizabeth's Hospital a number of patients can be tested simultaneously on different schedules. Printed circuit computer components make for an economy and flexibility of gear which would have been difficult to achieve with older devices. Moreover, a careful clinical study of the same patient and an enquiry into subjective states of mind during actual performance can proceed in parallel with the operant experiment. The data both warrant and are amenable to mathematical analysis.

Nonverbal and Verbal Behavior in the Dyadic Transaction, Cue and Expectation in Relation Response

There are thus some clinical responses in the single subject which —though unsatisfactorily—can be expressed in quantitative terms. It is significantly more difficult to measure a piece of behavior in an interpersonal field. The psychiatric interview or the analytical session are the prototypes of this situation. Much has been written on the nature and analysis of this transaction (Hilgard et al., 1952; Masserman, 1958); and it has, correctly, in my view, been described as a system of expectations as well as of communication (Lennard and Bernstein, 1960). The interaction is here created by a continuum of individual signals—gestures, non-verbal sounds, words, sentences—which carry symbolic meaning. These are subjectively perceived and put out behaviorally, there being a constant interplay between subjective and manifest elements. The moment-to-moment input into this system is thus enormous; and the devices developed to reduce randomness and sources of variance can, to date, but mark a well-intentioned beginning. The traditionally "neutral" attitude of the psychoanalyst is such a device. The study of nonverbal cues in a transaction is another.

Gestures have been viewed by some as the most economical way of communication (Critchley, 1939), and have been examined with a view to disturbances in communication (Ruesch and Kees, 1956; Ruesch, 1957). A notation system for analysis of body motion and gestures known as "kinesics" has been developed (Birdwhistell, 1952). Separate silent and sound film analysis of a transaction presents another approach. A method has recently been introduced for the analysis of motion picture records by accurate geometrical fixation in successive planes. (Dierssen et al., 1961). These techniques—because of the specialization and also the expense they involve—have so far been used only sparingly in psychiatry. Nevertheless, they may quantify cues which are of the oldest in the body of clinical medicine.

There are similar and more varied attempts to quantify aspects of verbal behavior; analysis of the nominative, connotative quality of words is but one of such analyses. There is suggestive evidence (through the use of appropriate filters) that the frequency spectrum alone—robbed of any connotative quality—can convey the affective quality of a speech sample (Hargreaves and Starkweather, 1962). Respiratory function during speech is another index (Goldman-Eisler, 1955) giving evidence of striking regularities in relation of patterns to speech production, and particularly in regard to verbal output (syllables) per expiration. An extension of this time-analysis of speech production is provided by the interaction chronograph (Chapple, 1940, 1949). Used in a standard, nondirective interview situation, this has already yielded valuable results. In essence, this instrument is an automatically controlled electronic stopwatch, measuring total speech time (irrespective of words) designated as action, pauses, silences, tempo, and other variables in both subject and observer. The coupling of the apparatus to data reduction devices increases the yield and makes possible the derivation of further measures, such as initiative and dominance. These measures have proved reasonably reliable (Matarazzo et al., 1956; Tuason et al., 1962), and there are indications that they may be sensitive to change, including drug-induced change (Tuason and Guze, 1961). *Time* of action thus emerges as an important element in communication, providing, with pitch, the matrix in which the detail of connotative meaning is embedded.

As in operant conditioning behavior, time analysis forms an important element in verbal behavior. Verbal behavior is, in fact, operant behavior, a probabilistic symbolic game in which a piece of behavior operates on one's environment and determines outcome of behavior; verbal conditioning (Luria, 1961) makes it possible to examine these contingencies experimentally. In this reciprocal feedback system of an interpersonal transaction it is not easy to separate patient behavior from therapist behavior; both therapist and patient are, in a sense, participant observers of each other, and the total transaction is the behavior of a two-group, or dyad (Lennard and Bernstein, 1960). It is in these contextual terms that the detail of verbal symbolic behavior must be viewed.

Some analysis of the naturalistic therapeutic transaction has been proceeding for some time and is beginning to bear fruit (Leary and Gill, 1959). The microscopic analysis of samples of speech with regard to word type, grammatical and syntactic structure, the themes referred to, and the context of such themes, suggests that the technique is sensitive to drug effects (Gottschalk et al., 1956). Moreover, it is possible to assess, in a preliminary way, the relationship between the specificity of a therapist's remarks and the expansion of constriction of the patient's statement which follows (Lennard and Bernstein, 1960). Patients talk more in response to verbalization of low structure. The more directive and constrictive the quality of activity, the more likely the negative reaction.

Buried in this obvious statement, there is another aspect of the same phenomenon. If linguistic transaction is in fact a system of mutual expectations, then expectation should influence subjective experience, as manifested in language. These expectations can be experimentally altered. There is, for example, some evidence (in need of much detailed study) that the mere presence of an observer in an experimental analytical situation significantly influences the imagery in psychoanalytic free association (Colby, 1960). In a more direct way, expectation, manipulated either by direct instruction or by implied association, can markedly influence the subjective effect of a drug. This is most obvious in the old, old remedy of the placebo (Beecher, 1959a, p. 65). Moreover, when a drug (e.g., pentobarbitone) effect is compared with *both* placebo and untreated control, diametrically opposite results have been reported leading to the conclusion that

> because of the several varieties of placebo reaction, as well as their potential for interaction with pharmacodynamic effects of drugs, this dynamic quality, which is inseparable from the act of drug administration in man, must be taken into account, and controls must be used which identify the direction as well as magnitude of the placebo effect. For this it may be necessary to use the *unblinded "no-drug-at-all control"** to complement the usual identical dummies in the double blind setting (Modell and Garrett, 1960).

A cognate approach is to examine the interaction between paradoxical instructive set and effect of a drug (for example, the administration of amphetamine with instructions appropriate to a barbiturate or vice versa). Such experiments are in progress (Fisher, 1962).

GROUP INTERACTION, WARD SETTING, AND THE CLINICAL TRIAL

It is obvious from the foregoing that forces which powerfully influence a dyadic social field are bound to be manifest in an amplified degree in larger groups. The subject of small group interaction has been thoroughly reviewed (Hare et al., 1955; Nowlis, 1960), and classified for such factors as group size, the communication network, the personal and social characteristics of members, role differentiation, initial expectancy

---

* Italics by present author.

of members with respect to each other, and setting, as important input variables. Various methods have been used to approach the subject. For example, the communication network can be controlled by varying the sequence of communication between subjects (Christie et al., 1952). A topographical system of notation—chain, wheel, star, circle—(Christie et al., 1952) has been introduced, and quantification is possible by means of devices such as the transmittance matrix (Roby and Lanzetta, 1958) linear graph analysis (Cartright and Harary, 1956) or measure of centrality (Leavit, 1951) or independence. The mathematical problems in the analysis of small group behavior have also been recently considered (Solomon, 1960). A physical task (e.g., getting a ball up a spiral plane) can be arranged to depend upon the collective skills and cohesion within a small group. In one such instance, such a task was found to be sensitive to sleep deprivation and medication (Laties, 1961). Even in the absence of a definitive task there are striking changes in the interpersonal field following medication. Thus one study (Rinkel et al., 1955) on the effects of LSD-25 reported a significant increase in avoidance, withdrawal, hostile, punitive, competitive behavior, while friendly reciprocal, equalitarian behavior was clearly reduced. The effect of a drug on behavior must thus be considered in a social field. The same drug, in the same dose, in the same subject will produce different effects according to the interpersonal and motivational situation in which it is given. This, particularly, applies to moderate doses of drugs.

It is much more difficult to study interaction in a large group, such as a ward population. Here both overt observation and observation by a participant observer assuming a patient role (Caudill et al., 1952) have been practiced. In our own laboratory, and arising out of the need of the clinical trial, a method known as the Social Interaction Matrix was developed by Kellam (1961). This device makes use of a suitably marked grid to record the amount and kind of social contact between patients on the basis of regular and frequent observations on the ward during the day. It is a scale deliberately designed to measure the amount of social mobility among patients, and one of the several instruments available to quantitate behavior on a psychiatric ward.

There are many such devices, and around them center some of the liveliest controversies in psychiatry. Should rating scales be used or should one rely on clinical observation only? If rating scales are to be used, who is to use them, how often, and why? Is the physician's rating based on a half-hour interview once a week more reliable that that of the Nursing Assistant, potentially having access to the patient for eight hours? How should raters be selected, and how trained? Upon whose vocabulary is the rating scale to be built? What are minimal criteria for scale validity in terms of content and construct? When do criteria become predictive? These and many other questions continue to be asked, and have been authoritatively reviewed (Lorr, 1960). One can draw comfort from such opinions. It is possible, for example, to record serially, and adequately, behavior in a metabolic unit (Beauregard et al., 1961). The reliability of some scales is high, so much so that by careful selection of items of high information content, a reliability of 0.9 can be achieved with as few as 12 items (Lorr, 1960). Moreover, when such scales are used in a formal controlled clinical trial of several phenothiazines (Casey et al., 1960; Kurland et al., 1961), the conclusions regarding rank order of the various compounds compare not at all badly with an open, non-blind, clinical assessment (Freyhan, 1959).

The native clinical experience evidently is still a match for artificial intelligence, and the computer we carry in our skull is at least equal to its metal counterpart. Somehow the experienced, sensitive, and skeptical clinician collates data for internal consistency and error simultaneously at many levels, arriving at a formulation which represents a creative act of very high order. It is humbling that, despite its limitations, ordinary language should be able to convey its message so clearly in such a for-mulation. Rating scales thus have their place, but should be used only where there is clinical judgment. It is, in fact, when rigid assessment precludes continuous observation of clinical process over time, when ob-servation of the outer shell of behavior presumes either to ignore or to infer subjective states of mind, that it is well to send one's young colleague back to the ward to write a long anecdotal history. Refined statistical manipulation will not mask poor case selection, or coarse rating-scales, or poor inter-rater agreement. Sooner or later truth will out. In this age of restless manipulation it is well to learn to stare at phenomena in the ward; to take up the fragment, and the detail, only after having had a sense of the subtlety of the whole.

ON THE NEED FOR NEW SYMBOLIC SYSTEMS IN
PSYCHOBIOLOGY AND PSYCHIATRY

In 1854, George Boole, a man who self-taught had risen to a Royal Society Medal and a Chair in Mathematics at Queens College, Cork, published his "Investigation of the Laws of Thought." In this work, as in an earlier one—"The Mathematical Analysis of Logic" (1847)—he examined the ability of symbols to express logical propositions, "the laws of whose combination should be founded upon the laws of mental processes which they represent." In searching for such outward representation, he invented the theory of classes and sets and the nonassociative relation between them, devising a symbolic algebraic shorthand for the expression of these relations in which concepts such as product, complement, inclusion, and a number of others are clearly represented.

Boole's path-breaking contributions led by way of Frege (1879), Jevons (1864), Peirce (1880) to Whitehead and Russell's "Principia" (1910-1913) in our day. One may note, in passing, the titles of some of these earlier works. Jevons named his work "Pure Logic, or the Logic of Quality apart from Quantity." Frege called his study a *Begriffschrift* —a "formula language, (Formelsprache)" of pure thought. Somehow the inexpressible, the suggestive qualities which in other circumstances we would call intuitive, grew into communicable notations and symbols of great propulsive power—and opened a world of relations hitherto considered closed. It is outside my competence to examine the influence of Boolean algebra on modern experimental physics. However, the relation of a theory of sets and classes to communication and information transfer is nearer at hand. For the very word "communication" (from "communicare") implies sharing—i.e., the sharing of properties; and any encoding process depends upon the apprehension of such shared properties among sets and classes. It is by this sharing, too, that redundancy, far from being wasteful, serves in the transfer of information. Redundancy provides context and thus minimizes error. It is a safety device in the flow of information (MacKay, 1961)—a reserve, incidentally, amply encountered in biological systems.

Yet how interdependent are the demands of a subject, and the demands of a language for a subject. When chemistry or electrical engineering needed appropriate symbolic forms of notation, such systems were duly invented: and when turn-of-the-century physics felt constrained by Newtonian mechanics, it was modified according to need. However, so young is biology as a science, and so much younger still is the biology of mental phenomena (which we will call psychobiology) that its great discoveries were made using a linguistic apparatus leased from chemistry and physics, and from the language of every day use. This hybrid arrangement has served for a time. No one will deny the many advances made so far. Nevertheless, it is clear that demands of quite a different order are pressing on the biology of our day. Interaction in macromolecular systems and the control mechanisms inherent in such systems are evidently of a different order from reactions between simple inorganic compounds. Any accounting for the flow of information in such systems (as, for example, in the obvious instances of the gene or the immunological specificity of proteins) demands a language in which mere chemical or descriptive language is no longer sufficient. Woodger (1952) has indeed attempted to define the elements of a concise formal language for some aspects of genetics and evolutionary theory: a difficult but enormously worthwhile task.

It is the fortunate, if embarrassing, feature of the phenomena of behavior and of mental life that by their very nature they brook less compromise in such matters than any other branch of biology. The purely physical and chemical analogies do not hold; and the psychochemical correlates demand, as we have seen, a much more detailed specification and description of behavior, and of concomitant chemical change, than is currently available. For behavior implies multiple simultaneous change of a system in time, and *form* in behavior is really a topology in time. Discursive, linear, metric language does not apprehend such patterns. Presentational, experiential language suggests intricate simultaneous relationships, but does not define them. Yet it is the characteristic of every culture that it has invented symbols for such subjectively experienced relationships. It is significant, too, that in its own evolution, physics (as well as the branch of mathematics known as topology) has developed a shorthand for the apprehension of cognate simultaneous relations in the so-called outside physical world.

Is it possible that in behavior and subjective experience we could see —if we wished to look long and hard—the "laws of thought" of which Boole spoke and which govern our understanding of the physical world? And is it possible that the two uses of language which we distinguished represent two mutually complementary ways—one multiple and simultaneous and the other serial and successive—by which the brain constructs its models of reality? I have elsewhere (Elkes, 1961b) tentatively examined the possible relation of schizophrenic thought disorder to information processing, or misprocessing, by the brain. In this scheme I suggested that transformations proceeded simultaneously at different yet closely interrelated neural levels, and distinguished between an ability to organize information serially in time—to structure in time—(in terms of the immediate adaptive demands of the "Here" and "Now") and a much more pervasive function of nervous tissue which depended upon its ability to organize simultaneously changing multiple inputs into a temporal topology of high information content. In this context the distinction between "serial" and "parallel" programming of computers concerned with pattern recognition is of special, if topical, interest (Selfridge and Neisser, 1960). Essentially, the distinction is one between asking questions serially one at a time, i.e., letting each answer determine the next question by successive elimination; or asking, as Neisser put it (1962), all the questions at once. It is found, for example, that in the recognition of patterns of letters of different calligraphic quality the multiple, parallel method is more economical and effective. The metal intelligence thus turns up with a familiar linguistic problem; and there is at least inferential evidence that, at one level of its organization, the nervous system has the capacity of asking many questions all at once.

The multiply connected reticular mixing-pool may provide a substrate for precisely such transactions. The illogical thought process of intense subjective experience, of the dream, and so-called "primary" process (Freud, 1900) may thus have its parallel in presentational language, in the "geometric" thinking of Clerk Maxwell, the principles of complementarity and coexistence of physics, and the multiple (or "parallel") approach of the modern computer; the logical, structured, sequential pattern of conscious deliberate action (sometimes called "secondary process") may be mirrored more closely in discursive language, the arithmetical approach, the scale, the serial analysis. Counting and pattern, rating and correlation, are thus at opposite ends. One feeds into the other, and science draws on them both.

This process is well illustrated in Harvey's famous passage in Chapter VIII of "De motu cordis" (1628) where, following the minute sequential observation described in the preceding parts, the "movement, as it were, in a circle' is first conceived. "Movement in a circle" implies an intuitive seeing of a relation in time. Indeed, time would appear to be the main axis around which we build our models of reality; and nowhere is this more apparent than in the models we construct to represent behavior, including human behavior.

It would seem advisable, in view of the foregoing, to give early thought to the development of adequate new symbolic systems in the study of interpersonal processes, and to relate such attempts, whenever possible, to existing instruments in the natural sciences. The creation of such new systems would require long-term planning within small groups. It would require highly trained observers and highly trained subjects, capable of self-observation, to whom unfamiliar phenomena have become familiar through practice, as foreign territories are to seasoned travelers, and who are capable of developing operational definitions of states experienced and observed. Such an endeavor would require close cooperation between psychiatrist, psychologist, mathematician, and communication engineer; it might require training of one discipline in the skills of the other, to ensure a most direct personal contact with the phenomena. It would require much debate, and much crude trial and error. Yet, the history of science suggests that once such a beginning is made progress can be quite rapid. It may be not too much to hope that concepts only partly or inadequately covered by present-day language may, before very long, find a more adequate expression in new symbolic systems of greater precision and power.

The usefulness of such systems may—and I would venture to say, will—not be confined to the study of behavior. For the phenomena of behavior pose some fundamental issues in biology—particularly in regard to the storage and transfer of information in living systems. Indeed, the chief merit of behavior may perhaps lie in its intolerance to facile analogies borrowed from other branches of science, and its compelling need for rules in its own right. The Behavioral Sciences, and that vast body of experience known as Clinical Psychiatry, thus need not look apprehensively over their shoulders; having been nourished by the natural sciences, they may well be in a position to repay a longstanding debt. It is one's hope—and, if pressed, would be one's contention—that a science of Clinical Psychiatry is in the making in our day; and that in its growth, it will enlarge the realm of the very sciences on which, quite properly, it still depends.

REFERENCES

Abramson, H. A., Jarvik, M. E., Kaufman, M. R., Kornetsky, C., Levine, A., and Wagner, M. (1955). *J. Psychol.* 39, 3-60.

Beauregard, R. M., Wadeson, R. W., and Walsh, L. (1961). *J. Chronic Diseases* 14, 609-628.

Beecher, H. K. (1959a). "Measurement of Subjective Responses." Oxford Univ. Press, London and New York.

Beecher, H. K. (1959b). *In* "Quantitative Methods in Human Pharmacology and Therapeutics" (D. R. Laurence, Ed.), p. 102. Pergamon, New York.

Birdwhistell, R. L. (1952). "Introduction to Kinesics." Univ. of Louisville Press, Louisville, Kentucky.

Boardman, W. K., Goldstone, S., and Lhamon, W. T. (1957). *A.M.A. Arch. Neurol. Psychiat.* 78, 321-327.

Boole, G. (1947). "The Mathematical Analysis of Logic." Combridge.

Boole, G. (1854). "An Investigation of the Laws of Thought." Walton and Maberly, London.

Breuer, J., and Freud, S. (1893). Neurologisches Zentr. 12, 4-10.

Carnap, R. (1959). "The Logical Syntax of Language." (Reprinting of 1st English edition, 1937, Routledge, Kegan and Paul, London.) Littlefield, Adams, Paterson, New Jersey.

Cartright, D., and Harary, F. (1956), *Psychol. Rev.* 63, 277-293.

Casey, J. F., Lasky, J. J., Klett, C. J., and Hollister, L. E. (1960). *Am. J. Psychiat.* 117,97-105.

Cattell, R. B. (1960). *In* "Drugs and Behavior" (L. Uhr, and J. G. Miller, eds.), p. 438. Wiley, New York.

Caudill, W., Redlich, F. C., Brody, E. B., and Gilmore, H. R. (1952). *Am. J. Orthopsychiat.* 22, 314-334.

Chapple, E. D. (1940). *Genet. Psychol. Monogr.* No. 22, 1-247.

Chapple, E. D. (1949). *Personnel* 25, 295-307.

Christie, L. S., Luce, D. R., and Macy, J., Jr. (1952). "Communication and Learning in Task Oriented Groups." Technical Rept. No. 32, Cambridge, Mass., Research Laboratory of Electronics, Massachusetts Institute of Technology.

Clyde, D. J. (1960), *In* "Drugs and Behavior" (L. Uhr and J. G. Miller, eds.), pp. 583-538, Wiley, New York.

Colby, K. M. (1960) *Behavioral Sci.* 5, 216-232.

Critchley, M. (1939). "The Language of Gesture." Edward Arnold, London.

Dierssen, G., Lorenc, M., and Spitaleri, R. M. (1961). *Neurology* 11, 610-618.

Ditman, K. S. (1960). *In* "The Use of LSD in Psychotherapy" (H. A. Abramson, ed.), p. 118. Josiah Macy, Jr. Foundation, New York.

Elkes, J. (1961b). *In* "Chemical Pathology of the Nervous System" (J. Folch-Pi, ed.), pp. 648-665. Pergamon, Oxford.

Fisher, Seymour. (1962). Personal communication.

Frege, G. (1879). "Begriffschrift, eine der Arithmetischen Nachgebildete Formelsprache des reinen Denkens." Halle.

Freud, S. (1900). "The Interpretation of Dreams." Reprinted (1938). *In* "The Basic Writings of Sigmund Freud," p. 525. The Modern Library, New York.

Freyhan, F. (1959). *Am J. Psychiat.* 115, 577-585.

Goldman-Eisler, F. (1955). *Brit. J. Psychol.* 46, 53-63.

Gottschalk, L. A., Kapp, F. T., Ross, D. W., Kaplan, S. M., Silver, H., MacLeod, J. A., Kahn, J. B., Van Maanen, E. F., and Acheson, G. H. (1956). *J. Am. Med. Assoc.* 161, 1054-1058.

Grinker, R. R., Miller, J., Sabshin, M., Nunn, R., and Nunnally, J. C. (1961). "The Phenomena of Depressions." Hoeber, Harper: New York.

Hamburg, D. A., Sabshin, M. A., Board, F. A., Grinker, R. R., Korchin, S. J., Basowitz, H., Heath, H., and Persky, H. (1958). *A.M.A. Arch. Neurol. Psychiat.* 79, 415-425.

Hamilton, M. (1960). *J. Neurol. Neurosurg. Psychiat.* 23, 56-62.

Hare, P., Borgatta, E. F., and Bales, R. F. (eds.), (1955). "Small Groups. Studies in Social Interaction." Knopf, New York.

Hargreaves, W. A., and Starkweather, J. A., personal communication.

Harvey, W. (1628). "Exercitatio anatomica de motu cordis et sanguinis in animalibus." G. Fitzer, Frankfurt.

Hilgard, E. R., Kubie, L. S., and Pumpian-Mindlin, E. (eds.) (1952). "Psychoanalysis as Science," Stanford Univ. Press, Stanford, California.

Hofmann, A., Heim, R., Brack, A., and Kobel, H. (1958). *Experientia* 14, 107-109.

Houde, R. W., and Wallenstein, S. L. (1953). "Drug Addiction and Narcotics Bulletin," Appendix F, p. 660, National Research Council, Washington, D.C.

Jevons, W. S. (1864). "Pure Logic, or the Logic of Quality Apart from Quantity." London.

Kellam, S. G. (1961). *J. Nervous Mental Disease* 132, 277-288.

Knight, R. A. (1963). *In* "Specific and Non-Specific Factors in Psychopharmacology" (M. Rinkel, ed.).

Kurland, S. A., Hanlon, T. E., Tatom, M. H., Ota, K. Y., and Simopoulos, A. M. (1961). *J. Nervous Mental Disease* 133, 1-18.

Lacey, J. I. (1956). *Ann. N. Y. Acad. Sci.* 67, 123-163.

Langer, S. K. (1942). "Philosophy in a New Key," 9th printing (revised, 1958). New American Library, New York.

Langer, S. K. (1957). "Problems of Art." Scribner, New York.

Laties, V. G. (1961). *J. Psychiat. Research* 1, 12-25.

Lasagna, L., and Beecher, H. K. (1954). *J. Pharmacol.* 112, 306-311.

Leary, T., and Gill, M. (1959). *In* "Research in Psychotherapy" (E. A. Rubinstein and M. B. Parloff, eds.), pp. 62-95, American Psychological Association, Washington, D.C.

Leavit, H. J. (1951). *J. Abnormal Soc. Psychol.* 16, 38-50.

Lennard, H. L., and Bernstein, A. (1960). "The Anatomy of Psychotherapy." Columbia Univ. Press, New York.

Lewis, T. (1942). "Pain." Macmillan, New York.

Lindsley, O. R., and Skinner, B. F. (1954). *Am. Psychologist* 9, 419-420.

Livingston, R. B. (1958). *In* "Handbook of Physiology," Section 1: Neurophysiology (J. Field, H. W. Magoun, and V. E. Hall, eds.), pp. 741-760. American Physiological Society, Washington, D.C.

Lorr, M. (1960). *In* "Drugs and Behavior" (L. Uhr and J. G. Miller, eds.), pp. 519-539. Wiley, New York.

Luria, A. (1961). "The Role of Speech in the Regulation of Normal and Abnormal Behavior." Liveright, New York.

Mach, E. (1886). "The Analysis of Sensations and the Relation of the Physical to the Psychical." Translated from the 1st German ed. by C. M. Williams; Open Court Publishers, Chicago, 1914.

MacKay, D. M. (1961). "The Science of Communication." Inaugural Lecture at University College, of North Staffordshire, University College of North Staffordshire, Keele, England.

Masserman, J. H. (ed.) (1958). "Science and Psychoanalysis." Grune & Stratton, New York.

Matarazzo, J. D., Saslow, G., and Guze, S. B. (1956). *J. Consult. Psychol.* 20, 267-274.

Maxwell, J. C. (1856) Transactions of the Cambridge Philosophical Society. *In* "Scientific Paper of J. C. Maxwell" (W. D. Niven, ed., 1890, Cambridge), Vol 1, pp. 155-229.

Modell, W., and Garrett, M. (1960). *Nature* 185, 539.

Neisser, U. (1962). Personal communication.

Nowlis, V. (1960). *In* "Drugs and Behavior" (L. Uhr and J. G. Miller, eds.), pp. 563-581, Wiley, New York.

Nowlis, V., and Nowlis, H. H. (1956), *Ann. N. Y. Acad. Sci.* 65, 345-355.

Peirce, C. S. (1880). *Am. J. Math.* 3, 15.

Rinkel, M., Hyde, R. W., Solomon, H. C., and Hoagland, H. (1955). *Am J. Psychiat.* 111, 881-895.

Roby, T. B., and Lanzetta, J. R. (1958). *Psychol. Bull.* 55, 88-101.

Ruesch, J. (1957). "Disturbed Communication." Norton, New York.
Ruesch, J. and Kees, W. (1956). "Nonverbal Communication." University of California Press, Berkeley, California.
Russell, B. (1927). "Philosophy," p. 265, Norton, New York.
Selfridge, O. G., and Neisser, U. (1960). *Sci. American* 203,60-68.
Skinner, B. F. (1938). "The Behavior of Organisms." Appleton-Century, New York.
Solomon, H. (ed.) (1960). "Mathematical Thinking in the Measurement of Behavior." Free Press of Glencoe, Illinois.
Solomon, P., Kubzansky, P. E., Leiderman, P. H., Mendelson, J. H., Trumbull, R., and Wexler, D. (eds.) (1961). "Sensory Deprivation." Harvard Univ. Press, Cambridge, Massachusetts.
Szara, S. (1956). *Experientia* 12, 441.
Szara, S., and Rockland, L. H. (1962). *Proc. 3rd, World Congr. Psychiat.* 1, 670-673. Univ. of Toronto Press, Toronto.
Taylor, J. A. (1953). *J. Abnormal Social Psychol.* 48, 285-290.
Tuason, V., and Guze, S. B. (1961). *Clin Pharmacol. Exptl. Therap.* 2, 152-156.
Tuason, V., Guze, S. B., McClure, J., and Beguelin, J. (1962). *Am. J. Psychiat.* 118, 438-446.
Uhr, L., and Miller, J. G. (eds.) (1960). "Drugs and Behavior." John Wiley, New York.
Weiner, H. (1962). *J. Exptl. Anal. Behavior* 5, 201-208.
Whitehead, A. N., and Russell, B. A. W. (1910-1913), "Principia Mathematica," 3 vols. Cambridge Univ. Press, London.
Whorf, B. J. (1956). "Language, Thought and Reality. Selected Writings (1927-1941)." Wiley, New York; and the Technology Press, Massachusetts Institute of Technology, Cambridge, Massachusetts.
Woodger, J. H. (1952). "Biology and Language." Cambridge Univ. Press, London and New York.

11

HENRY BROSIN, M.D. with
WILLIAM S. CONDON, Ph.D. and
WILLIAM D. OGSTON, M.D.

> *It is an honor to participate in this ceremony to pay our respects to our beloved friend, Dr. Leo Bartemeier. Although he has contributed much more than most men as a scientist, clinician and administrator of the welfare of his fellowman during a long lifetime, and has received many honors for his public achievements, I would like to express my deep personal gratitude to him for his steadfast example of a life-style which is admirable and worthy of emulation. In periods of rapid transition of socio-economic and related value systems, it is popularly said that we do not have adequate models for "the good life." While the indictment is all too true for many, I believe that Dr. Bartemeier has lived the good life honorably and even with distinction, and we need not despair. He offers hope as well as accomplishment.*

Film Recording of Normal and Pathological Behavior

ONE OF THE GREATEST obstacles to a systematic study of living human interaction is the inadequacy of methods of recording the multiple levels of signal systems which make up the totality of human communication. The relatively easy availability of sound-film and audio-visual tape has made possible much more detailed study of these signal systems, and provides us with a technique analogous to the microscope, which has opened up new fields for study, particularly in the clinical interactions between patients and therapists.

Human behavior has been recorded and studied since men could talk, draw and write. Over the centuries many varieties of specialists came into being to analyze and dissect the methods of recording behavior, in contrast to the generalists in the humanities and social sciences. However ingenious and imaginative the students of the methods of that vital sphere of human behavior known as "communication" were, and we applaud their achievements, we are not much better off than Plato or dozens of poets and philosophers who lament the inadequacy of the written word as a vehicle for the thousand subtleties for conveying human feelings. "It is not what you say, but the way you say it," is a common reproof in "misunderstandings." In spite of these insights, written descriptions using dictionary words and punctuation marks remained our principal method of recording behavior until recently. With the exception of dance notations and the work of a few students of "expressive movement," there had been no notable progress in relating linguistic, paralinguistic, kinesic (body movement), or visceral components of the communication stream of signals between people until sound film became easily available at relatively reasonable prices. This is all the more remarkable because Charles Darwin, perhaps the greatest genius of his age, wrote a monograph, *The Expression of the Emotions in Men and Animals* in 1872, in which he outlined five strategies for studying human behavior: (1) child development; (2) psychoses; (3) myths and art work; (4) animal behavior (ethology); (5) and the use of photographs. We were far into the Twentieth Century before the full meaning of these recommendations was appreciated by scientists, and only in the past decade are there genuine, large-scale efforts being implemented by professional workers in child development and communication. It is equally curious that the tremendous impact of Freud upon our culture did not result in a greatly increased systematic investigation of both these areas in view of his insistence upon the vital importance of the early years of life, and upon the kinesic elements (body motion, posture, gestures, facies) in the exchange of messages between people. Knapp has reviewed this development in the introduction to the book *Expression of the Emotions* of which he is the editor.[25] Knapp's book, a collection of papers and discussions from a symposium on the Expression of the Emotions in Man, held at the 1960 meeting of the American Association for the Advancement of Science, is an excellent general introduction to the subject. Another helpful survey is found in the volume edited by Thomas S. Sebeok, Alfred S. Hayes and Mary Catherine Bateson called *Approaches to Semiotics*.[39] This comprises transactions of the Indiana University conference on paralinguistics and kinesics held in 1962, and furnishes the reader with some of the concepts and methods being developed at that time. More recent guides are the books, *Methods of Research in Psychotherapy*, edited by Gottschalk and Auerbach[24] (1966), and the third volume in the American Psychological Association's series, *Research in Psychotherapy* (1968)[40], and articles and monographs by A. E. Scheflen (1965).[34-38]

To be sure, there were a few psychoanalysts who followed Freud in his excellent case studies and essays, especially *The Psychopathology of Everyday Life* (1901) which stressed the body motion, linguistic or somatic components of messages, but there were no sustained systematic experiments.[22] There were also psychologists who understood the need to study human communication as a unified complex of signal systems carrying a wide variety of messages including internal modulations to alter meanings, or even contradictions or negations, but only recently have there been systematic studies.[40]

Linguists, particularly those with an anthropological background, opened the door to an understanding of linguistic systems *as they actually occur in spoken language*, in contrast to studies of written words. We usually associate the names of Leonard Bloomfield (1933) and Edward Sapir (1949) as significant leaders in this field, both due to their own work, but also from the work of their highly influential pupils.[33] In 1942 Kenneth Pike devised methods of written notations for pitch, stress and juncture of spoken sentences, which along with other properties of speech made something approaching reliable transcription of ordinary speech possible.[31] His large volume *Language in Relation to a Unified Theory of Behavior* (1967), while very difficult to read because of the technical vocabulary, describes many of the problems inherent in the analysis of the spoken word and attempts rational solutions.[31] Particularly significant is Pike's effort to grapple with the concept of a "unit" in his discussions of "etic" and "emic" which will be evident in our discussion.

Another important theoretical consideration in the study of language as a biological phenomenon, although not of immediate practical importance, is Lenneberg's *Biological Foundations of Language*.[29] Our attempts to study communications systems as cultural systems which are in harmony with our biological heritage can be enriched by studies which clarify the workings of the human central nervous system and its evolutionary development.

The long path by which the following studies came into being since December, 1955 has been told in other places and need not be repeated here.[8-12] My co-authors Doctors William S. Condon and William D. Ogston have provided me with samples of their recent investigations, not previously reported, which will be of interest to clinical psychiatrists. I should mention that the energy and time required for microstudies of film and tape are so great that I do not expect practicing therapists to enter this field. Film viewing of patient-doctor interviews with a focus on large unit transactions can be very rewarding to clinicians and students, especially in supervisory situations, but the necessarily slow, patient, frame-by-frame checking, rechecking and cross-referencing requires very large segments of time.

The natural history approach, as used by ethnologists, has led to a fuller description of the life styles of many species, revealing patterns which many species share and others which only exist within a single species. The varied courting, territorial, and aggressive behaviors of many species have been examined carefully and complex forms of shared communicational behavior were found to exist.

This use of complex, shared patterns of behavior also appears to be (along with speech) an important aspect of human communication. The ways in which human interactants share posture together and move together, including the rhythmic variations of such movement, conveys important statements about their relationship. This also applies to group processes. There seems to be constant behavioral feedback at many levels that a listener or listeners are attending to what one is saying. Varied degrees of intimacy, distance, and hostility can be expressed through these behavioral relationships, Much of this, however, appears to occur out of awareness. Scheflen has studied intensively the postural relationships among interactants and has found that they convey many clues about the nature of the on-going relationships among these interactants.[36,37]

Interactants also move together in a very intricate dance-like fashion. The body of a speaker was found to move in configurations-of-change which are (hierarchically and organizationally) isomorphic with the articulatory segmentation of his own speech. Further, the body of the *listener(s)* moves in configurations-of-change which are isomorphic with speech/body motion configuration of the speaker. This synchronous behavior occurs in normal human interaction from the micro level up to and including the phrasal level. It may occur at still higher levels.

The following illustration is taken from a film in which a man and a woman appear to engage in a precise courting dance, seemingly without being aware of it. In the film both man and woman (who are sitting in chairs) begin to lean toward each other at the same frame (1/24 of a second). This continues for approximately fifteen frames. They then stop at the same frame, raise their heads together for three frames, then lean back into their chairs together, again stopping at the same frame. They then reverse direction together and come forward slightly. Most of these intricate moves occur in the absence of speech. There appear to be many degrees of interactional synchrony and this heightening or lowering of the relationship (again apparently out of awareness) is in some sense responded to by the participants.

The woman says, "Yeh, I said what was that and then I said well. . . ." The man and woman sit relatively quietly across the emission of the first phrase, "Yes, I said." She is moving her head and her left arm while her right hand is cupped under her chin. The man is moving his right arm, while his left leg is crossed over the right and is still. At the onset of "what was that" the woman's right hand rapidly leaves her chin and her hand comes down to the table during the emission of this phrase. At the onset of this same phrase the man's left leg begins to extend rapidly horizontally, leaving its position of rest across the right leg. He thus begins to uncross his legs exactly at the onset of the phrase and synchronously with the right arm movement of the woman. Across "and then I said well . . ." the woman twists in her chair toward the table and moves her feet on the floor. Across this same phrase the man puts his left leg down to the floor and also twists toward the table.

The total utterance, then, is broken up into three phrasal elements which are accompanied by sustained body-motion configurations on the part of both. They move relatively slowly across the first phrase, speed up together across the second phrase, and then slowly together across the third phrase. Their bodies were also moving together synchronously across the syllables and words of this same total utterance. This same precision of sharing of movement has been observed in many films of human interaction.

All aspects of movement and posture appear to be utilized in these interactional "statements." All are part of and function together within the on-going stream of behavior. Posture and movement are not separate forms of communication, but function reciprocally and cooperatively within the total matrix of the interactional process.

And as they convey statements of degrees of togetherness so also, it seems, they can convey statements of degrees of exclusion and rejection. This is particularly so in groups. For example, a sharing of posture and movement by two people in a group of five people indicates that they are probably, at that moment, interactionally closer to each other than to the other three. It is also, simultaneously, an exclusion, in a certain sense, of the other three. In this fashion complex subgroup relations can be detected within a larger group.[27]

In a film of a group of four persons discussing a topic, a segmentation into two subgroups was possible in terms of the shared movement patterns. When either subject A or B would speak (they agreed on a point), the other member would move more than either subjects C or D. Conversely, when either C or D spoke, the other would move more than either A or B. Thus the sharing of movement together served to distinguish subgroups. There was little sharing of posture in this particular sequence.[27]

An area which deserves much further study is the family communicational structure.

In Pittsburgh a sound-film study is being conducted with twins. Mothers with their "normal" twins and mothers where one twin is mentally ill are being filmed. Each of the mothers is filmed interacting with her twins. At the present time only a few films have been studied so the tentative findings are only suggestive.

One film is of a mother and her fourteen-year-old twin girls (one of whom is schizophrenic) being interviewed by a psychiatrist. In this film the "well" twin and the mother are almost constantly either sharing posture together or moving together. They also move in serial contiguity, i.e., if the mother moves, the twin almost always immediately follows suit and conversely. They even adjust their skirts together at the same 1/24 of a second. They laugh and smile together. It almost looks as if they are partners in a communicational conspiracy.

On the other hand, the mother and the ill twin very seldom share either posture or movement together. Several times when this twin adopts a posture similar to that of the mother, the mother immediately changes posture. It is as if she avoids engaging in communication at this body motion level.

Another film shows eight-year-old twins (a normal girl and her ill brother) interacting with their mother. A similar conspiracy between the girl and the mother seems to occur. The mother and the girl each successfully and laughingly create a tower out of blocks after the boy fails awkwardly. She tends to widen her eyes, raise her brows, bite her lip, stiffen her shoulders, and not smile when she looks at or talks to the boy. She tends to relax her body, lower her head and smile when she talks to or interacts with the girl. This mother also exhibited some evidence of micro self-dyssynchrony; there were also several relatively clear occurrences of micro-strabismus.

A third film, which shows "normal" eight-year-old twin girls interacting with their mother, was examined as a contrast. The mother appeared to give an almost equal amount of attention to each child and without marked difference. There was some indication of a slight preference for one twin. A fourth interaction, of normal thirteen-year-old twin girls and their mother, was similar to that of the preceding film of normal subjects. There was an absence of marked difference in relating to the twins.

This is limited data at present and many more films need to be studied. Analysis thus far seems to suggest that the ill twin may exist in a markedly different communicational structure than the normal twin in the same family. Much of this is ostensibly out of awareness. However, one cannot infer that this is the cause of the illness. It does accent and possibly perpetuate the communicational isolation. A similar communicational isolation may occur with patients in non-twin families.

If the behavioral-communicational factors described earlier *are* basic, interactional aspects of human behavior, they deserve study by the psychiatrist. Verbal content is almost always accompanied by these parenthetic nonverbal commentaries. Schizophrenic patients, at least in the limited population (50 patients) thus far studied, tend to move differently during interaction. In most of the cases studied, some part of the body tended to remain excessively still for a long period of time. They do not participate in the moving, rhythmic dance of normal interaction. One hypothesis might be that they have been excluded from participating in the shared patterns of normal behavior for so long that they do not know how or are reluctant to try. The communicational behavior of the sick twins seemed related to the structure of the communicational situation in which they lived.

Body motion is emerging as a significant area of interactional commentary. For example, there are some tentative indications that dominance-submission may be an important background aspect in much ostensibly civilized male-male interaction. Four films have been made, each one of two males interacting. In each of these films the dominant male (in that situation) picked up his chair and moved it so that it sliced into the space of the other male. The dominant male also tended to control the conversation.

In one film the submissive male lowered eye-gaze first every time gaze contact was made except near the end of the film. At this point the dominant male made a prearranged, joking, verbal attack designed to startle the other. From this point on the dominant male dropped eye-gaze first.

The above hints were the result of passing observations which were not further explored. The idea emerged again in the following context. Many young, Negro males in South Chicago were given job training, but they were later failing their job interviews. The following tentative hypothesis was formulated. Suppose that the black man went into the interview with the white boss with the "set" that he was equal to the white man. But in the animal kingdom there is a pecking order, or dominance-submission hierarchies. In reality, perhaps, he should be sending submissive signals. The white boss may have been angry out of awareness that his dominant status was being subtly challenged. The following set of three films was made in order to try and explore some of the above reflections.

In the first film subject A, a lower-middle-class Negro male of about 30 (who is working on his master's degree in computer science) talks with subject B, a white male president of a Chicago corporation. They are not told what to talk about but only that we are interested in human interaction. Subject A has brought two books and sets them beside his chair in camera range. He could easily have left them in the outer room.

In the second film this same subject A interacts with subject C, a high-status Negro male who holds an important job in community relations. (He is a Y.M.C.A. executive earning $20,000 a year or more).

In the third film subject A interacts with subject D, a male Negro janitor.

Thus in this series of films subject A interacts with an older white executive, an older Negro executive and an older Negro janitor. Subject A's behavior changes in each of the films. The content of the conversations also seems to reflect the relationship. In the first film subject A and the white executive have a mild difference of opinion. Subject A defends higher education and the executive feels that more skilled labor needs to be trained.

In the second film, subject A talks about his boyhood in the Y.M.C.A. and calls the black executive "Sir." He never calls the white executive "Sir."

In the third film, subject A and the janitor talk about the role of the Negro male in the family and about how difficult it was for a male Negro to get a job, but how this is now changing. The janitor indicates that he is a "custodian," and both laugh at some of the high sounding names used to conceal the word *janitor*. Subject A tells the janitor that he is in charge of a library computer complex.

The first film of subject A and the white executive is most interesting. Subject A reclines back in his chair with a slight smile on his face in a mildly provocative manner. He and the executive voice their opinions on the merits of education *vs.* skilled training. The body motion structure seems to reflect the content. First one and then the other make slapping movements and kicking movements toward each other. These occur as emphasis gestures accompanying speech. But from another perspective they resemble very much the threat gestures of male animals. At one point, about five minutes into the film, the white executive makes a very vehement striking motion (the most intense kinesic movement in the film) with his raised hand and bares his teeth in a grimace. The verbal content is as follows. "Course I . . . I want . . . I don't wanna be misunderstood. I . . . I firmly (the slap occurs across the word "firmly") believe this education is so important."

Precisely as the executive begins his slap and synchronously with it, subject A comes up out of his chair, sits up straight and leans forward attentively. At this point the subject matter changes and the executive asks how he can use computers in his business. There is some indication that subject A and the executive were engaged in a dominance-submission struggle out of their awareness. It would appear that almost one-third of the time was spent in getting this settled before other forms of communication could begin. On the other hand, when subject A and the other Negroes converse, there appears to be little of this. These explorations are only tentative, but, again, they suggest the possible importance of body motion in human communication.

As mentioned earlier, in passing, a long-range hope of the research was that an increasing discovery of order in normal behavior might be useful as a contrastive basis for the examination of pathological behavior. In contrast to the harmonious integrity of normal behavior, pathological behavior displayed various degrees of self-dyssynchrony. Tentatively, self-dyssynchrony is observed as a change, usually by one or two body parts, occurring within and in contrast to other movements being smoothly sustained at that time. For example, the right fingers may be extending smoothly for two frames, while the mouth opens smoothly for those two frames, yet the left index finger may flex and extend during that same interval. A film of *one* aphasic patient, studied frame by frame, revealed that his speech delayed behind his body motion by approximately 1/24 of a second. There were also other self-disharmonies as well. An analysis of a film of a stutterer indicated that he became self-dyssynchronous at the points of stutter. Examination of yet another film, this time of a young boy with petit mal seizures, also revealed self-dyssynchrony.

Two examples of divergent behavior will be of interest. The first involves a portion of film of a three-and-one-half-year-old girl referred because her mother was concerned that the child was not talking. The child had begun to talk about the age of a year but had discontinued talking at age of eighteen months, after being able to say a few words like *brush, button* and *duck*. Crawling, walking, and toilet training had occurred at the usual time, and there had been no regression in these activities. Psychiatric and audiometric tests raised the question of possible deafness. The girl was then brought to our attention to see if we could determine whether or not she was deaf. A frame-by-frame analysis of a film made of the child in interaction led to the surprising finding that the little girl moved synchronously with ambient noises in the surroundings. If someone were speaking to her and a sound would intrude, she would move in response to that sound, rather than the person. Normal children, filmed in a relatively similar situation, almost totally disregarded such noises, even when they were quite loud.

The second example of divergent behavior is that of "Eve Black" of the *"Three Faces of Eve"* (1957), originally described by Doctors C. H. Thigpen and H. M. Cleckley of Augusta, Georgia, who also made a thirty-minute sound film of the actual patient in her three different personalities and at various stages of her therapy. Actually, four personalities were reported by the authors, since the last personality to emerge, "Jane," revealed two aspects. The initial presenting personality was "Eve White," a demure, shy, well-mannered woman, although sadness and tension could be seen behind her reserve.

"Eve Black," the first of the multiple personalities to emerge, was wild, irresponsible, and mischievous. "Jane" who revealed two aspects, "Jane I" and "Jane II," appeared to be a mature, capable person. She emerged late in therapy and ultimately became the dominant personality. A frame-by-frame analysis revealed a transient asymmetry in the patient's face and in particular a transient yet rapid and pronounced strabismus which was not observable at normal projection speed. Thigpen and Cleckley do not refer to this in their writings. These observations raise questions about whether or not they are the basis for "fleeting impressions or subliminal perceptions which form the basis for" clinical intuition.

When examined frame by frame, three characteristic types of divergent eye movements emerged. 1) One eye would move horizontally to the left or the right, while the other remained still. The eye might then shortly move back to its original position or remain in the divergent state. In several instances, for example, the eye would move right in one frame and then move back left again in the next frame, giving the appearance of a rapid bobble of the eye. 2) Both eyes would diverge; this often occurred quite rapidly. For example, the right eye would move right, and the left eye would move left simultaneously at the same 1/24 of a second, and only at that 1/24 of a second. 3) While both eyes are moving in the same direction one eye would move markedly faster than the other eye. In normal behavior the eyes appear to move together at approximately the same speed. This presentation will deal primarily with the number of times strabismic *movements* occur with respect to the different personalities. The actual divergent movement of one eye in relation to the other, the going into or out of divergence, is presented rather than sustained divergent states.

In this film there were approximately 73 detectable occurrences of strabismus. "Eve White," who was on film for seven minutes, had eleven occurrences of strabismus, largely of the left eye. "Eve Black," on the film for nine minutes, had 56 occurrences, predominately of the right eye. "Jane I," on the film for four minutes, revealed six instances. And finally, two years later, "Jane II," who was shown for two-and-a-half minutes, displayed no instances of strabismus. On the contrary, her behavior seemed quite self-synchronous. There are no references in the literature to transient strabismus as described above, as far as we can discover.

Another famous case of multiple personality, "Miss Beauchamp," a patient of Morton Prince (1906), was described as having headaches and visual disturbances along with many other symptoms.[32] Sally Beauchamp, the personality almost identical to that of "Eve Black," was described as having a peculiar form of anaesthesia in that, with her eyes closed, she could feel nothing. Prince likens this anaesthesia to hysterical monocular amblyopia in which a subject cannot see with the "blind" eye if the other is closed, yet sight returns to the affected eye as soon as the opposite eye is opened. More significant is the statement by Sally that while Miss Beauchamp is concentrating her mind on central vision, she, Sally, need not pay attention to that, but can concentrate her own mind on peripheral vision and recognize things in the periphery.

Anna O., the famous case of Freud's colleague, Breuer (1895), was described as being split into two personalities, one of which the patient called "her bad self."[23] At the onset of her illness she showed the following visual disturbances: a convergent squint with diplopia, deviation of both eyes to the right so that when her hand reached for something, it always went to the left of the object.

Such clinical selections suggest the possibility of a more than purely semantic relationship between the dissociation of a personality and the dissociation of normal oculomotor parallelism. A somewhat similar, but less marked, dissociation of normal oculomotor parallelism has also been noted by Dr. Condon in several films of schizophrenic patients. This is a very tentative finding which will require further study. Strabismus of this form has not been observed thus far in any normal behavior (over 100 films analyzed frame by frame). However, a rapid convergence lasting 1/48 of a second occurred in a normal subject under delayed auditory feedback.

The literature relating to oculomotor inbalance indicates that divergence of one eye from its parallel axis with the other eye is varied in its nature. Both systemic and local conditions may affect ocular neuromuscular mechanisms. The oculomotor disturbance may be intermittent, as in the condition known as intermittent exotropia, in which the two eyes appear for the most part to be well coordinated, yet one eye may suddenly turn out, often through a rather large angle of divergence. The patient is really not aware that the eye has turned out nor does he experience double vision. The mechanism whereby coordinated binocular vision is interrupted is not known.

These examples illustrate the clinical relevance of close-grained studies of human interaction by means of sound film. There are now available many other samples of interactions, both normal and pathological, which strongly suggest that some aspects of the mental status of the patient and the therapist, and their external synchrony with one another can be examined in depth. Although it is most difficult to predict if such studies will ever become mechanized via computers so that they will be useful to practicing clinicians for the purpose of diagnosis, prognosis, compatibility, cultural barriers, measurement of progress, and description of ongoing process, the possibility exists and should be explored. Not only are ample resources and talented workers required, but an openminded willingness to deal with complex "units" which are appropriate for dealing with complex systems in two or more living people.

REFERENCES

1. Birdwhistell, R. L. *Introduction to Kinesics. An Annotation System for Analysis of Body Motion and Gesture.* Washington, D.C., Dept. of State, Foreign Service Institute, 1952.
2. Birdwhistell, R. L. The Frames in the Communication Process. Paper presented at the American Society of Clinical Hypnosis, Annual Scientific Assembly, October 10, 1959.
3. Birdwhistell, R. L. *Paralanguage; 25 years after Sapir. In* Brosin, H. W. (ed.) *Lectures on Experimental Psychiatry.* Pittsburgh, University of Pittsburgh Press, 1961.

4. Birdwhistell, R. L. Chapter for *Conceptual Bases and Applications of the the Communicational Sciences.* Berkeley, University of California Press, April 1965.
5. Birdwhistell, R. L. *Some Body Motion Elements Accompanying Spoken American English. In* Thayer, Lee (ed.) *Communication: Concepts and Perspectives.* Washington, D.C., Spartan Books, 1967, Chpt. III.
6. Birdwhistell, R. L. *A Kinesic-Linguistic Exercise, June 1967. In* Mc-Quown, N. A. (ed.) *The Natural History of an Interview.* New York, Grune & Stratton, to be published.
7. Bloomfield, L. *Language.* New York, Holt, Rinehart and Winston, 1933.
8. Brosin, H. W. *Contribution of Linguistic-Kinesic Studies to the Understanding of Schizophrenia; Discussion of Ray L. Birdwhistell's Paper. In* Auerback, A. *Schizophrenia; An Integrated Approach.* New York, Ronald Press, 1959, pp. 118-123.
9. Brosin, H. W. *Implications for Psychiatry. In* McQuown, N. A. (ed.) *The Natural History of an Interview.* New York, Grune & Stratton. Chpt. IV. To be published.
10. Brosin, H. W. *Linguistic-Kinesic Analysis and Psychiatry.* Paper presented before the San Francisco Psychoanalytic Society, San Francisco, October 8, 1956.
11. Brosin, H. W. Linguistic-Kinesic Analysis Using Film and Tape in a Clinical Setting. *Amer. J. Psychiat. (Suppl.)* 122: 33-37, 1966.
12. Brosin, H. W. Studies in Human Communication in Clinical Settings Using Sound Film and Tape. *Wisc. Med. J.* 63: 503-506, 1964.
13. Charny, E. J. Psychosomatic Manifestation of Rapport in Psychotherapy. *Psychosom. Med.* 28: 305-315, 1966.
14. Condon, W. S. and Ogston, W. D. A Method of Studying Animal Behavior. *Journal of Auditory Research* 7:359-365, 1967.
15. Condon, W. S. and Ogston, W. D. A Segmentation of Behavior. *Psychiat. Res.* 5:221-235, 1967.
16. Condon, W. S. *Linguistic-Kinesic Research and Dance Therapy.* Paper presented at American Dance Therapy Association Convention, October 1968. To be published.
17. Condon, W. S. and Brosin, H. W. *Microlinguistic-Kinesic Events in Schizophrenic Behavior.* Paper read at Conference on Schizophrenia, November 14, 1968. To be published.
18. Condon, W. S. and Ogston, W. D. *Speech and Body Motion Synchtrony of the Speaker-Hearer. In* Kjeldergaard, P. (ed.) *Perception of Language,* Columbus, O., Charles E. Merrill Books. To be published 1969.
19. Condon, W. S. and Ogston, W. D. Sound Film Analysis of Normal and Pathological Behavior Patterns. *J. Nerv. Ment. Dis.* 143:338-347, 1966.
20. Condon, W. S., Ogston, W. D. and Pacoe, L. V. Three Faces of Eve Revisited; A Study of Micro-Strabismus. To be published in *J. Abnorm. Psychol.*
21. Darwin, C. *The Expression of the Emotions in Man and Animals* (1872) New York, Philosophical Library, 1955.
22. Freud, S. *The Psychopathology of Everyday Life* (1901) *Standard Edition* 6. London, Hogarth Press, 1960.
23. Freud, S. *Studies of Hysteria* (1896) *Standard Edition* 2:21-47, London, Hogarth Press, 1955.
24. Gottschalk, L. A. and Auerbach, A. H. *Methods of Research in Psychotherapy.* New York, Appleton-Century-Crofts, 1966.

25. Knapp, P. H. (ed.) *Expression of the Emotions in Man.* New York, International Universities Press, 1963.
26. Kendon, A. Some Functions of Gaze Direction in Social Interaction. *Acta Psychologica.* 26:22-63, 1967.
27. Kendon, A. *Some Observations on Interactional Synchrony (Pub scene)* Pittsburgh, Western Psychiatric Institute and Clinic, August 1967. Unpublished papers.
28. Kendon, A. *Some Relationships between Body Motion and Speech; An Analysis of an Example.* Revision of a paper presented at the Research Conference on Interview Behavior, University of Maryland, Institute of Psychiatry, Baltimore, April 22, 1968.
29. Lenneberg, E. H. *Biological Foundations of Language.* New York, Wiley, 1967.
30. Loeb, F. F. The Microscopic Film Analysis of the Function of a Recurrent Behavioral Pattern in a Psychotherapeutic Session. *J. Nerv. Ment. Dis.* 147(6): 605-618, 1968.
31. Pike, K. *Language in Relation to a Unified Theory of the Structure of Human Behavior.* The Hague, Mouton, 1967.
32. Prince. M. *The Dissociation of a Personality.* New York, Longmans, Green, 1906.
33. Sapir, E. *The Selected Writings of Edward Sapir.* Berkeley, University.
34. Scheflen, A. E. Human Communication: Behavioral Programs and Their Integration in Interaction. *Behav. Sci.* 13:44-55, 1968.
35. Scheflen, A. E. On the Structuring of Human Behavior. *Amer. Behav. Sci.* 10:8-12, April 1967.
36. Scheflen, A. E. *Strategy and Structure in Psychotherapy.* Philadelphia, Eastern Pennsylvania Psychiatric Institute, 1965. (Behavior Studies Monograph, v. 2)
37. Scheflen, A. E. *Stream and Structure of Communicational Behavior.* Philadelphia, Eastern Pennsylvania Psychiatric Institute, 1965. (Behavior Studies Monograph, v. 1)
38. Scheflen, A. E. The Significance of Posture in Communication Systems. *Psychiatry* 27:316-331, 1964.
39. Sebeok, T. A., Hayes, A. S. and Bateson, M. C. (ed.) *Approaches to Semiotics.* The Hague, Mouton, 1964.
40. Schlien, J. M. *Research in Psychotherapy.* Vol. III. Washington, D.C., American Psychological Association, 1968.
41. Thigpen, C. H. and Cleckley, H. A Case of Multiple Personality. *J. Abnorm. Soc. Psychol.* 48:135-151, 1954.
42. Thigpen, C. H. and Cleckley, H. *The Three Faces of Eve.* Kingsport, Tenn., Kingsport Press, 1957.

12

JULES H. MASSERMAN, M.D.

One of life's deep gratifications is being thought deserving of an enduring friendship, and when that friendship has been accorded to me by a personage as scientifically respected and universally loved as Leo Bartemeier, the satisfaction is great indeed. Dr. Bartemeier needs no new accolades from me to add to the many richly deserved ones he has already received throughout the world; instead, it is I who am being honored by being asked to join in this Festschrift.

Biodynamic Psychiatry

I AM AWARE that in recent psychiatric texts Biodynamic Psychiatry has been accorded segregation as a "new school of thought," despite my own oft-repeated plea that the term "school" better applies to aggregations of fish than to congregations of scientists. Let me affirm, then, that Biodynamics is neither doctrine nor cult, but attempts to integrate current understandings as to how and why living things behave, and what may be done to ameliorate their adverse reactions to internal and external stresses. As in all other branches of sciences, then, the heuristic sources of Biodynamic Psychiatry are threefold:

First, the study of the evolution of animate behavior, ranging from micro-protoplasmic reactivity to the macro-transactional intricates of human conduct.

Second, a search for significant common denominators in ostensibly antithetical theories of the etiology and therapy of deviant conduct.

And third, the formulation of the postulates and practices thus derived in operational terms, so that they can be tested and further clarified by laboratory and clinical methods analogous to those used in other scientific disciplines.

One conative coherence may be noted immediately with regard to each of these historical, comparative, and experiential-experimental vectors: namely, that possibly all living things, and certainly man, have always *behaved as if* (to use Hans Vaihinger's philosophic term) they had three ultimate (Ur-) goals or entelechies:

First: to retain individual well-being and longevity;
Second: to develop whatever conspecific hegemony was necessary for
　　　　　group survival and,
Third: to seek creativity and existential significance.

Let us briefly examine the means by which we have perennially endeavored to attain these three Ur-objectives.

I.　EVOLUTIONARY-HISTORICAL PERSPECTIVES

Physical: Ever since our Pleistocene origins as *homo sapiens*, we have tried to mitigate our fears of our inimical universe through our one talent of prime survival value: our capacity for developing sciences and technologies. In two of the most important of these—medicine and surgery— we have sought to find means to cure our ills and restore our skills by various medicaments ranging from useless or poisonous herbs and minerals to advanced antibiotics, and by various surgical procedures from the ancient splinting of fractures and trephining of skulls to the current transplantation of livers and hearts. Fortunately neuro-psychiatry, as a re-coordinated branch of medicine, is once again developing physical, pharmacologic and operative as well as communicative-social modes of relieving man's material fears and their somatic resonances.

Socio-cultural: Nevertheless, scientific advances alone have proved inadequate in our quest for security, for our expanding knowledge has repeatedly revealed mysteries and challenges beyond our ken, and warned us that the technology which our possibly unfriendly neighbors might develop could be more lethal than our own. Because of this latter awareness we have learned to seek more inclusive human alliances, ranging *from* primary maternal ties *through* extended familial loyalties and allegiances to the clan, tribe, city and state toward international compacts. Within all of these aggregations specially selected men have been given specific tasks designed to enhance group welfare: kings* and constables are made

---

* Our term "king" (German *Koenig*, head of state) is derived from Anglo-Saxon *cyning*, head of kin. (Perry, 1966)

responsible for internal government; soldiers are made responsible for collective security (which, in accord with our perennial paranoia, we often view as dependent upon external conquest) and medicine men are relied upon for the treatment of physical illnesses or for the correction of excessive deviations from locally accepted norms of conduct. Once again, this reintegration of medical and social functions is being revived as "social psychiatry."

Philosophic-Theologic: But these irregular and sometimes inchoate strivings, even when combined with our pyramiding technical capacities, have still not been effective in allaying a third and even broader concern, since no cabal of human scientists, however large or learned, has ever been able to control the heavens, secure the future, explain the nature, values or meaning of life, or mitigate the inadmissibility of death. We have therefore perennially erected cosmic *metaphysical* systems presumably within our ken, or operated by supernatural beings whom, as we once controlled our parents, we can influence directly by appeals, bribes, or putatively prescribed behavior—or indirectly by employing medicine men or priests who, in their temples and attached sanatoria were wishfully charged not only to minister to our physical needs and to arbitrate our mundane relationships, but also to alter in our favor the mystical workings of the universe, and so to fulfill our yearnings for transcendent omnipotence. Thus do our patients still attribute to us, as physicians and psychiatrists, thaumaturgic as well as physical and social powers.

II. COMPARATIVE-DYNAMIC APPROACHES

Despite their seeming diversity, all of the successful methods employed to alleviate our Ur-anxieties in all times, places and cultures have had the same three dynamic vectors in common: to restore our physical wellbeing, to promote our ethno-cultural adaptations, and to foster our theophilosophic serenity. As one whimsical illustration of this in a peripatetic dialogue with my psychiatric residents and psychoanalytic trainees, I have occasionally proposed some outrageous postulate such as: *resolved, that electroshock therapy and classical psychoanalysis are essentially more alike than different in their therapeutic actions and effects.* In the past—though not as much recently—this usually evoked a storm of protest that, as both an analyst and a neuropsychiatrist, I should know that the two methods are manifestly and incomparably different, *inasmuch as*:

EST is "enforced," "physical," "impersonal," "stereotyped," "rigidly conducted," "suppressive," *whereas*, in diametric contrast, psychoanalysis is "voluntary," "psychologically dynamic," "exquisitely interpersonal," "flexible," "evocative," "restorative of memory," and "designed to explore the Unconscious so as to develop to the full the patient's cognitive and adaptive capacities through *'insight.'* "

At this juncture, I appropriately point out that the last catechism directly begged the question since, in the historical and comparative contexts in which I have posed the question, "insight" itself could be operationally defined only as that temporarily ecstatic state in which patient and therapist transiently share approximately the same illusions as to the cause and cure of each other's difficulties. With such additional goads, my residents began to explore subtler dimensions of therapeutically significant similarities between electroshock and analysis, and came up with the following disconcerting symmetries:

Physical parameters: Both EST and psychoanalysis offer a clinical escape from the mundane stresses of external reality onto a sensorially isolated bed or couch (Greek: *klinikos*) presided over by a certified and trusted parental surrogate for about the same average number of recumbent hours. Both methods serve to disorganize current patterns of deviant behavior: EST by direct cerebral diaschises followed by at least partial synaptic reorganization; analysis by semantic and symbolic dissociations and subsequent alterations of concept and reaction.

Interpersonal influences: In each case, the patient elects, under more or less overt "external" pressure, the physician and the method of therapy he regards as most suitable for his needs. In every instance, the patient is sympathetically accepted as "ill" and in need of help by a therapist who is convinced of the special validity of his own theories and the efficacy of his techniques—and thus rounds out a *folie à deux* that is nevertheless often operationally effective.

Social Parameters: Both methods entail covert physical, economic, social and other sanctions: in EST, persistence in disapproved conduct on the part of the patient subjects him to more incarceration, more quasi-lethal experiences, more post-ictal headaches, continued exclusion of visitors and other penalties; in analysis, resistance to the analytic process entails more time, more expense, more depreciating and disillusioning "interpretations" given without privilege of effective contradiction, plus the induction of a disruptive "transference neurosis" and the final insult of being accused of having an "unanalysable character disorder" (i.e., being, in the therapist's social judgment, incurably obnoxious). Conversely, there are highly desirable rewards for changes in the patient's behavior more in accord with the therapist's standards (the "patient compliance" of Ehrenwald): e.g., after "successful" EST, expanded hospital privileges, escape from institutionalization, and restored familial and social status; or, after analysis—at least until recently—an assumption of cryptic wisdom privy only to the initiate, acceptance in the sophisticated elite of the "thoroughly analyzed" in the suburban cocktail circuit, and—for Institute trainees—ecstatic admission to, and referrals from, the local Psychoanalytic Society.

Mystical: Finally, in both methods, patient and therapist join in an essentially worshipful belief either that Bini and Cerletti on the one hand or Freud on the other brought providentially inspired salvation to ailing mortals, attainable through differently prescribed rituals of suffering, expiation, enlightenment and reacquisition of metaphysical grace. Any agnostic who, at national meetings, has attended the Section on Electro-Convulsive Therapy or—usually at another hotel at a discreetly noncommunicative distance—a Seminar of Psychoanalytic Theory and Therapy will have experienced the unmistakable aura of sacerdotal devotion as well as the purportedly scientific import of both proceedings.

Within the bounds of reductionist sophistry, then, objective analyses of the therapeutically operational factors in each method may help clarify the common vectors we have been considering, viz: to help the patient realize that his formerly cherished patterns of "neurotic" (i.e., transactionally irritating) or "psychotic" (i.e., culturally incompatible) conduct in the three spheres of physical, social and philosophic adaptation are no longer either necessary or profitable, and concurrently to learn (through implicit or explicit guidance, personal re-exploration and culturally reorientating experiences) that new modes of adaptation can prove more physically pleasurable, socially advantageous and existentially fulfilling— and therefore preferable.

III. BIODYNAMIC CONCEPTS TESTED BY EXPERIMENTAL AND CLINICAL INVESTIGATIONS

Since this aspect of biodynamics has been my especial concern for the last third of a century, I shall order the remainder of this paper as follows: first, a comment on the relevance of animal research to psychiatric theory and therapy; next a statement of four propositions as to normal and abnormal behavior in experimentally testable form; third, brief descriptions of significant laboratory observations; and finally, a discussion of current and future clinical applications.

Significance of Animal Experiments to Biodynamics

Two preliminary questions may still sometimes arise at this juncture—to wit: "Are animal experiments *really* applicable to the subjective and social complexities of human behavior?" Or, in a more subtly patronizing vein: "Must we not be careful about "anthropomorphizing" animal data and be on guard against drawing false clinical inferences?" Such questions are now seriously raised far less frequently than formerly, but in briefest riposte may be respectively countered thus:

Neurophysiologically, just as the human central nervous system, although manifestly more highly developed in some respects, is nevertheless of the same basic design as that of other chordates, so also is human conduct more responsive to communicative and social influences—and thereby more contingent and versatile than the behavior of the lower animal, not essentially different in basic adaptational patterns.

Epistemologically, no "datum," whether labelled "material," "experiential," "experimental," "intuitive" or whatever, is ever really "given" in pristine purity by a gracious cosmos; instead, since "data" can never be more than man's incomplete, exceedingly fallible and artificially categorized perceptions of his supposed universe, terms such as "real," "objective," "subjective," "anthropomorphic," etc., become tautologic shibboleths, meaningless to the modern logical-positivist rationale of science.* Possibly out of misplaced pride in their own species, some psychiatrists may continue to insist on the precious uniqueness of human neuroses, but even they may find the following studies in animals disconcertingly reminiscent not only of the development of individual and social conduct in man, but significant to the therapy of his neurotic and psychotic deviations. Since "science" is but a testing and refinement of contingent premises, can such postulates be formulated for the most complicated field of all—animate behaviour?

Biodynamic Theses

I have essayed to test in our own work the following four hypotheses, respectively applicable to motivation, learning, adaptability and neurotigenesis, and operative in both animal and human conduct:

1. *Motivation*: The actions of all organisms are directed toward satisfying physiologic needs, and therefore vary with their intensity, duration and balance.

---

* Cf. Once more the extension of Kantian philosophy by Hans Vaihinger.

2. *Perception and Response*: In seeking these fulfillments, organisms conceive of and interact with their milieu not in terms of an absolute "external reality," but in accordance with their genetic capacities, rates of maturation, and unique experiences.

3. *Range of Normal Adaptation*: To maintain adequate levels of satisfaction, higher animals develop a broad range of adaptive techniques by employing versatile methods of coping with difficulties or by modifying or changing goals as necessary.

4. *Neurotigenesis*: However, when physical inadequacies, motivational-adaptational conflicts and environmental stresses (especially *unpredictabilities*) exceed an animal's innate or acquired capacities for adaptation, internal tension (anxiety) mounts, neurophysiologic (psychosomatic) dysfunctions occur, and the organism develops over-generalized patterns of avoidance (phobias), stereotyped behavior (obsessions and compulsions), deviant conspecific and extraspecific transactions (social deviations), and regressive, hyperactive, hostile or bizarrely "dereistic" (hallucinatory, delusional) responses analogous to those in human neuroses and psychoses.

These inferences, always subject to modification by further data, have emerged from the work conducted by my associates and me during the past three decades. Permit me to review our principal observations.

Ontologic Studies

Phases of development: Our records and films of individual animals of various species from infancy to adulthood have confirmed the thesis that the young of all organisms (as Piaget and others have shown for the human) normally evolve through an orderly succession of stages during which sensory modalities are distinguished and resynthesized; integrated *individualized* concepts of the environment are developed; manipulative skills are refined; early dependencies on parental care are relinquished in favor of exploration and mastery; and peer and sexual relationships are sought through which the animal becomes normally "socialized" in its group.

Formative experiences: Infants given a stimulating early milieu and opportunities for continuously nutritive and protective contacts with parents or their surrogates and later with peers, manifest progressive self-confidence, acquire motor and social skills, and develop "group acculturations."

Learning and Symbolism: Animal young show patterns of dependency, exploration, play, "tantrumy" rebelliousness, fetishism (i.e., continued attachment to objects such as rubber gloves used in early feedings), gradually more effective psychomotor adaptations, and other characteristics significantly parallel to those in human children. In this process, the parents or surrogates involved, (even when the latter are not of the animal's species) impart their own traits to the adopted young. For example, a young rhesus raised from birth in the investigator's home learned to respond sensitively and adequately to many intonations of language and patterns of human action, but never acquired some of the aversions (e.g., a fear of snakes) supposedly "innate" in rhesus monkeys raised by their own mothers.

Early deprivations: In contrast, young animals subjected to prolonged periods of solitary confinement, even though otherwise physically well cared for, do not develop normal initiative, physical stamina or adequate social relationships.

Character deviance: Unusual early experiences may engram peculiar characteristics which persist through adulthood. For example, if a young animal is taught to work a switch and thus subject itself to increasingly intense but tolerable electric shocks as a necessary preliminary to securing food, for the rest of its life it may continue to seek modalities for eliciting such shocks even in the absence of any other immediate reward and may thus appear to be inexplicably "masochistic" to an observer unacquainted with its unique experiences.

Neonatal brain injuries: a remarkable finding was that adequate care and training could in large part compensate for extensive brain damage in the newborn. Monkeys subjected to the removal of both temporal or parietal cortices at birth, but given a protective and stimulating home environment thereafter, suffered minor kinesthetic and affective impairments which could be revealed by specific tests or during periods of sensory deprivation, but developed otherwise adequate individual and social adjustments. On the other hand, in the absence of such special care and training, bilateral lesions in the thalami, in the amygdalae, or in cerebral areas 13, 23 and 24 impaired adaptive capacities more seriously in young than in adult animals, and did not ameliorate experimentally induced neurotic behavior as effectively as in the case of adults.

Early "psychological" traumata: These were even more devastating: if the young animal was subjected to unpredictable or exceedingly severe conflicts among counterposed desires and aversions, or even between mutually exclusive conditional satisfactions, it developed deeply ingrained inhibitions, fears, rituals, somatic disorders, social maladjustments and other aberrations of behavior which became highly elaborate and more difficult to treat than those originating in adulthood as described below.

Social Relationships

Animal societies in the laboratory as well as in the feral state organize themselves in hierarchies of relatively dominant and submissive members, with leadership and privileges generally pre-empted not by size or strength alone but in accordance with special aptitudes and "personality" skills. However, these relationships could be modified in the following significant ways:

Parasitism, Industrial Strife and Technological Solutions

Cooperation: Each of a pair of cats or monkeys could be trained alternately to operate a distant mechanism to produce food for its conspecific partner; however, when one became preemptive at the food box, a fairly stable worker-parasite "industrial" relationship could be established in which the other operated the feeder sufficiently frequently for both while receiving only part of the profits. Significantly, two such workers among fourteen pairs proved to be sufficiently "intelligent" (i.e., possessed of unusually high perceptive-manipulative capacities) to jam the mechanism which supplied food to both animals so that it operated continuously, thus solving the social problem by one form of technological automation.

"Altruism": Some monkeys continued to starve for many hours— though never more than a day or so—rather than pull a lever to secure readily available food if they had learned that this also subjected another monkey to an electric shock. Such "succoring" behavior was apparently less dependent upon the relative age, size or sex of the two animals than on (a) their individual "character" and (b) whether or not they had been mutually well-adjusted cagemates.

Aggression: Conversely, actual fighting between members of the same species to establish various relationships was minimal; primacy and dexterity manifested by only occasional gestures of pre-emption were nearly always sufficient to establish dominance and privileges. Indeed, physical combat appeared only under the following special circumstances:

(a) When an animal accustomed to a high position in its own group was transferred to one in which it came into direct conflict with new rivals themselves accustomed to dominance.

(b) When a dominant animal was subjected to a conjoint territorial rebellion by an alliance of subdominants.

(c) When a female with increased status derived from mating with a dominant male thereafter confidently attacked members of her group that had previously dominated her.

(d) When a dominant animal, by being made experimentally neurotic, fell to a low position in its own group and thereafter expressed its frustrations by physical attacks both on animate and living objects in its environment.

Experimental Neuroses and Psychoses

Methods of induction: In accordance with the fourth biodynamic hypothesis, marked and persistent deviations of behavior could be induced by stressing the animal between mutually incompatible patterns of survival: for instance, subjecting a cat to an *unpredictable* electric shock during conditioned feeding, or requiring a monkey to secure food from a box in which, on several occasions, he had unexpectedly been confronted with a toy snake (an object as representationally dangerous to the monkey as a live, poisonous one). Yet counter to early Freudian doctrines of neurotigenesis, "fear" in the sense of dread of injury need not be involved at all; i.e., equally serious and lasting neurotigenic effects can be induced by facing the animal with difficult choices among mutually exclusive satisfactions—situations that parallel the disruptive consequences of prolonged hesitations among equally attractive alternatives in human affairs. More recently Dr. Marvin Woolf and I have employed variably delayed auditory feedback of the animal's conditioned vocalizations or irregularly timed food or shock signals as other methods of rendering its physical milieu unpredictable and thereby anxiety-provoking and neurotigenic. Any of these stresses, when they exceeded the animal's adaptive capacities induced physiologic and mimetic manifestations of anxiety, spreading inhibitions, generalizing phobias, stereotyped rituals, "psychosomatic" dysfunctions, impaired social interactions, addictions to alcohol and other drugs (v.i.), regressions to immature patterns of behavior, and other marked and persistent deviations of conduct.

Constitutional influences: Animals closest to man showed symptoms most nearly resembling those in human neuroses and psychoses, but in each case the "neurotic syndrome" induced depended less on the nature of the conflict—which could be held constant—than on the constitutional predisposition of the animal. For example, under similar stresses spider monkeys reverted to infantile dependencies or catatonic immobility; cebus developed various "psychosomatic" disturbances including functional paralyses, whereas vervets became diffusely aggressive, persisted in bizarre sexual patterns, or preferred hallucinatory satisfactions such as chewing and swallowing purely imaginary meals while avoiding real food to the point of self-starvation.

Methods of Therapy

After the trial of scores of procedures only nine general techniques proved to be most effective in relieving experimentally induced neurotic or psychotic symptoms in animals. The methods, here tachistoscopically reviewed with only a glance at their human analogies, were these:

1. *Satisfaction of a biologic need* such as frustrated hunger, thirst or sex in a conflicted organism. (Analogous in humans to feeding a starving Quaker fearful of stealing essential sustenance.)

2. *Removal of the animal to a more favorable environment.* (In man, to a better home, climate, job, or spouse.)

3. *Resolving of a motivational impasse* by measured rewards and/or stresses kept within the organism's tolerance. (As in conducting an acrophobic patient by moderate stages to increasing heights in "behavior therapy.")

4. *Furnishing opportunities for the utilization of acquired skills by which to reassert control over a previously threatening environment*; e.g., restoring manipulative predictability by providing another device by which the animal could relearn to obtain food. (In clinical parallel, inducing a crashed but unhurt airplane pilot to recover his acutely shattered feeling of mastery by flying another plane immediately and successfully.)

5. *Providing an exemplary group of well-adapted ("normal") organisms*: i.e., putting a food-inhibited aggressive cat among cooperatively conditioned feeders.* (Or sending a "problem child" to a "good" school where children behave in the desired manner.)

6. *Retraining the animal by individualized care and guidance*, the experimenter acting as a "personal therapist" conversant with the nature of its experiential traumata and their neurotigenic effects. (In effective psychoanalysis, helping the patient recall and re-experience conflicts and dispelling their current residues by "corrective emotional experience" vis-à-vis the therapist and elsewhere in the world.)

---

* Recent work with Dr. Marvin Woolf has demonstrated that untrained "observer" monkeys will imitate distant "demonstrator" monkeys in manipulating specific objects. It seems true indeed that "what monkey sees, monkey does."

7. *Employing electroshock or other methods of producing cerebral anoxia and diaschisis* to disintegrate the neural basis of undesirable patterns of behavior. (A method that may be utilized in humans, although never without some impairment, however subtle, of future capacities.)

8. *Performing various brain operations* to induce similar neuropsychologic disorganization. In monkeys, lesions in regions corresponding to cortical areas 12, 23, and 24 were, as noted, most suitable for this purpose. However, the after-effects of any brain operation depended not only on its site and extent but also on the preceding experiences and characteristics of the animal. For example, bilateral lesions of the dorsomedial thalamic nucleus impaired the learning capacities of a normal animal but left it gentle and tractable; in contrast, the same operation rendered a neurotic animal irritable and vicious.

9. Finally, *various drugs could also be used for the temporary disorganization of disturbing perceptions and conflictful reactions,* thus facilitating other methods of therapy. Additional pharmacologic observations were as follows:

(a) Effectiveness: Most of the commercially promoted "ataractics" (meprobamates and phenothiazines) were less generally effective than drugs long tested in clinical therapy; e.g., alcohol, paraldehyde, and the barbiturates and bromides.

(b) Preventive action: Such drugs, if administered in mildly obtunding doses *before* subjecting an animal to stress or conflict, would also partially prevent the after-effect of an otherwise traumatic experience. (By analogy, humans, too, are apt to take an alcoholic "bracer" or a trusted "tranquillizer" before asking for a raise, proposing marriage or contemplating some other supposedly hazardous undertaking.)

(c) Addiction: However, a neurotic animal permitted to experience the relief from fear and inhibition produced by alcohol would then prefer alcohol to non-alcoholic food and drink, and thus develop a dipsomania which would persist until its underlying neurosis was relieved by other means.* (In man, similar psychopharmacologic effects of addictive drugs are demonstrably operative but are, of course, complicated by highly individualized ethnic and culturally symbolic influences.)

Human Correlates

These experiments, then, added to those of Sechenov, Pavlov, Gantt,

---

* The author's motion picture film, "Neurosis and Alcohol," is illustrative (distributed by the Psychological Cinema Register, State University, Pennsylvania. USA).

Delgado, Skinner, Mirsky, Brady and many others, may have helped to clarify basic issues relevant to both "normal" and "deviant" behavior; however, since man's perceptive, mnemonic, symbolic and adaptive capacities are undenably much (though not by necessity "infinitely" or "by quantum jumps") more complex than that of any other animal, it is obvious that mice in mazes, cats in cages, and monkeys in pharmacologic hazes cannot furnish data that completely "explain" human conduct. To return to our opening theme then, man most obviously seems to differ from all other animals in having developed three ultimate axioms, or Ur-functions, that are uniquely immanent in human motivations and transactions—namely:

To seek physical strength and technical omnipotence, with which to assert progressive control over the material universe and eventually to deny his own mortality;

To develop human relationships leading *from* the primal mother-child dyad *through* loyalties to the family, clan, tribe, state and nation, *to* a growing imperative toward the brotherhood of man;

To sustain an existential faith that man's being has an enduring dignity and significance in some universal teleologic, theologic or eschatologic system that extends beyond the here-and-now into eternity.*

Applications to Clinical Therapy

We have always implicitly known that, although no sentient human can ever be completely certain of his health, friends or philosophy, *adequate modicums* of security in each of these spheres are essential to his welfare; consequently, all methods of medico-psychiatric therapy have been effective only in so far as they restored physical well-being, fostered more amicable interpersonal relationships, and helped parochial man amend his beliefs so as to render them more locally acceptable and useful without stultifying his individuality, infringing on his essential freedoms, or stereotyping his intellect, imagery and creativity.

How, then, with this background of genetic-physiologic-ethnic-cultural

---

* In this triplicate context, the experimental analogs of our technics of psychiatric therapy may be correspondingly regrouped as follows: *Physical*: Gratification of somatic needs, relief of stress, environmental pressure to adapt, reassertion of manipulative skills, and the use of drugs, electroshock or other cerebral alternatives (Experimental methods 1, 2, 3, 4, 7, 8, and 9). *Social*: Dyadic restraining or conspecific group rehabilitation. (Experimental methods 5 and 6). *Metaphysical-Existential*: Implicit in a primal joy in life, and some animals' faith in, and devotion to, their glorified human Master.

(i.e. biodynamic) understanding, shall we emancipate ourselves from some of the more stultified therapeutic rituals of our recent past?

Transactionally, if patients are to continue to come to us as physicians for the care they seek, we must regain, cherish and augment public regard for us not only as skilled technicians but also as dedicated humanitarians deserving the highest respect and confidence—in other words, to try to merit the traumaturgic role imposed upon us. Differences of professional opinion, as in my scientific field, are acceptable, but public polemics, a trade-union facade, and blatant economic, forensic or political partisanships diminish our stature and impair the trust we need if we are to serve our patients to their and our best advantage. No one of us can alone undertake this essential restoration of our former prestige and influence; it is a task—and an important one—for all of us.

Next, in our direct handling of individual patients, we must discard our cold armor of aloof "professionalism" and accept each supplicant not as a "diagnostic challenge," or as a faceless vessel of stereotyped psychopathology (a repulsive solecism)—and least of all as only another economic research item—but as a troubled human being seeking comfort and guidance as well as mere relief from physical suffering. These larger requirements can be met as follows:

Regardless of whether the patient's complaints are considered as primarily "organic," "psychosomatic" or "neurotic," bodily discomforts and dysfunctions should be ameliorated by every medical and surgical means available. When indicated, conservatively prescribed and frequently changed sedatives and hypnotics can be used to dull painful memories, diminish apprehension and quiet agitation. For these purposes I continue to find clinically as well as experimentally that the barbiturates, bromides, aldehydes and other well-tested drugs will in many cases be found preferable to some of the widely promoted but dubiously effective "ataractics" and "tranquilizers." Our first concern then, should be Ur-objective I—to restore our patients' zest and joy in living.

But since no man is an "Islande intire of Itself," the therapist must also recognize that his patient may be deeply concerned about financial, sexual, marital, career and related interpersonal problems that may also seriously affect his physical as well as his social well-being. This involves an exploration, always discerning and tactful rather than unnecessarily disruptive and prolonged, of:

the patient's characterologic assets and vulnerabilities;

the attitudes, values and incentives he derived from his past experiences;

the channelling effects of past successes or the disruptive remains of past and current tribulations;

the residues these experiences have left in patterns of effective (normal), socially ineffective (neurotic), or bizarrely unrealistic (psychotic) conduct;

the ways in which these patterns relieve or exacerbate the patients' current difficulties; and finally,

which of them are most accessible to various methods of rationally clarified and effectively guided individual, familial, occupational and social re-orientations and re-adaptations.

It has been my gratifying experience that in many cases a properly trained, sensitive and dedicated physician can, in the time he can easily make available if he wishes, conduct the essential psychotherapy required. In brief, this will consist of using gentle reasoning, personal example and progressive reorientative experiences to help the patient re-examine and correct his prejudices and past misconceptions, abandon infantile or child-like patterns of behavior that have long since lost their effectiveness, revise his values and objectives, restore his initiative, recultivate his occupational social and creative skills, acquire new ones and in general adopt a more realistic, productive and lastingly rewarding ("mature") style of life. In this skillfully directed re-education (and good psycho-therapy is about as "non-directive" as good surgery), the enlightened cooperation of family, friends, employer or others may, with the patient's consent, be secured and utilized to the full. By such means, the patient's interpersonal readjustments (Ur-objective II) will be strengthened by renewed communal solidarity and security—a *sine qua non* of compre-hensive treatment.

To mitigate the third or cosmic Ur-anxiety, the patient's religious and philosophic convictions should, instead of being deprecated and under-mined, be respected and strengthened insofar as they furnish him with what each of us requires: a belief in life's purpose, meaning and value. In this inclusive sense, medicine, being a humanitarian science, can never be in conflict with philosophy or religion, since all three seem to be designed by a beneficent providence to preserve, cheer and comfort men, and thereby constitute a trinity to be respected by any physician deeply concerned with man's health and sanity. Indeed, with respect to these latter concepts, it is of historic-philologic significance that the term *sanatos* implied to the ancients the indissolubility of physical and mental functions (*mens sana in corpore sano*) and that the very word "health" can be traced to the Anglo-Saxon root *hal* or *hōl,* from which are derived not only physical *haleness* and *healing,* but the greeting, *"Hail, friend!"* and the concepts of *wholeness* and *holiness.* Ergo, once again Greek, Roman and Gaul have bequeathed to us, in the rich heritage of our syncretic language in which wish and "reality" merge, their penetrating recognition of the indissoluble physical, social and philosophic components of medical and psychiatric therapy.

History Teaches That History Cannot Teach Us; and yet—with so many consistencies between past and present, can we also extrapolate the future? Let us group a few predictions around our now familiar categories.

Ur-objective I re the Technology of the Future: Despite the perennial legends of Pandora, Golem, Frankenstein, et al. in almost every mythology —and the knowledge that we now have a plethora of materials for a nuclear holocaust to kill every human on earth ten times over, I doubt— since I *must* doubt—that our race is really hell-bent on suicide. Rather, in pursuit of our first Ur-illusion, we shall discover dimensions and forces yet unconceived; we shall distill the ocean and desiccate its fish for tasteless food; we shall conquer cancer and induce new diseases; we shall explore the planets and find them lethal; in short, we shall continue to match our puny technologies against a universe ever beyond man's finite ken or control—and probably be more bewildered by the endless cosmos than ever.

Ur-objective II re the Society of the Future: A world community is the only alternative to Armageddon, and since *homo sapiens* is a single, universally fecund species, differences of "race" or color will eventually become about as distinguishable as Lombard, Hittite, or Etruscan strains are now in their mixed Mediterranean or Australian descendants. We shall become more alike and, in accordance with Ur-illusion II, perhaps become a bit more inclusively friendly.

Ur-objective III as the Theology of the Future: Finally, we may develop a sense of cosmic being that will transcend the dogmas, rituals and theocracies of our current religions further than we have progressed from the animistic superstitions of our savage ancestors. And when man achieves this breadth of vision and depth of understanding, he may also become humbler, kinder, wiser—and possibly, a bit happier.

13

DAVID M. LEVY, M.D.

Homage to a very dear friend and colleague, to a pioneer in the field of psychiatry who has widened its dimensions in so many ways. Always the beneficent "participant observer" whom I have cherished so many years. This article is my tribute also to the members of his family.

Maternal Feelings toward the Newborn

MATERNAL FEELINGS toward the newborn can be investigated in various ways. Mothers may be asked about such feelings during their stay in the hospital or at a later date. But direct inquiry has numerous pitfalls. Since the maternal state is so prone to feelings of guilt, direct questions about feelings toward the baby are potentially too "threatening" to be generally useful. For that reason, among others, when a method of inquiry into this subject is selected, reliance is best placed on indirect questions.

Free association—as in psychoanalytic therapy—is one of the most fertile sources of data on human feelings. But in this study the data were derived from reminiscences, inasmuch as the feelings were so limited in time (the first neo-natal week) as to be especially vulnerable to rationalization and reconstruction. Furthermore, the differentiations of feeling from day to day, following childbirth, are often lost to memory. For the psychiatrist's purpose it is sufficient to attain the patient's emotional response to the early experience with the infant as an entirety. The minutiae of the experience are enlightening but not indispensable.

Daily introspective records furnish another source of data for our subject. They require, however, special cooperation and skill on the part of the mothers employed and special problems, as I have learned, in interpreting the results. This method has not been sufficiently exploited.

So far I have mentioned the methods of direct inquiry, of free association, and of introspection. Since the specific data of this investigation are derived largely from observations it will be best to forego further enumeration of other procedures and consider some aspects of the method I have employed.

The observations were made in five different hospitals in New York City by three observers, each one working separately. An observer, after the necessary cooperation was secured, stood at the foot of the bed and made a written record of observations of mother and baby, from the time the baby was brought in by the nurse until the baby was taken away. Each mother was observed for two or three periods during the first neonatal week. Each period lasted, with some exceptions, twenty to thirty minutes. There were, in all, forty-four mothers. The observed activity was, in general, breast-feeding.

The group may be described as heterogeneous. Different religions, color, cultural and economic levels were represented. The group contained primiparae and multiparae. The age range was chiefly between twenty and thirty years.

Now the most careful description of the data of observation and the most refined method of collecting, classifying and correlating them cannot pinpoint feeling, which can be inferred only from differences of behavior toward the baby.

For example, when we compare the methods mothers employed in stimulating their babies to suck (patting the back, jiggling the breast, pushing the nipple into the baby's mouth, etc.), we noted a marked difference in the early and the later days of the week. The difference lies in the strength of the stimulation. To make the comparison valid we must compare the different classifications of sucking activity with each other. That is, we must know how the method of stimulation changes as the baby's sucking changes, and how, under the same or similar conditions, the method changes. The same mother, for example, whose baby sucked poorly during an observation period in the first three days of the week would be much more sparing of a forceful stimulation than on a later day.

From such findings we infer that mothers are more tender with the baby during the early days. Tenderness is inferred from a difference in behavior. We have other sources for such an inference. They are seen in a certain softness of movement, in differences of maternal response when feedings are frustrating and when they are painful. In all such instances we must rely on observed differences of behavior, on the variation of patterns of response under comparable conditions.

Why is this display of tenderness not so apparent in the later days of the neonatal week? Why does the first display of tenderness during stimulation not continue? On this point our inference is further removed from the immediate data of observation. We would say that the change in attitude toward the baby takes place in regard to his weakness and helplessness. By the third, certainly by the fourth day, after more than twenty feedings, the mother has had increasing evidence of the baby's powerful sucking equipment, also his power to resist the mother's stimulation to suck, by clamping his jaws and refusing the nipple. The word *refusal*, used by doctors, nurses and mothers, implies motivated behavior. Certainly, in their remarks to the baby, "Why won't you suck?," "You naughty baby," etc., the mothers act as though the baby knows clearly what he is doing. (This is a kind of projection that must be hard to resist in the nursing situation when the baby is so intimately part of oneself.)

For the mother of a first-born the change in the concept of "baby" after the first few days would theoretically be more striking than for the multiparous mother. This inference could be proven more readily by inquiry than by observation. There are other factors to consider in regard to the change in the stimulation pattern. One of them applies to the open ward in which a competitive attitude towards successful feeding may arise. Another applies to wards in which the feedings are scheduled and limited to thirty minutes. The mother often feels an urgency to get all the milk into the baby she possibly can within the limit of time allowed.

Such factors, however, are present also in the early days. Also the difference in the patterns early and late are quite significant. The rough stimulations not only differ from the common variety in a quantitative way. They may include some that are also qualitatively different, like hard shaking of the body, or quick rolling of the head.

Now suppose we find two mothers who use rough stimulations on the first or second day? Suppose we find also that they differ consistently from the others in all situations which offer a differential for roughness? Can we say then that their lack of tenderness for the baby is evidence of some lack of maternal feeling? One may argue that their eagerness to make sure the baby gets enough milk overrides all other considerations, that this ambition for the baby explains everything. One may argue also that they have high standards. When they take on a job, of feeding the baby or anything else, the job is the important thing. Nothing else counts. Or one may argue that their persistency is evidence of unconscious hostility, that behind the screen of their zeal and industry they are vindictive. For a solution of a problem of this kind we have two procedures.

One is to study a mother's behavior toward her baby in situations in which the problem of persistency does not present itself (as in the end phase of the feeding period when a halt has been called to the breast-feeding and the pair are merely waiting for the nurse to return). The other procedure is a tentative one, though found to be very useful as a preliminary device.

By means of a standardized interview which has to do with previous interests in babies and in mothering, we can select those mothers who are the most and the least maternal. Using their behavior as guides we can match against them those mothers whose persistency we wish to analyze in every comparable situation. In that manner we learn that in the case of one of the very persistent mothers there is a consistent diminution of maternal feeling; in the case of the other, though affectionate on the average in most situations, her feeling for the baby gives way to her determination to ensure continuity of sucking whenever the baby is not avid for the breast. From these cases and others we have learned that a high maternal feeling has a modifying effect on what we may presume to be typical personality attributes when they are in conflict with a positive feeling for the baby, at least in the neonatal week. That is, in situations in which all mothers give evidence of annoyance, impatience, or frustration, they reveal it in a milder form, and this mildness, as analysis of the observations indicates, does not always mean that they are less provoked. It is achieved in certain situations by exerting greater control. Thus as proof of maternal feeling we may add—to the manifestations of tenderness in a positive way—the diminution and control of negatively charged feelings.

Using the same method of analysis on all the activities to be found in relational behavior we were able to delineate about twenty situations that contained what we may call a differential for maternal attitude. That is, in these situations there were variations of the pattern of behavior in a positive or negative direction that could best be explained as the result of maternal feeling. The behavior patterns included among others: the manner of greeting the baby, indifferent or distracted behavior like reading a book during the nursing, absently gazing about the room, immediate and later response to the baby during painful feedings, passivity in the form of failure to aid the baby's sucking under a variety of conditions, display of affection, etc.

The influence of maternal feeling in some instances determined the presence or absence of a pattern. In most instances it determined the form of the pattern—its shape, so to speak—as depicted by the variety and number of its components. Thus in greeting the baby, the components of the pattern included one or more of the following items—words, smiles, laughter, cuddling, patting and stroking—arranged in an ascending line of positive feeling.

When all the patterns of maternal response to the infant were analyzed in order to discover if and how they were influenced in any way by maternal feeling, we found that the effect of this feeling was to sustain the work involved in the care of the infant, intensify the relational behavior in terms of interest and affection, and inhibit any potentially harmful impulse. The effect of the feeling-determinant on maternal behavior is thus both binding and restraining. For the tiny and helpless infant activates all the nourishing, sustaining, and protecting qualities of the relatively giant mother and helps to neutralize or modify her potentially harmful tendencies whether in the form of indifference, neglect or physical force.

The work involved in breast-feeding can be measured in terms of *persistency* or *continuity*, which is also a measure of devotion to the task, in a number of ways. We can study the time that elapses before the baby, after arrival, is brought to the breast, the time taken out when there is a break in the sucking, whether due to the baby's release of the nipple or the mother's withdrawal of it because of pain or other reason, and also the relative proportion of time used for or on behalf of the baby's sucking in the time available during each feeding period observed. Comparisons of the mother's devotion to the task by means of the time factor must be made with due regard to the conditions under which a feeding takes place. On one occasion the baby's sucking may be so strong and regular that the mother need hardly exert herself to ensure continuity of sucking throughout the feeding period. On another occasion the baby's sucking because of its slow, weak and irregular quality or because of the baby's propensity to sleep instead of to suck may sorely tax the mother's energy, endurance, and patience. The baby may be brought in for a feeding when the mother herself is falling asleep. She rouses herself and under the conditions of sleep and fatigue may have to contend with a baby crying with hunger whose first five or even ten minutes at the nipple may consist of rapid, powerful sucks with a vice-like grip. The mother's feeling for the baby is then put to a severe test. What will happen after she withdraws the breast because of pain? How long before she will resume the feeding? In order to render situations of this kind comparable we have tried to get a measure of the severity of pain by the use of such criteria as the sucking strength, the mother's quickness of withdrawal, her vocalizations of pain, facial expression, shifting of limbs, and excoriation of the nipples. There is a marked variation of response featured at one end of the scale by quick restoration of the breast and also display of affection regardless of pain or fatigue; at the other end of the scale, withdrawal and failure to continue the feeding even when the movement of the baby's lips present a clear indication of readiness to go on.

However difficult a *painful* breast-feeding may be, there is little if any evidence of the mother's provocation in terms of anger or annoyance with the baby or retaliatory behavior. The situation is quite different when the feedings are *frustrating*. In such feedings when the baby has to be aroused from sleep and numerous efforts are made to initiate the sucking, the baby responds in a manner that encourages the mother to continue her striving because success appears to be imminent. The baby opens an eye, moves his head, makes a seeking movement for the nipple, puckers the lips, finally secures a real purchase on the nipple, even holds on to it firmly, and then, after gradually and slowly progressing to the stage of sucking, nothing occurs. Under such conditions all the mothers revealed evidence of annoyance, irritation, impatience, and, in some cases, definite retaliatory behavior. Now we were concerned not with the presence or absence of a frustration pattern, since the pattern was always there, but with its magnitude and its influence on the mother's persistency. In regard to the latter, the variation was—as in the case of painful feedings—a continuity of effort regardless of the severity and frequency of frustrating experiences at one end of the scale, and at the other end a yielding of all effort after one such experience.

You see that we can utilize clearcut observations as a basis for determining the persistency of effort, and thereby arrive at a measure of devotion to the task of nursing the baby. You will remember also that earlier in this lecture it was noted that persistency of effort can go too far. Its modification also gives evidence of maternal feeling.

Now the measure of devotion by the measure of persistency of stimulation, the duration of time-intervals and the amount of passivity will be understood more clearly.

The mother's interest in the infant is evidence of her relatedness, of her continued awareness of him, regardless of distractions that may arise from boredom, states of fatigue, painful or pleasurable body sensations, or feeding difficulties, or external stimuli such as happenings in the ward. Interest is conveniently measured by lapses, evinced in conversation with mothers in adjacent beds, reading a book or newspaper, gazing into space, and also failure to observe the baby's sucking needs. We have learned that in analyzing the differential value of distraction in the neonatal week we must take special cognizance of painful feedings. During the experience of pain, highly maternal mothers may reveal evidence of distraction. It seems likely that during such periods they use distracting conversation as a means of tolerating, or reducing the painful sensations and thereby inhibit the impulse to withdraw the breast. As observed in feeding periods, acute pain is the strongest obstacle to relational behavior. Regardless of her devotion, the mother's rapport with the newborn is temporarily interrupted.

Alertness to the baby is best observed in those feedings in which the baby's sucking needs constant activation. In such cases a response follows whenever the mother exerts some effort to keep the baby going; otherwise it ceases entirely. The sucking, once started, gradually weakens and slows down. Stimulation at the right moment starts another series, and the sucking goes on. The mother applies her ministrations at the slow-down point of each series of sucks. The continuity of sucking is achieved largely through her constant vigilance.

This type of feeding is in marked contrast to one in which continuous sucking is achieved with hardly any effort on the mother's part. Such feedings, though more frequent later on, are seen also in the neonatal week. The performance on the part of mother and infant is so well geared, so well are both attuned to the nursing period, that the performance is smooth and flawless. There is no evidence of fatigue or pain or frustration. Both are so wedded to the act that it appears to transcend the actors. One then has the impression of observing a nursing as a thing in itself rather than a mother nursing or a baby being nursed.

In both types of feeding—the one characterized by constant effort and alertness to the baby, the other characterized by seemingly effortless behavior—the mothers may be equally interested and absorbed in their babies as far as our observations reveal. In both, no evidence of distraction may be discerned.

The observational proof of devotion and interest may best be followed by consideration of tenderness, since it is found in the same kind of behavior. We have referred previously to evidence of tenderness in the mother's manner of stimulating the baby's sucking. It was seen in the softness of some of the components of the stimulation pattern and in the control of rough movements. These were possibly hostile reactions during specially trying situations. The more positive expression is seen in the first few days and at the beginning of the stimulation pattern at other times in the neonatal week. It is seen in the sequence of stimuli beginning with light movements of nipple over lips, light patting of back or stroking the cheek with gradual increase in strength and tempo. When as a result of impatience or annoyance or for whatever reason a harsh stimulation, hard shaking or pushing or slapping, has finally erupted, one may infer from the mother's recoil, and a quick shift to gentler movement, that her outburst of energy has occasioned a feeling of guilt and a kind of reconciliatory behavior. This inference seems more convincing when a direct display of affection accompanies the gentler movements which follow the rough ones.

The crescendo of movements that rises to a peak of highly charged activity occurs almost exclusively in frustration feedings. The baby's manner of response to the mother's persistent stimulation is an important factor in bringing it about. The mother's problem is the double one of rousing the baby from sleep and overcoming his resistance to sucking activity. If he persists in sleeping and furnishes no sign of awakening after she has run through her gamut of stimulations, she is very likely to let him have his way. When he gives a sign of arousal she is encouraged to go on. When encouraging signs follow one after the other—the partial opening of an eye, the movement of a cheek, puckering of the lips and so on—they add momentum to her efforts. The overcharged activity of the mother and her angry retorts occurred only after a series of five or more increasingly encouraging signs from the baby led her to go on and on to a final defeat. Such frustration occurred after prolonged and exhausting effort when there seemed every reason to anticipate a successful outcome. The mother's perturbation under such circumstances can be well understood. She seems then to forget entirely that she is simply trying to nurse a baby who is too sleepy at the time to respond. She acts as though the baby purposely trapped her, luring her on. Sometimes also she adds insult to her injury by saying angrily, "He won't take my milk."

In the frustrating situation, the measure of control can be observed in the sequence of the pattern of stimulation, in the remarks made to the baby at the height of frustration, and the attenuating behavior that follows. The situation serves our purpose as an example in which even a mother who has more maternal feeling than the average must exert control. The less maternal mothers were still sufficiently controlled to prevent the reaction of rage. However, the hospital setting is itself a restraining influence.

The notion that a mother carries within her potentially harmful impulses to her own baby may be regarded by some readers as an exaggerated conception applicable only to special cases of psychoneurotic or psychotic mothers who suffer from infanticidal impulses. That even infants commonly arouse hostile impulses which are stronger than the usual kind released by sarcastic rejoinders or other verbal discharge can be comprehended more easily by considering the incessant crying of babies with colic. More maternal mothers are able to absorb a difficult experience of this kind with little effect on maternal attitude. Those who respond to their newborn with less than the average degree of maternal feeling may be affected quite adversely. The constant crying, especially in the case of a firstborn, blights the rosy anticipation of joyous motherhood, denies to the mother the pleasure and the binding value of cuddling, and is a sore tax on physical endurance. It is a tax also on the exertion of constant control over retaliatory feelings and impulses.

The control of such feelings during breast feedings and the control also of the mother's strength, simply in an adaptive way, to conform to the baby's comfort and welfare, were regarded as evidence of tenderness. The word *tenderness* is not well suited to the connotation of control in the physical sense of reducing the strength of a stimulus to its minimal effective application. The term seems appropriate enough, however, when the mother is seen protecting the baby from too strong stimulations, when strong ones are called for, protecting the baby also from harsh words in spite of pain, and rendering any necessary manipulation of the baby's body into a gentle act devoid of brisk movement or roughness.

The observational source of the evidence for maternal devotion, interest, and tenderness has been presented. Now we may consider a direct display of affection for the baby, an expression of maternal feeling usually regarded as its most characteristic feature.

It is probably for that reason that the task of measuring maternal feeling by its most obvious expression is so elusive. In our culture everyone is so well imbued with the stereotypes that constitute affectionate behavior towards a baby that the face one makes, the vocalizations, and the baby-talk may operate like the reflexes of conventional behavior. Mothers of newborn babies readily indulge in kissing sounds and baby-talk regardless of positive or negative feeling.

Actually the differentials of maternal feeling can be revealed adequately in the study of devotion, interest, and tenderness alone. One hypothesis underlying the choice of differentials was the belief that, in mammals generally, retrieval—which constitutes, besides a protecting response, a way of giving body warmth—was an action analogous to cuddling. Cuddling, however, was not as valid a differential of maternal feeling as certain movements of patting and stroking, when employed as independent bits of behavior, especially during intervals of time apart from nursing behavior.

Of least value as evidence of affection were talking and kissing sounds. Since, in all the hospitals in which our observations were made, mothers wore a mask when the baby was present, actual kissing was rarely performed.

Display of affection was observed also as concurrent behavior while the baby was sucking. Most difficult was the analysis of such behavior when it appeared to be inextricably bound with the nursing, as in such activities which served to initiate the sucking and at the same time reveal affection.

The display of affection under special conditions may give discriminating value to the more conventional forms. Thus any display of affection to the baby after withdrawing the breast during painful feedings may have special meaning. A mother diverted her glance from the baby and for several minutes gazed at the ceiling, then glanced back and displayed affection to him. The gazing was due, it was inferred, to pelvic discomfort. The affectionate display was inferred to be the result of some feeling of guilt for the moments of separateness. Such subtleties of inference are based on a careful study of sequences of behavior with reference to the mode of response characteristic of each individual and each comparable situation.

The display of affection that immediately followed the mother's transient neglect of the baby as indicated by distraction, breast withdrawal, passivity, etc., could be accounted for only as some kind of reparation for something that should not have happened. If its root can be traced to a feeling of guilt, the more maternal mothers had more of it than others. Given a more positive maternal feeling it would appear more likely that any assumed hurt or neglect of the baby would be taken more seriously. Obviously guilt arises from hostile feelings, from ambivalent feelings and also from lack of feeling. Guilt may also arise, if my inference is correct, as a consequence of a highly positive feeling for the baby, with its increased sensitivity to the baby's response.

When the observations that underlie the inferential terms we have used are analyzed for magnitude and consistency, we find that they come closer to each other, the higher or the lower their position on a scale of appropriate values. That is another way of saying that the "high" maternal mother is very likely to be consistently high in devotion, interest, tenderness, and affection and that the "low" maternal is very likely to be consistently low in regard to those attributes. Variations are more likely to be found in the midgroups and, generally, in the observation of maternal behavior in the later weeks. Thus we are all familiar with a type of mother who has devotion, interest, and affection to a high degree, but is lacking in tenderness. She is the "roughhouse" type of mother who seems nevertheless quite maternal.

Numerous constellations of maternal patterns can be derived by combining the measures of the four attributes in different ways. For our purpose, however, it is sufficient to indicate that each attribute stresses a special kind of relational behavior and must exert therefore a special kind of influence on the baby. Our own observations in the neonatal week, as well as numerous clinical studies of maternal behavior, led us to believe that a good measure of protective behavior is much more likely to be found in the maternal response to the infant than affectionate behavior. That may be a characteristic expression of the law of survival. Those maternal activities which ensure the viability of the child have the highest priority. The least maternal members of the group of women we studied gave no evidence of affection as expressed in the manner we have described. They gave slight evidence of tenderness, relatively more of interest and most of what we have called devotion to the task of nursing. We can say of them that by virtue of application to the task, and the modification of roughness, they enabled the baby to survive, in spite of apparent deficiency of relatedness and affection. However, even from the point of view of survival alone, it can be shown that relatedness and affection also have survival values, or at least, that the care and protection of the infant are so reenforced by them that they are more likely to survive. Thus, from a purely evolutionary or adaptational viewpoint it may be argued that maternal, social and emotional responses are basic elements in relational behavior, and that, besides enhancing the baby's life, they help to make it possible.

The function of feeling in maternal behavior may thus be regarded as a powerful reinforcing agent, strengthening and intensifying every component in the mother-infant relationship in a positive way. A recent inquiry may indicate one of the factors involved in this process. Each of several hundred mothers was asked the question: "How soon after the baby was born did you have the full maternal feeling?" A number were able to tell us the day, sometimes even the minute in which this feeling occurred, as an acute and well-defined event. The most frequent description of the feeling was one of possession—"The baby is all yours." The strength of the possessive feeling alone may explain some of the components of the maternal response.

Emotional privation is a clinical term that refers in a specific sense to a lack or diminution of the affectional phase, of emotional warmth, in the mother-child relationship. A mother may be highly conscientious in her devotion to and interest in the baby, yet give no demonstrable evidence of affection. Numerous studies of such cases reveal characteristic difficulties, particularly an inordinate need of love. They represent in the emotional sphere our best examples of deficiency diseases.

Further studies of this type may yield knowledge of the effect of other forms of deficiency, or of excess, derived from a careful analysis of the functional value of each of the main components of maternal behavior.

We may now consider some applications of our findings to the field of mental health. In regard to breast feeding, a safe inference can be made that it is a more severe test of maternal attitude than bottle feeding when special difficulties arise. These have to do particularly with the frequency of painful and frustrating feedings. The less maternal the mother, the more likely her attitude towards the baby may be affected by such experiences. The tendency to project the feelings aroused onto the baby is an important consideration. Unless the mother is above the average in maternal attitude, it would seem wiser not to endanger her relationship to the baby by insisting on breast feeding, when it is consistently difficult. On the other hand, for mothers who find the experience of nursing a pleasant and easy one, there is every advantage in continuing it.

We are concerned particularly with those mothers whose feeling for the infant is of that degree that the experience of breast-feeding itself may raise or reduce it. In that case we would propose that, when feedings are arranged on schedule, the time for each feeding be extended and that, more importantly, the mother be encouraged to accept a wide latitude in the infant's propensity to suck. The main trouble arises when the mother tries desperately to make every minute count until the nurse returns for the baby. Those arrangements where the baby is left full time with the mother solve a number of these problems. However, the effect on mothers who are average or less than average in maternal feeling has not been studied, as far as I am aware.

More important than these considerations, from a mental health viewpoint, is the tendency on the part of the clinicians to blame mothers for not possessing a high degree of maternal feeling. Our own clinical studies indicate that the psychiatrist's notion of "average" maternal feeling is way above the average. As a result of this error, he is prone to search in the life history of his patient for the kind of experience that would explain a distortion in the growth of maternal feeling. Since a fertile source of such distortion arises from unconscious hostility, he is very likely to find confirmation of his inference in that area. As a result he may unwittingly arouse a feeling of guilt in his patient because she is not more maternal than most women. Mothers are especially vulnerable to maternal guilt, probably because the demands of rearing the infant commonly evoke at times hostile feelings.

In bringing this paper to a close it is important to note its limitations. I have not considered the psychological influences on maternal feeling which are derived from studies of the life-history of the individual. Rather, I have tried to measure maternal attitudes as they appeared when the observations were made and to determine the psychological response to comparable events during the same period of time. This, clearly, has not been a study of psychogenesis. It has been my task rather to demonstrate the value of a psychological study based on ordinary observations of on-going behavior limited to a short span of time. I hope that I have demonstrated that the usual inferences concerning the play of emotion on human behavior have left out of consideration a number of factors, and that it is possible to make the analysis out of which our clinical inferences are made a more careful and objective procedure.

Part III

PSYCHIATRY'S COMMITMENT IN THE COMMUNITY

Hope is a passion for what is possible.
—KIERKEGAARD

The sense of community is inherent in man's nature. He has an eternal awareness—paradoxical in view of his frequent internecine strife—remarked by Goethe:

Even from the lowest company one burrows
A sense that one's a man like all the rest.

Recent developments in our society have forcibly reminded psychiatry of the inter-relatedness of men, despite race, creed, or nationality. They have punctuated history with tremendous tumult. As William Godwin writes in *The Rights of Man and the Principles of Society,* "We are not connected with one or two percipient beings, but with a society, a nation, and, in some sense, with the whole family of mankind. Of consequence that life ought to be preferred which will be most conducive to the general good."

This section of *Hope—Psychiatry's Commitment* centers on community in change. It is divided into two sections— the religious community and the secular society. The religious community is included especially, for reasons already mentioned in the introduction. And as Moltmann says, hope makes religion "the source of continual new impulses toward the realization of righteousness, freedom and humanity." More effective treatment of the mentally ill is only part of the hope psychiatry struggles to offer humanity. Primary prevention, better education, and a concern for the whole range of social issues are also part of psychiatry's concern for the community.

Part III

Section One

THE RELIGIOUS COMMUNITY

The cultural-social origins of psychiatry and religion are identical with those of the witch doctor. Some say that this bit of history has as little relevance to psychiatry and religion's roles today as has the seventeenth-century barber's art to the modern surgeon's skill. But, although it is true that history is ill-served by the attempt to fuse the concepts of the clergyman's and the psychiatrist's roles, it is, at the same time, undeniable that the minister and the physician share similar concerns in their service to the human community.

David Bakan and other modern writers have speculated at length upon the relationships between the two concerns, conjecturing about the links between psychoanalysis and Jewish mysticism. In this section of *Hope—Psychiatry's Commitment,* Dr. Schnaper explores some of the analogues between modern psychiatric thinking and the teachings of the Talmud. Doctor Whitehorn pointed out in his chapter (Part I, section 1, chapter 3) that the "useful meaning of maturity or immaturity is centered . . . on the humanly inescapable problems of leadership, authority and responsibility" because men live in communities. Father Burghardt discusses the ongoing evolution of authority in a religion, and some of the psychological implications of the authority "crisis" in religion. Doctor Reidy analyses sensitivity groups and their use by religious communities. And Doctor Hirschberg discourses on those factors which contribute to effective group-living in a religious community of women.

Thus—in the section which follows—theologian, educator, and clinician join to clarify the boundaries and interfaces of religion and psychiatry.

14

NATHAN SCHNAPER, M.D.

> *It was a singularly moving experience for me to share the speakers' platform on one particular occasion with Leo Bartemeier. The audience was a very large group, the women's auxiliary of a Jewish hospital. Prior to the presentations, we were led to a room to be served lunch. We were all seated with spoon poised over fruit cocktail. I leaned toward Leo and asked if he would like to say grace. He did. After he finished there was a short, dramatic silence, then the meal and conversation began.*
>
> *Following the lunch, a group of excited women surrounded me and in awe and amazement, and in almost a single voice exclaimed, "He's a psychiatrist? And religious, too? How can that be?" Very simple, when the "that" is Leo Bartemeier.*
>
> *There are many facets that combine to make this great and wonderful man—to which this* Festschrift *is testimony. To that aspect of Leo, his deeply religious conviction, I dedicate this article and with love.*

The Talmud: Psychiatric Relevancies in Hebrew Tradition

CURRENTLY, WE TAKE for granted many psychological structures and concepts that we assume to have evolved during the past century or so. Almost two thousand years ago, the talmudists were developing thoughts and ideas analogous, if not similar, to those of today. The significance of their thinking has had a subtle influence on present-day psychiatry.

Dynamic, as opposed to descriptive, psychiatry came into its own in

---

* An earlier version of this article was published in the *Journal of Religion and Health*, Academy of Religion and Mental Health, Vol. 6, No. 3, July 1967, and reprinted by permission.

the nineteenth century and received impetus and dominance here in the twentieth. Ecclesiastes tells us "and there is nothing new under the sun" (Eccles. 1:9); and indeed this is so. Poets, ancient and modern, anticipated Freud, particularly in the areas of the unconscious and psychic determinism. So it is not surprising to learn that a series of scholars some two thousand years ago debated psychological issues in the course of investigating and understanding the Bible. What is remarkable, however, is their sensitive insights into psychological concepts and attitudes of their day that would be analogous, if not applicable, to those of today.

The Talmud (*lamad*—study, teach), next to the Bible, is the most important compilation of Judaic religious and civil law. It consists of two interwoven parts: The Mishnah (*shanah*—to repeat in an oral sense) and the Gemara (*gemar*—to complete). There are two Talmuds: the Palestinian, developed by the teachers and scholars resident in Palestine; and the Babylonian, representing the ideas of those in Babylonia. While both include the Mishnah, the Babylonian Talmud is larger and fuller. (This paper deals only with the Babylonian Talmud.)

The Mishnah is an expansion of the Laws enumerated in the Pentateuch, plus the text of the law and lore handed down orally by teachers through generations, and it encompasses the years 450 B.C.E. through 200 C.E.* As is to be expected, the cultural mores, influences, and historical events of those years had their effects on laws, ideas, and opinions expressed in the Mishnah, and of that matter in the Gemara as well.

The Gemara, the exegesis of the Mishnah, evolved slowly over the next three centuries (200 C.E. to 500 C.E.). It "completes" the Mishnah to form the Talmud by two seemingly divergent paths. The core of the Gemara is the Halakah (from *halak*—literally, walking). It follows the Mishnah carefully, developing an expositional interpretation of religious law, and thus becomes the legalistic structure of the Talmud. The other constituent of Gemara is Haggadah (literally, narration), which includes all interpretation of the Scriptures that is not halakic. These are nonlegal, but provide a rich storehouse of common sense, legend, allegories, tales, reminiscences, poems, personal reflections, and more. It is an error to consider the two parts of the Gemara as rigidly separate or independent. They represent the interests and philosophies of the same men, each man traveling both routes, and therefore should be considered as a teaching whole.

With the foregoing as background for orientation, we are now ready

---

* B.C.E., Before the Common Era (B.C.). C.E., the Common Era (A.D.).

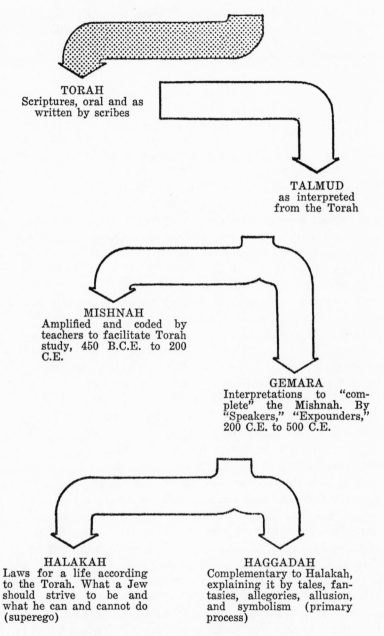

TORAH
Scriptures, oral and as
written by scribes

TALMUD
as interpreted
from the Torah

MISHNAH
Amplified and coded by
teachers to facilitate Torah
study, 450 B.C.E. to 200
C.E.

GEMARA
Interpretations to "com-
plete" the Mishnah. By
"Speakers," "Expounders,"
200 C.E. to 500 C.E.

HALAKAH
Laws for a life according
to the Torah. What a Jew
should strive to be and
what he can and cannot do
(superego)

HAGGADAH
Complementary to Halakah,
explaining it by tales, fantasies, allegories, allusion,
and symbolism (primary
process)

Figure A.   Evolution of the Talmud

to consider the similarities between the Talmud and present-day psychiatry. For the purpose of clarity, the following presentation will be in three parts: 1) techniques, 2) theory, and 3) psychological ideas and attitudes of the Talmud.

TECHNIQUES

In an over-all way, the techniques for interpretation of the Bible and Mishnah suggest the techniques utilized in psychotherapy. The approach used in both appears, at first glance, informal and less than well-organized. Studies and discussions over the centuries gradually built a reference work consisting of six divisions (*sedarim*—Orders), each subdivided into 7-12 Tractates (*Massichtoth*), and these into chapters and finally sectional paragraphs. This is analogous to the seemingly undirected hours of work by patient and therapist, the culmination of which is a vast repository of facts, fantasies, and memories. In effect, the patient, with his therapist's help, writes (and *is*) his own best "text-book," which he can use as his guide to more comfortable living.

No subject in the Talmud is fully treated in any one passage. A tenet must be put together from many parts, and a superficial reading is inaccurate as well as inadequate. This seeming lack of order and system applies to treatment. A surface view is frequently misleading. Patients may agendize their problems and their psychopathology on the first visit; they frequently do so without conscious awareness. Then piecemeal over the ensuing months the same material evolves, but in a fragmentary way and with the patient's increasing understanding of dynamics. (This is one of the major factors necessitating long-term treatment; fortunately, it does not take centuries, as was the case with the Talmud.)

The patient's direct presentation of problems and complaints represents the basic framework around which the therapy is built. In the Talmud, this is the analogous function of the Mishnah and Halakah insofar as the legal problems are delineated and structured. Haggadah is a process of elaboration, utilizing narrative reasoning in much the way the patient does. The technique for building Haggadah and amassing patients' productions is one and the same: free association. We ask our patients to tell us, as freely as they can, "what comes to mind." The scholars of the Talmud would associate to a scriptural passage, offer an interpretation, then associate to a reminiscence, then to an allegorical story, etc., and others would join in. This led at times to going far afield, as it occasionally does today with patients, and even in seminars, post- and post-post-graduate.

Technically, the psychiatric interview is oriented toward encouraging and furthering understanding of what the patient means on all possible levels. This was the ultimate desire of the talmudic teachers and scholars —to analyze a verse for all possible meanings. For the most part, four methods of exegesis were used: *Peshat*—the simple, literal explanation; *Remez*—allusion, allegorical, philosophical interpretation; *Derash*—seeking, investigating, expositional commentary; *Sod*—secret, symbolic meaning. The Zohar (Splendor),* the gospel of Jewish mysticism of the Middle Ages, combines the beginning letters of the four words to form the word PARDES (Paradise, garden). Intentionally or otherwise, it is obvious that therapists employ the same approaches to the patient's verbal and non-verbal productions. Certainly, patient material is perceived on its simple, allegorical, and secret (unconscious) level, and the searching process is constant. In dream interpretation, the literal (manifest) and the allegorical and secret (latent) meanings are sought. *Derash* is in every respect similar to the therapeutic attempts at clarification and then confrontation. The esoteric meanings are, in treatment as in the Talmud, significant interpretations to be dealt with.

It is axiomatic in the psychotherapeutic process that the therapist take nothing for granted. This includes verbal redundancy in the service of wished-for conviction. Shakespeare's insight was reflected in the Queen's statement in *Hamlet*: "The lady doth protest too much, methinks." This was the rule in biblical interpretation. For example, in Exodus XX. 9: "Six days shalt thou labor and do all thy work." Since there could be no tautology "labor" and "work" must have different meanings. After much discussion, it was decided that "labor" must refer to livelihood and "work" to avocation. This differentiation indicated purpose: that a man should busy himself with an avocation; "a man only dies through idleness" (ARN XI). In the treatment setting, when a patient proclaims "my childhood was happy, *very* happy" or "I love my husband, *really* love him," substantive doubt is immediately evoked in the therapist's mind.

In treatment, the therapist and patient are confronted by many ideas

---

* Compiled by Moses de León in Spain about 1300. Legend attributes it to Simeon ben Yochai in the second century C.E. It concerns itself with mystic concepts about the world, nature, and the soul (transmigration). It influenced many Christian philosophers and thinkers, particularly during the Renaissance.

that seem contradictory. So it is in the Talmud, with many opposing thoughts expressed by the commentators through the years. However, in both situations, these contradicting ideas, thoughts, and attitudes inherently stimulating further thoughts rather than immediate acceptance lead to mature evaluation. In this way rational choice is accomplished. It may not be rapid, nor is it always the ideal preference, but it is worked through.

Finally, in treatment as it is in the Talmud, everything is "grist for the mill." In both, seeming irrelevancies, non-sequiturs, and even the unimportant are significant. The Talmud considered religion, ethics, business, the physical life (health, disease, marriage), dreams, the universe and cosmos, politics, social and moral life, jurisprudence, superstitions (which were frowned upon but tolerated, for people would be "unhappy" without them)—in short, anything and everything. It is noteworthy that when patients feel they can talk of everything, the discerning therapist who alertly accepts "everything" as suitable material to be analyzed earns for himself an intellectual by-product—a large fund of general information—some useful, some not.

THEORY

In 1923, Freud delineated three "structures," each having a functional relationship to the other.[1] He referred to them as the id, the ego, and the superego. According to Freud, the id is the precursor of the other two. (More recent authors postulate a common, undifferentiated matrix present at birth, from which all three structures develop.[2]) The id, assumed to be present *at birth*, contains the psychic representatives of the drives, sexual and aggressive. The ego, developing during the first year of life, consists of a series of functions. Included in this series are those having to do with co-ordinating the individual's relationship with his external environment and reconciling the demands imposed on the individual by the id and the superego. The superego begins to develop at the age of five or six, but is not firmly established until the age of ten or eleven.[3] This structure of the mind functions as the individual's moral sense and sets the standards for the ideal he should strive to attain.

Almost two thousand years prior to Freud, the talmudic rabbis analyzing the passage, "Then the Lord God formed man" (Gen. II.7), constructed a theory of good and evil urges to be found in every human being. They began with the question of why the word *wayyitzer* ("and He formed") was spelled with two *y*'s. Their conclusion was that each *y* represented a *yetzer* (impulse, imagination) and that God created two impulses in man, one good (*Yetzer Tov*) and the other evil (*Yetzer Hara*) (Ber. 61a). Although this may suggest casuistry, and indeed some of their subsequent reasoning was primitive, the application of their ideas has strong parallels with the theory cited above.

The evil impulse (like the id) is present at birth.* By common agreement, this impulse is construed as sexual drive. It is not necessarily bad, as God creates only that which is good, and is evil only if abused or misused. "Were it not for that impulse, a man would not build a house, marry a wife, beget children or conduct business affairs" (Gen. R. IX.7). If there were no evil impulse, there would be no wrongdoing, being "good" would be without meaning, and hence no moral sense could exist.

The good impulse (like the superego) is manifested at a later age. This is age thirteen, when a boy can fulfill the Commandments and assume responsibility for his actions. The good impulse implies moral consciousness and functions by saying "no" to the particular inappropriate urge of the moment—very much as a child, having learned "no, no" from his parents, says the words to himself when about to transgress, thus forming a primitive superego.

Both impulses are in constant struggle, and the one that dominates affects the psyche of the individual and manifests his character. The psyche, according to talmudic opinion, is composed of two of the five names for the soul and functions much like the ego, arbitrating between the two impulses. The two applicable names are *Ruach* (spirit or breath) and *Neshamah* (disposition). Significantly, these are man's, exclusively.

Physiologically, the evil impulse is located in the heart and leads to the following: "The wicked are under the control of their heart (evil impulse) but the righteous have their heart under control." (Gen. R. XXXIV.10) Here the individual's needs and impulses are acknowledged but the mature, healthy ego remains in control. That drives need to be curbed if the individual is to become civilized is also recognized. The evil impulse is first like a spider's web, but in the end like a rope (Suk. 52a). "The evil impulse is at first like a passerby, then like a lodger, and finally like the master of the house" (*ibid.*, 52b). Also, self-discipline de-

---

* The rabbis sought to establish the exact moment and debated the issue. Rabbi Judah *Hanasi* (Judah the Prince, Patriarch, c. 200 C.E., credited with compiling the *Mishnah*) tells of a discussion with Antoninus—Marcus Aurelius or his general—believing that the evil impulse began with conception. The latter argued that if this were true, then the fetus could kick its way out of the womb at will. R. Judah then agreed that it must begin with emergence since (Gen. IV.7): "Sin coucheth at the door." The "door" must mean "the opening of the Mother's body" (Sanh. 91b).

velops strength, as one who conquers his impulse becomes "mighty" (Aboth. IV.1).*

Many suggestions, courses of action, and admonitions are offered by the talmudists to combat this powerful and controlling basic urge. Nonetheless, in their wisdom they were cognizant of the force of compulsion and the "irresistible impulse." For the person who struggled sincerely but unsuccessfully with his impulse, they offered advice (Chag. 16a). He was to dress in black (as a sign of mourning) and go to a strange place where no one would know him and discharge his desire. Although it was acknowledged that God was aware, even when one sinned in secret, a man was admonished to sin in a place where he was not known, lest he set an example and encourage others to sin (Sifra *ad hoc.*).

SOME TALMUDIC CONCEPTS WITH PSYCHOLOGICAL ORIENTATION

Heredity and free choice. Although man may be born with the evil impulse and even be burdened by the consequences of the wrongdoings of his fathers, he alone is responsible for any wrongs he may commit. Man does not inherit sin, original or otherwise. He may be influenced by family or friends, but he must assume personal responsibility as he molds his life according to his inner desires. "Man can act virtuously or viciously" (Antiq. XVIII.1.3.).** The entire human race shares *one* common ancestor. Therefore, none can plead heredity and claim a wicked or righteous ancestor to justify his particular character (Sanh. 38a).

In Deut. XI.26 it is stated: "Behold, I set before you this day a blessing and a curse." The sages understand this and other portions of the text to mean that God offers the individual free choice as to how he directs his life, asking only that he give careful consideration to the consequences.

The parallel in treatment is evident, albeit the therapist is no god. The patient comes into this world with certain constitutional and familial

---

* The force of each of the two impulses is expressed allegorically in Ecclesiastes IV. 13: "Better the poor wise child than the old foolish King." Interpreted (Eccles. R. *ad loc.*), the good impulse and the evil impulse respectively are contrasted: the good impulse is poor, because none pays it attention; wise, because it shows the proper way; and a child because it appears later in life. On the other hand, the evil impulse is old as it begins at birth; foolish, because it encourages one to go astray; and a king because all heed it.

** An interesting talmudic legend: The angel responsible for conception is named *Lailah* (night). He sets a seminal drop before God and asks whether it will become a person who is strong or weak, rich or poor, wise or foolish. At no time is there mention of wicked or righteous (Nid. 16b).

assets and liabilities. However, it is incumbent upon him to understand himself (inner desires and drives), as well as his relationships. When he does, he can then resist blaming his parents, begin to weigh his own actions and their consequences. At this point he is free to choose what he wants to do with his life.

Self-preservation. The instinct for survival is primary in all species. Man's struggle in this direction is manifested by his heroic as well as his less heroic actions. Not infrequently, the suicide reflects a fantasied resistance to submission, or an "escape" into a death that represents a reunion with mother. Daily, psychiatrists are faced with the machinations and the lengths to which patients go in the service of self-preservation. The rabbis, too, took a realistic point of view toward this need. They pondered the responsibility of the Jew toward his religion in times of stress. "In connection with all the prohibitions mentioned in the Torah (Holy Scriptures), if a man is told, 'Transgress and be not killed,' he may transgress and save his life, with the exception of idolatry, unchastity and bloodshed" (Sanh. 74a). If his choice is between living and one of these three, there is no alternative but death. In subsequent discussions they added a fourth cardinal sin: slander. This sin was considered by some to be a most grave one. The tongue ". . . slays three persons: the speaker, the spoken to, and the spoken of" (Arach. 15b). Also, "The Holy One, blessed be He, says of such a person, I and he cannot dwell together in the world" and "whoever speaks slander magnifies iniquities equal to the three sins of idolatry, unchastity and bloodshed" (*ibid.*). It is startling to note that when patients begin to be critical of their parents during treatment, their guilt mounts to a degree suggesting that they knew all the time what the rabbis were talking about.

Hope and Faith. The Talmud is replete with references, discourses, advice and anecdotes concerning hope and faith. This is proper. Hope is implicit in that fathers plant for their children and children plant for their children. Hope (*tikvah*), the expectation of something desired, implying faith and trust, and characteristic of all religions, is particularly essential to the Jewish religion. (*Hatikvah*, The Hope, conceived as a Zionist hymn in the late 1800's, has been the anthem of the State of Israel since its inception.)

Faith (*emunah*), corresponds to the kinship between God and man. (There is no word in the Bible or in the Talmud for the concept, religion. Thus, when necessary, the word, *Emunah,* is used.) Hope and faith meet on the common ground of trust in the Lord. Through centuries of pain, despair and persecution, one conviction has comforted and sustained every Jewish father and, in turn, his son: faith in the continued hope for the coming of the Messiah.

In man's relationship with and to his God, he must have sufficient faith in Him so that his theology then becomes a way of life. In turn, God, the Creator of the world, controls all things for man's special benefit. " 'The Lord is my portion,' saith my soul; 'therefore will I hope in Him.' " and " 'It is good that a man should (hope and) quietly wait for the salvation of the Lord' " (Lamentations III, 24, 26).

The Lord is the moral Judge of the world, and in the long run virtue will triumph. "The hope of the righteous shall be gladness; but the expectation of the wicked shall perish" (Prov. X.28).

The Prophets never despaired. Nor did the talmudists. The bleaker and darker this day, the brighter tomorrow. While the present may be empty, the future is full of hope. "Those who have faith in God need not worry about the coming day" (Sot. 48b). "To him who puts his hope in God, will the Lord be a protection in this world and in the world hereafter" (Men. 29b).

These concepts have application in psychiatric treatment. Faith and hope in God requires man to have faith in himself. Otherwise, his faith consists in merely making prayerful petitions without any sense of personal commitment. Treatment demands that the patient make such a personal commitment—not the kind that subscribes to psychiatry cultishly, but rather the kind that presupposes the hope (expectation) that the patient can be more comfortable if *he* works at it.

In the two-way exchange that makes for meaningful therapy, the therapist has to share this faith. It is a constant source of revelation to see patients, who seemingly have no faith and no religion, develop one or the other or both. Wherein this faith lies hidden would require metaphysical conjecture.

Hope is particularly important to those dealing with the dying person. No mortal can say when anyone is going to die, and to take away hope is to destroy that person. In Kings II.20, we read that the prophet Isaiah tells King Hezekiah to "set thy house in order; for thou shalt die, and not live." The talmudists point out that God heard Hezekiah's prayers and spared him, and they chide Isaiah for trying to take away hope.

Suicide. Until the Talmud, there was no word for suicide. Then the word employed was *hitavdoth,* from the root word *avod,* to lose. There are at least six recorded suicides in the Bible, only one with God's permission, Samson.* The talmudists considered suicide repugnant, based on the verse, "And surely your blood, and the blood of your lives, will *I* require" (Gen. IX.5). Hence the person committing this act was to be denied public mourning and eulogy. A suicide would be defined as one who announces how he intends to kill himself. A child is never termed a suicide, as he is not responsible. Judges were cautioned to be alert to individuals confessing to a crime, without witnesses, which would require the death penalty. The confessor might be mentally unbalanced and seeking a way to die. In later writings, it was decided that one who commits suicide under great mental or physical strain, or not in full possession of his faculties, or in order to atone for past sins is not a sinner. Thus, suicide as resistance to persecution is sanctioned. There is very little that present-day psychiatry can find to differ with in these thoughts (Keth. 130b; A.Z. 17a, 18a; Taan, 29a and Midrash Gen. 65:22).

Insanity. Psychosis, gross or implied, was recognized in the Bible and in the Talmud. If one is out of contact with reality, tears his clothes without reason, is intoxicated to the extent of being unconscious, or exposes himself to unnecessary danger, he is considered insane (*shoteh*).

It is of interest, in view of present-day discussions as to whether mental retardation is properly the concern of the psychiatrist or the pediatrician, that the talmudists decided the question on the basis of competency. The imbecile, the idiot, the minor (*katan*), the deaf-mute (*heresh*), and the insane were legally not responsible. The rabbis were aware of periods of remission and ruled that the insane could be held accountable for acts committed during periods of lucidity (Chag. 3b).

The understanding that the psychotic is not a volitional person, but "has action but no thought" (Maksh. III.8), resolves the issue of competency. These people cannot enter a transaction that requires consent; can give no testimony; are not criminally culpable; cannot participate in civil action (the court acts as trustee for the incompetent); and cannot marry, or married, cannot divorce (Yeb. 112b).**

* The others: King Saul; his armor bearer; Ahithopel; Zimri; and Abimelech. Saul was a depressive, at times delusional. When his armies were about to be destroyed by the Philistines, he killed himself with his sword. In contrast, Abimelech received a cracked skull when a woman knocked over a stone. He felt he was dying and asked a soldier to run him through with his sword so as "not to die at a woman's hand." There were two suicides recorded in the Apocrypha: Razis, and the mother of seven sons tortured by Antiochus.
** The Bible denies the deaf-mute the prerogative of marriage and divorce. However, the rabbis amended this by stating that if a deaf-mute, by the use of signs, could show comprehension, e.g., could answer questions

As to the matter of the married psychotic entering into divorce (*Get*) proceedings: In theory, only the husband could obtain a divorce and for such reasons as sterility, adultery, or improper conduct. This was relatively easy to accomplish. In practice, the wife's interests were protected, although the husband's consent was required. She could divorce for nonsupport, loathsome occupation, impotence, or refusal to consummate the marriage. To restrain a hasty divorce, the man was required to pay the *Kethubah*—marriage settlement. (Yeb. 63b; *ibid.*, VI.6; Keth. XIII.5; Ned. XI.12; Keth. 77a) (How many divorces are aborted in these times by the threat of alimony?) Insanity was not considered grounds for divorce by either party. "If a wife becomes insane, the husband cannot divorce her; and if the husband becomes insane, he cannot give a divorce" (Yeb. XIV.1). (This is in contrast to earlier Mosaic law, which stated that a psychotic woman could be divorced.) The rabbinical reasoning was that a psychotic woman without protection would soon fall prey to lustful and evil-minded persons. A husband could, in lieu of divorce, take another wife if he were willing to go through considerable "red tape" in getting rabbinical approval. In the case of the husband suffering insanity, and since a divorce could be accomplished only through his conscious consent, his illness precluded this possibility.

In summary: There is little recorded as to etiology. There are talmudic references to folk-lore that holds "demons" responsible for "sinfulness." Treatment, as implied in the foregoing material, was not unlike that of today. The mentally ill were not isolated from the community as were the lepers, but rather were given a kind of protective parental concern. The legal aspects are particularly significant in the modernity of their views. This kind of thinking could be a model for needed progressive mental health laws in many states today.

Women and marriage. As students of female psychology, the rabbis showed a masculine bias. They had an eye for beauty and used it, they regarded men and women as equal (B.K. 15a). However, in the realm of equality, they considered themselves to be "more equal." Women were not permitted to study the Scriptures, as they had too many responsibilities in the home. They were accused at times of being loose-tongued, jealous, lazy, querulous, and garrulous (Gen. R. XLV.5). Other (majority) opinions were in opposition and more to the point. Women were credited with

---

requiring positive as well as negative answers, he was competent to marry or divorce.

great capacity for tenderness, mercy,* inspiration, and influence. Wives and mothers could make scholars out of their husbands and sons (Ber. 17a). Women were noted for their passion for beauty, clothes, treating their eyes, curling their hair, rouging their faces, and occasionally being light-minded. This love and concern for the self in women was regardless of age. In reply to the statement that these characteristics were permitted only to the young, R. Chisda said: "By God, it is even permitted with your mother and your grandmother, and even if she stood on the brink of the grave; for as the proverb tells 'A woman of sixty, the same as a girl of six, runs to the sound of the timbrel'" (Keth. 65a, 59b, and M.K. 9b). The same manifestations observed today would be referred to as narcissistic and perhaps phallic exhibitionistic, but would be sadly devoid of impact.

The Pentateuch has no term referring to marriage specifically, but includes it in the category of "covenant." The Talmud, in turn, deals with marriage in many passages, labeling the relationship between husband and wife as *kiddushin* (sanctification). In this way, the *Yetzer Hara* (sexual drive, desire) is channeled in a constructive direction. Sexual relations are governed by *taharah* (purity) of the family outlined in Lev. XV. 19-28. The laws found in these verses are elaborated in the Talmud. A successful marriage is not predicated upon an ideal sexual relationship, but disturbance in the latter can subtly interfere with or destroy an otherwise "good" marriage. While there are many urgings on the part of the rabbis for man to marry, a note of caution concerning sociological and characterological considerations is injected: "Young man, lift up thine eyes, and consider what thou wilt choose for thyself as a wife. Do not set thine eyes upon beauty, but look at the family" (Taan. 26b.).

According to the Talmud, women need and should enjoy sexual relationships as much as men do, but always in the confines of marriage. Also, their conjugal rights are carefully spelled out. Examples: A man, with his wife's consent, may take a vow not to have intercourse with her for two weeks against the will of the wife; a student may abstain for thirty days while he studies the Torah, laborers for one week. A woman has the right to expect sexual relations every day if her husband is unoccupied; twice a week if he is a laborer; once a week if he drives a donkey (they would travel to near villages); once every month for camel-drivers (who would go longer distances); and once every six months for sailors. If the

---

* The Hebrew word for mercy is *rachamim*, from the root word *rechem*, meaning uterus.

husband failed to comply, she could take him to the Rabbinical Court. Sex on the Sabbath was, and is, considered a *mitzvah* (good deed). (Keth.).

Contraception. The Scriptures demand "Be fruitful and multiply" (Gen. I.28). However, this is incumbent upon men and not women. Onan, Jacob's grandson, who "spilled his seed upon the ground," was not killed for masturbating, but for practising coitus-interruptus. (Also, for not fulfilling the Levirate ceremony of marrying the widow of his older brother.) Where pregnancy might endanger the woman's life, she is permitted and even urged to use contraceptives. Three situations are noted in particular: where the woman is a minor and a pregnancy could be fatal; where the woman is pregnant and might abort; and where the woman is a nursing mother and might have to wean her child prematurely if she became pregnant (Yeb. 12b). The latter clause reflects the sagacious awareness of these men of the requirements for the child's healthy physical and emotional development.

Therapeutic Abortion. This is an emotionally-charged topic today for lay and medical groups. The psychiatrist is frequently asked to sit in judgment as to who shall or shall not be entitled to such an operation. This is reflected in the statistics. Sixty per cent or more of therapeutic abortions are done for "psychiatric indications." Unfortunately, because of stringent statutes, there are times when the psychiatrist is asked to pre-empt the law.

The Judaic point of view, as expressed in the Talmud, was decided in a characteristic manner. First, there is no question of entry of the soul before birth or the claim of salvation after death. Secondly, the mother has rights, as the fetus is an organic part of her (like her appendix). Therefore, if the woman is in "hard travail," the fetus is to be cut up in her womb. Once the head is delivered, the child has equal rights. Another justification, if the mother's life is in danger, is the defense against an aggressor: "If one comes to kill you, be first and kill him" (Sanh. 72a).*

Children. It is in this area particularly that the psychological perspicacity of the talmudists is most evident. Having children is regarded by the Talmud as a two-way street. There are responsibilities incumbent upon parents and upon children. The child must honor the parent and the latter must love the former. The Old Testament commands: "Honor thy father and mother" (Exod. XX.12) and "Fear thy mother and father" (Lev. XIX.3). These two statements were searched by the rabbis for

---

* Justifiable homicide, the one exception to the interdiction concerning bloodshedding.

meaning. Their explanation: The father is given precedence in the first phrase because it is known that the young child has greater affection for his mother; and in the second phrase the mother is given precedence because it is the father, primarily, who is feared (Kid. 30b-31a). Applying the "no tautology rule" to the seeming repetition in these verses, the rabbis concluded that both parents are thus "equal." A child, when the parents are of different faiths, should follow that of the mother, as his needs and his well-being are dependent upon her.

What about the requirements placed upon the parents? One who "loves and well nourishes his children is blessed" (Pes. CVI.3). Children should not be terrorized (Git. 6b). On the other hand, they should receive merited punishment. If a child is not punished, he may grow up to be "utterly depraved" (Exod. R.I.1). The concept here is that the indulged child is actually the deprived child. So that a child may not become frightened "to the degree he might take his own life," "Never threaten, but punish him at once or say nothing" (Semachoth II.6). The ideal course with children (and women) is "to push away with the left hand and draw them near with the right hand" (*ibid.*).

It is unwise to make promises to children and then not keep them, as this "teaches the child to tell lies" (Suk. 46b). Parents are warned to be careful of their talk in the house as "the talk of the child in the street is that of his father or his mother" (*ibid.* 56b).

In their astuteness, the rabbis knew that love for one's children comes before affection for one's parents: "A father's love is for his children, and the children's love for their children" (Sot. 49a). Nonetheless, they stressed man's need for children, not only for his individual immortality, but for society's benefit as well. The Hebrew word for children is *banim;* for builders, *bonim.* With this play on words, the profound statement is made that children are builders; not only do they build the future of the family, but also of the community.

There was agreement that at least two children constituted a family. One school of rabbis (Shammai) took the view this meant two sons, another school (Hillel) believed one son, one daughter. The Talmud contains many arguments, pro and con, voicing the preference for male progeny. A few samples of the arguments stress continuance of the family name, support in old age, and that sons could study the Scriptures, whereas girls could not. One particular bit of reasoning attributed to Ben Sira is both amusing and revealing in its keen insight into the unconscious. "It is written,—A daughter is a vain treasure to her Father. From anxiety about her he does not sleep at night, during her early years lest she be seduced, in her adolescence lest she go astray, in her marriageable years lest she does not find a husband, when she is married lest she be childless, and when she is old lest she practise witchcraft" (Sanh. 100b).

CONCLUSION

The Talmud is a testimonial to man's capacity to think and to build toward reason. It is true that these men saw life through the vision of their particular culture. This thought has been used as a criticism against other thinkers—Freud, for one. However, these scholars, in succession, labored over a period of many centuries, each influenced by his own particular time. Yet, despite the changing character of their various cultures, they saw "human nature" as we see psychology today; only the jargon is different.

It is also true that fundamentally the Talmud is a religious treatise. This fact does not detract from its wisdom, but rather made it possible. Beginning with the concept of a God who was very concerned and involved with human events, the talmudic scholars could then ponder the problems of mankind. The history of those years and their vicissitudes taught them psychology. Therapists struggle with the issue of whether or not to consider value judgments of their patients. The scholars saw man as having individual rights, but also as a social being. Therefore, such matters as love, justice, peace, charity, mercy, education, and morals were his personal responsibilities, if he was to be inwardly comfortable. Man, they felt, could not separate mind from body and experience well-being. One affects the other as does the individual and his society. If this be so, then it behooves the psychiatrist to consider not only the interpersonal relationships of his patient, but his relationships to the community as well, and in the context of realistic value judgments. This implies more than intellectual insight on the part of the patient. (According to the talmudists, no amount of prayer or confession is meaningful unless it is accompanied by a change of conduct. "If a man is guilty of a transgression, makes a confession of it but does not amend his behavior, to what is he like? . . ." Taan. 16a). The therapist can shrug the matter off by placing the responsibility on the patient. Hidden in this same context, and even more subtle, is the question of therapeutic results. An example is the so-called skilled and sharply-honed theoretician who abhors practicalities as they relate to the world around him and the patient. Technique is then not the means to a goal, but a goal in itself. If the technique of therapy has been orthodox within the limits of the therapist's particular school, the application of insight becomes the responsibility (and the burden) of the patient. This is true; the patient does have free choice as to what he wants to do with his life. But it is incumbent upon the therapist to investigate *all* areas. It is also free choice, if either the patient or the therapist is unwilling, for each to seek another partner.

The construction of the Talmud reflects dynamic thinking rather than descriptive. Like treatment it is concerned with struggles, not labels. On cursory examination, one might dismiss much of the Talmud as being akin to primary process thinking, and obsessional at that. Certainly it contains much that is allusion, allegory, symbolic and primitive; but so does psychiatric treatment—and both deal with the difficulties in life and living. The work of the talmudists was *process* in the sense of continuing development involving many changes. Each generation and each century utilized the past, made its contribution to the present, and reached out to the years and people to come. This is the way in psychotherapy. Through his work with his therapist, the patient learns the meaning of his past, what he can give to the present, and what he wants to do with his future. The writing of the Talmud has ceased, but its effect has not. The patient's treatment can come to termination, but the process never stops.

REFERENCES

1. The Divisions of the Talmud:
   First Order: Zera'im (Seeds) ; Tractates, eleven
       Topics: Liturgy, laws dealing with farm products, tithe, Sabbatical year, etc.
   Second Order: Mo'ed (Season) ; Tractates, twelve
       Topics: Sabbath, Holydays, taxes, etc.
   Third Order: Nashim (Women) ; Tractates, seven
       Topics: Marriage, Levirate marriage, marriage detail, infidelity, vows, divorce, etc.
   Fourth Order: Nezikin (Torts) ; Tractates, ten
       Topics: Property rights, crimes, idolatry, testimony, courts, etc.
   Fifth Order: Kodashim (Sanctities) ; Tractates, eleven
       Topics: Sacrifices, offerings, food and drink, dietary laws, etc.
   Sixth Order: Teharoth (Purities) ; Tractates, twelve
       Topics: Defilement of utensils, corpses, lepers, menstruation, animals, water purity, cleanliness, etc.

(Within the six Orders there are 523 chapters. Customarily, religious texts and portions thereof were titled by the opening word. E.g., the book, Genesis, is named *"B'resheet"*—"in the beginning.")

Apocryphal Tractates (Post-mishnaic): Ten, plus four late small ones. Topics: Writing the Scrolls, mourning and burial, chastity, ethical conduct, conversion, etc.

Tosephta (Supplement), unofficial code, paralleling the Mishna and of uncertain authorship, dating somewhere third to fifth century, C.E.

Abbreviations: (Tractates)

Ber.: Berakoth	Men.: Menachoth
B.K.: Baba Kamma	Ned.: Nedarim
Git.: Gittin	Sanh.: Sanhedrin
Chag.: Chagiga	Suk.: Sukkah
Yeb.: Yebamoth	Aboth.: Pirké Aboth
Nid.: Niddah	A.Z.: Aboda Zara
Sot.: Sotah	Pes.: Pesahim
ARN: Aboth d'R. Nathan	Kid.: Kiddushin
Keth.: Kethubboth	Taan.: Ta'anith
Maksh.: Makshirin	Arach.: Arachin
M.K.: Mo'ed Katan	R.: Rabba; R. Gen., R. Lev., etc.

Talmudic references in body of paper are cited by tractate, chapter, and paragraph.

2. Freud, S., *The Ego and the Id*. London, Hogarth Press, 1927.
3. Hartmann, H.; Kris, E.; and Loewenstein, R. M., "Comments on the Formation of Psychic Structure." *Psychoanal. Study Child.* 1946, 2, 11-38.
4. Brenner, C., *An Elementary Textbook of Psychoanalysis*. New York, International Universities Press, Inc., 1957, pp. 41-67.

15

WALTER J. BURGHARDT, S.J.

It is with affection and gratitude that I offer this essay on authority *to Leo Bartemeier. Rarely have I met anyone who weds so successfully the qualities that make authority credible: competence in his field, awareness of human weakness, sweet reasonableness, and strong love for the men and women whose lives intersect his own.*

The Authority Crisis in Catholicism: Analysis and Prognosis

I ASSUME THAT for a psychologist or psychoanalyst or psychiatrist one of the critical areas in human relations, one of the recurring sources of psychic disturbance, is the problem of authority. It should be of interest to the professional, therefore, to see the shift that is gradually taking place within Catholicism in the concept and uses of authority. In this paper I shall suggest the way in which the inevitable tension between authority and freedom in the Church promises to become creative in a context of community. Concretely, I shall do three things: (1) I shall cast a quick glance over my shoulder, to see where Roman Catholics were before the Second Vatican Council opened in 1962; (2) I shall look long into the present, to find the insights that represent progress over the past; (3) I shall peer warily into the future, to prophesy what all this may hold for the individual and the community in the decade to come.

I

My first main point: a swift glance into the past, to grasp the Catholic stance on authority before 1962. To shorten the story, I go back to the relatively recent past, to the nineteenth century, to Pope Leo

XIII. The late John Courtney Murray brought out three pertinent aspects of Leo's thought touching authority and freedom.[1] First, there is Leo's retrospective reading of history. I mean the famous "Once upon a time" paragraph in the encyclical letter *Immortale Dei*. In Murray's fine summary:

> Once upon a time there was a Golden Age, the medieval period. It was the age of Christian unity, of the alliance of the Two Powers, of the obedience both of princes and of peoples to the authority of the Church. Then came the Reformation. Essentially it was a revolt against the authority of the Church, and in reaction to it the Church laid heavy, almost exclusive, emphasis on its own authority. Later, by a sequence that was not only historical but also logical, there came the Revolution. It was essentially a revolt against the authority of God Himself, launched by the revolutionary slogan: "No one stands above man." . . . Again in polemic reaction, the Church rallied to the defense of the sovereignty of God, of the "rights of God," of the doctrine that there is no true freedom except under the law of God.[2]

Second, there was Leo's conception of the political relationship between ruler and ruled in civil society. It was a vertical relationship: the ruled are subjects; their single duty is obedience. The contemporary notion of citizen—someone not merely subject to but also participant in the processes of government, a human being with political and civil rights—such a notion does not come through in Leo.

> His emphasis falls on political authority, which is invested with a certain majesty as being from God, and which is to be exercised in paternal fashion in imitation of the divine sovereignty. In turn, the submission of the subject is to exhibit a certain filial quality. Moreover, society itself is to be built, as it were, from the top down. The "prince" is the primary bearer and agent of the social process. *Qualis rex, talis grex*. The ruler is to be the tutor and guardian of virtue in the body politic; the whole of the common good is committed to his charge. The people are simply the object of rule. Leo's political doctrine was plainly authoritarian. . . .[3]

Third, there was Leo's ecclesiology, his theology of the Church. Here the encyclical *Satis cognitum* is a profound commentary on Vatican I's Constitution on the Church, *Pastor aeternus*.

> The portrait of the Church that emerges is really a portrait of the role of the apostolic office, and in particular the Petrine office, in the

Church. In consequence, the ecclesial relationship . . . is the simple vertical relationship between ruler and ruled. The function of the faithful appears simply as obedience to the doctrinal and jurisdictional authority of the Church.[4]

These three aspects of Leonine thought—historical, political, ecclesiological—may strike the casual reader as dreadfully narrow, frightfully myopic. But it would be a mistake to judge the past purely by the present, to damn Leo XIII because he was not John XXIII. The Church, like any institution, fashions its doctrine under "the signs of the times." And for the nineteenth-century Church the historical signs of the times were the Reformation and the Revolution; the political signs of the times were the laicist conception of the state and the Jacobin conception of the sovereignty of the people; the ecclesiological signs of the times were the divine institution of a hierarchical Church and the submission of flock to shepherds in faith and order, in life and work.

It was within these perspectives that the classical Catholic doctrine on the freedom-authority relationship was fashioned. John Courtney Murray summed it up in one of his many magisterial paragraphs:

> Those who hold office make the decisions, doctrinal and pastoral. The faithful in the ranks submit to the decisions and execute the orders. The concept of obedience is likewise simple. To obey is to do the will of the superior; that is the essence of obedience. And the perfction of obedience is to make the will of the superior one's own will. In both instances the motive is the vision of God in the superior, who is the mediator of the divine will and the agent of divine providence in regard of his subjects, in such wise that union with his will means union with the will of God. The further motive, to be adduced when obedience means self-sacrifice, is the vision of Christ, who made Himself obedient even unto death.[5]

This, I assure you, was the conception of authority under which I grew up: in the home, in the school, in the Jesuits, in the Church. Parent, teacher, rector, bishop—decision-making was theirs. This was their task, their responsibility, God-given, with a corresponding grace of office— God's help to fulfil their mission. My task, my responsibility, was to act in harmony with their commands (save where sin was obviously present), eyes open if possible, eyes closed if necessary. Where authority was legitimate, the decision was presumably binding. Christian virtue lay in finding within the superior's will the will of God.

II

The classical conception of the freedom-authority relationship had much to recommend it: a vivid awareness of God, of the charism that accompanies authority, of obedience as a sharing in the humanness of Christ. There are elements of Christian truth in this vision which should not be mocked by antihistorical caricatures. The problem is, the classical conception is not good enough *for us*. And this brings me to my second main point: a long look into the present, to find the insights that represent progress over the past.

Briefly, the times are new, and the new times call for a new vision. The times are new. The Protestant-Catholic cleavage is yielding to an anguished quest for oneness. The Church-world segregation is crumbling before a massive yearning for compenetration. Today's Church is looking not behind but before, not to a putative Golden Age but to the coming-to-be of the kingdom.

Vatican II was keenly sensitive to the new thing. Two signs of the times it recognized as crucial—man's growing consciousness in two areas. I mean, first, man's growing consciousness of his dignity as a person. Pertinent here are the programmatic sentences that open the Council's Declaration on Religious Freedom: "A sense of the dignity of the human person has been impressing itself more and more deeply on the consciousness of contemporary man. And the demand is increasingly made that men should act on their own judgment, enjoying and making use of a responsible freedom, not driven by coercion but motivated by a sense of duty."[6] I mean, second, man's growing consciousness of community. Contemporary man is dissatisfied with the fifth-century, Boethian conception of the person as "an individual substance of a rational nature,"[7] with the emphasis on self-subsistence, incommunicability, independence; he insists that, to be fully a person, to be fully human, a man must be *with* the others and *for* the others—a vision that harmonizes splendidly with the Christian understanding of the Trinity, where the Persons are constituted by their relationship one to another.

Given this twin consciousness, the classical conception of authority is inadequate. Contemporary man is saying that sheer submission to a superior's will and mere execution of his orders do not satisfy the demands of personal dignity. "They do not call into play the freedom of the person at its deepest point, where freedom appears as love."[8] Nor do they give sufficient play to each man's responsibility to participate fully in community and to contribute actively to community.

Of John Courtney Murray's insightful contributions to the Church and the world, one of the most remarkable was his insistence that we must view the authority-freedom issue

within the context of the community, which is the milieu wherein the dignity of the person is realized. Community is the context both of command and of obedience. Community is also the finality both of command and obedience. Authority is indeed from God, but it is exercised in community over human persons. The freedom of the human person is also from God, and it is to be used in community for the benefit of the others. Moreover, since both authority and freedom stand in the service of the community, they must be related not only vertically but also horizontally. . . .[9]

It is impossible to express in some universal formula the relationship that should obtain between the ruler and the ruled in any and every community. Communities differ. Family, political society, Church—there is a uniqueness to each. With reference to the authority-freedom tension within the Church, four facets of Vatican II's ecclesiology are highly important as context for a solution.[10]

First, the Church is primarily the People of God. The basic condition of this People is equality—an equality in dignity and freedom—equality because all possess, are possessed by, the one same Spirit. This involves a charism, a charismatic quality, in the members; for through the Spirit God distributes to the faithful special graces for various tasks, converses ceaselessly with them, leads them into all truth, makes the word of Christ dwell abundantly in them.[11]

Second, the Church is a communion, a koinonia. Its inner form is the Holy Spirit, who is God's presence in the midst of His People. In the first instance, therefore, the Church is an interpersonal community, united to the Father and to one another through Christ in the Spirit. This is its primary purpose, indeed its ultimate purpose, already realized here, in time, but destined to endure hereafter, beyond time.

Third, as interpersonal community, the Church has a service to perform towards all humanity. Its function is to reach out, through the love that is its inner form, so as to draw all men into the communion of love, so that they too will respond in faith and love to the love whereby the Father loves His own People. The People, therefore, are essentially a missionary people, with a catholic mission of love.

Fourth, the Church is a visible society; therefore it has a structure of authority and a juridical order. Note, however: "The societal aspect of the Church is not alien or extrinsic to its communal and functional aspects, but essential to both of them and inherent in each of them."[12] The authority and juridical order stand in the service of the community, to help it be what it is (a community of love) and realize its function (a mission of love).

These four ecclesiological themes (People of God, interpersonal community, service of love, visible society) are not new, but Vatican II gave them a new order, a different emphasis. Leo XIII came to the notion of the Church as community from the notion of the Church as society; in consequence, he stressed the structure of authority in the Church, gave little play to the functions of freedom. "Authority seems, as it were, to stand over the community as a power to decide and command."[13] Vatican II came to the notion of the Church as society from the notion of the Church as community. "Authority therefore stands, as it were, within the community, as a ministry to be performed in the service of the community."[14] In this way the functions of Christian authority and of Christian freedom emerge with fresh clarity. In each instance, three functions, all in the service of the community.

Take the functions of authority. In Murray's vision, these functions are: unitive, directive, and punitive.[15] The primary function of authority is to unite, to establish communion, by initiating and sustaining Paul VI's "dialogue of salvation," to elicit from the charismatic community the insights of each of the faithful into the faith, to stir the love of the members for the community, to solicit their missionary concern—and all this with as much freedom as possible and only as much restriction as necessary. The second function of authority is directive, decisive, to insure that the deposit of faith is preserved, that the Body acts as one in the actions of its members—a function best achieved when the directives and decisions of authority are, through dialogue, the directives and decisions of the community. The third function of authority is corrective—an accidental function necessary for a sinful People, a function of service to the unity of the community, to be performed under the "due process" demanded by Christian dignity and freedom.

To these three functions of Christian authority correspond three functions of Christian freedom. In Murray's vision, these functions are: charismatic, executive, and self-corrective.[16] The charismatic function is the free response of the community to the unitive function of authority, to the call to participate lovingly in the dialogue of salvation—an exercise in obedience yes, but in its horizontal dimension. The executive function is the free response of the community to the directive function of authority—

a free acceptance of directives and decisions, free because I am doing what I know I ought to do, in consequence of loving dialogue, in order that the community may come together in a new way. The self-corrective function of freedom is the free response of the community to the corrective function of authority—a free refusal to be enslaved to self, to act against community.

Briefly, within Catholicism today the traditional vertical relationship of command-obedience needs to be supplemented by the horizontal relationship of dialogue between authority and the free Christian community.

The practical problem is: the Catholic Church is in a period of transition. The older authority-freedom relationship, excessively vertical, is not always recognized as inadequate; even where it is so recognized, the structures are not yet available for a satisfying horizontal relationship. And within Catholicism I must be constantly aware that the exclusively horizontal would be as destructive of the Catholic community as the exclusively vertical. As with authority and obedience, so with the vertical and horizontal: tension there must be, but the tension must be increasingly creative, so as to fashion progressively the community of faith and hope and love.

At the present moment we are hurting. Growth is a painful process, especially where the valid movement deep within is not discerned, is not recognized because it is veiled by the violence, the rebellion, that is its surface manifestation. In consequence, Rome and the States still betray some enslavement to the outmoded, a fear of the new mode. There are those in high places who do not see the implications of Vatican II, or who seeing the implications regret them. They have not come to grips with the problem so bluntly put by the Jesuit Scripture scholar John L. McKenzie in a provocative book:

> Who determines that what authority commands is the right thing to do? If it is authority alone, then we have absolute power; what authority commands is right because it is commanded. If it is those under authority, then we seem to reduce society to a chaos of individual decisions. Since both conclusions are intolerable, we have no solution except to repose the judgment of the reasonableness of the command both in authority and in the governed. Whatever the channels through which this common judgment is achieved, it can be said definitely that the society which has no means of reaching a common judgment is weak in its structure of authority.[17]

Despite the hurt in so many hearts, despite the drag of so many feet, the promise is rich. The reasons for hope are many. There is, in the first instance, Vatican II, which accepted the movement away from the so-called mentality of classicism (truth "already out there now," apart from people, severed from history) to historical consciousness (objective truth yes, but inescapably involved in history, ever in the anguished, quicksilver grasp of changing human beings).

There are, second, influential prelates like Léon-Joseph Cardinal Suenens, with his recent blueprint for tomorrow's Catholicism, splendidly titled *Coresponsibility in the Church*.[18] It is a program, founded on profound theological insight, to regroup the Church into an organic body with a shared responsibility. Without denying the validity of function or office, this vision of the Church stresses the profound truth that all power is directed to service, that what is of primary importance is the People of God. Or, as Suenens insists, the greatest day in the life of a pope is not his coronation but his baptism, the day of his mission "to live the Christian life in obedience to the gospel."[19]

There are, third, the canon lawyers within Catholicism. On October 5-6, 1968, the Canon Law Society of America (until fairly recently a highly conservative body in the respected tradition of law) sponsored an interdisciplinary Symposium on a Declaration of Christian Freedoms. Out of that symposium came a remarkable preliminary statement formulated against a background of theological, historical, and legal understanding. The Declaration affirmed, among others, the following inalienable and inviolable rights and freedoms of persons in the Christian community: the right to freedom in the search for truth, without fear of administrative sanctions; the right to freedom in expressing personal beliefs and opinions —in particular, the right of competent persons to express dissent from authoritative but noninfallible doctrines; the right of access to objective information, in particular about the Church's internal and external operations; the right to develop an individual's unique potentialities and personality traits without fear or repression by the Christian community or Church authorities; the right to work out one's salvation in response to the unique challenges of each age, each society, each culture; the right of all members of the Church to freedom of assembly and of association; the right to participate, according to each one's gift from the Spirit, in the Church's teaching, government, and sanctifying function; the right to effective remedies for the redress of grievances and the vindication of rights; due process in administrative or judicial procedures in which penalties may be imposed—including the right not to be a witness against oneself, the right to a speedy and public trial, the right to be informed in advance of the specific charge, the right to confront witnesses, the right to expert assistance and to counsel, the right of appeal. And all this on the basis of Christian existence!

There is, fourth, the growing awareness, insight, and sophistication of the Catholic laity. On the one hand, they sense increasingly the truth in the recent words of a young Catholic theologian:

> When we realize that the guidance of the Holy Spirit does not imply a theological "hot-line" which delivers correct answers to any and every pressing question; when we realize that the Holy Spirit guarantees the superior insight of the Church's authoritative teaching authority, in general and where the presumption is in its favor, not by a numinous inspiration but by providing the Church with individual human beings who possess the burning concern, the lack of prejudice, mental acumen, enthusiasm, and other qualities required to climb to this superior vantage point—then we realize that such guidance does not in every single instance eliminate those elements which can also hinder such a position being reached [excessive distance from the fundamental given of a problem—e.g., usury and carriage; premature systematization; cultural blindness; prejudice; fear of undermining one's own authority by a change of policy, etc.]. We can then better understand the sources explaining some of the errors present in the history of the Church's authentic teaching.[20]

On the other hand, they are increasingly aware of the implications in St. Paul's affirmation to the Corinthians: "A spiritual man is able to judge the value of everything" (1 Cor. 2:15), because the man with the Spirit has the mind of Christ. It is becoming clearer that the spontaneous judgment of a considerable number of theologically unschooled faithful represents a valid theological datum. Not that such judgment is necessarily correct, but that there are times when "such connatural knowledge speaks with genuine authority even while seeming to stand in conflict with authoritative teaching."[21]

The point I am making is this: despite the persistence of the older command-obedience perspective, there are strong signs of authority's horizontal dimension. I rarely predict with confidence, but one thing seems clear: authority in the Church will never again be what it was before Vatican II. Man is different; his world is different; and we have grown to a more profound understanding of what Christian responsibility, Christian freedom, demands in our time.

III

I have cast a quick look into the past, to see where Roman Catholics were before Vatican II. I have looked long into the present, to find the insights that represent progress over the past. Now my third point: I shall peer warily into the future, to prophesy what all this may hold for the individual and the community in the decade to come.

First, the area of personal responsibility will be significantly broadened for the average Catholic. The all but total dependence on authority which made sense for a relatively untutored populace is difficult to justify, impossible to sustain, in today's highly sophisticated society. From Lenten abstinence to contraception, in discipline and doctrine, the field of reflection, of group discussion and individual decision, has already expanded far beyond expectation; and the end is not yet.

Second, the psychic effects of this development will vary—grossly and subtly. There are those (mostly, but not all, under thirty) for whom authority's new look is a breath of fresh air which helps make Catholic existence endurable, even joyful, because it frees them for genuinely responsible action. There are those (mostly, but not all, over thirty) for whom the new approach to authority is a threat, either because it seems to subvert an essential ecclesiastical structure, or because it imperils an acquired security, or because it compels decision-making for which their Christian past has not prepared them. And there are those (of all ages) whose situation is ambivalent, because they see intellectually the need for the new, but built into their whole make-up is the older command-obedience relationship from which they cannot escape at all or only with inner violence. For these the agony is compounded by the realization that many of those who hold authority in the Church suspect the new development, that some even condemn it.

Third—and in consequence—the decade to come will find the Catholic community increasingly divided on major issues, because so many of these issues are intimately linked to a conception of authority and its uses. The reaction to Pope Paul VI's encyclical *Humanae vitae* (July 29, 1968) condemning contraception may well prove prophetic. Two divergent views quickly formed on what it means to say that a Catholic must form his or her conscience "in the light of the encyclical." For some, the encyclical is the decisive element in the formation of a Christian conscience on contraception; for others, the encyclical is one factor, important indeed but not necessarily determinative. It may be that we must go back to the Reformation to discover so dramatic, so traumatic a polarization of authority and conscience.

Fourth, there will be rifts not only within the community as such but within the individual psyche—particularly within the man or woman who "wants" to change but "cannot." Here, as I see it, there is a critical need for understanding, compassion, and patience; but the tragedy I foresee is that the advocates of radical restructuring will see no point in wasting these virtues on the unchangeable. A perceptive psychologist, John J. Evoy of Gonzaga University in Spokane, has phrased forcefully the position of the New Front:

> We refuse . . . to engage in agonizing attempts to communicate with those of you who will admit no need for substantive change. And we are reluctant to talk with you people who regard yourselves as middle-of-the-roaders. Why so? Are we afraid to listen to you? Maybe we are. Perhaps it is that we have too much at stake; we dare not risk losing it by listening to what you regard as balanced views. . . . In our quest for the meaningful in life we cannot afford the distraction of keeping an eye out for what might be imprudent. . . . Let prudence wait for tomorrow; adventurousness is today's need. . . .[22]

Fifth, I am reasonably confident that the contemporary crisis of authority can prove creative, need not be destructive. I am not at all blind to the many tragedies, personal and communitarian, which the authority-freedom conflict has occasioned since Pope John XXIII opened his famous windows (some would say, his Pandora's box). But neither am I blind to the calamities which an exclusively vertical approach to authority has generated over the centuries. The new vision of authority, with its stress on personal dignity and service to community, is profoundly insightful, basically biblical, splendidly Christian. How to implement this vision in a Church whose structural model has long been the pyramid (pope at the apex, bishops and all manner of clergy down the broadening sides, laity the base) will be a neuralgic problem of the seventies.

Finally, let me say that I feel about the authority syndrome somewhat as John Courtney Murray felt about the total Catholic problematic. With his singular insight, he predicted the course of events soon after Vatican II. He compared the experience of today's Catholic with the experience of the fathers at the Council. As was the experience of Vatican II, he said, so must be the postconciliar experience: the contemporary Catholic, like the bishops at the Council, must begin with a good deal of confusion and uncertainty, will therefore pass through a period of serious crisis and tension, but can expect to end with a certain measure of light and of joy and of hope.

REFERENCES

1. John Courtney Murray, "Freedom, Authority, Community," *America* 115 (1966) 734-41.
2. *Ibid.*, pp. 734-35.
3. *Ibid.*, p. 735.
4. *Ibid.*
5. *Ibid.*
6. Second Vatican Council, *Declaration on Religious Freedom* (Dec. 7, 1965) 1 (English translation from Walter M. Abbott, ed., *The Documents of Vatican II* [New York: America Press, 1966] p. 675).
7. Boethius, *De persona et duabus naturis* 3 (*Patrologia Latina* 64, 1345); cf. Thomas Aquinas, *Summa theologica* 3, 16, 12, ad 2.
8. Murray, *art. cit.*, p. 736.
9. *Ibid.*
10. For the four facets, I am deeply indebted to Murray's analysis, *art. cit.*, pp. 736-37.
11. Cf. Second Vatican Council, *Dogmatic Constitution on the Church* 9; *Dogmatic Constitution on Divine Revelation* 8.
12. Murray, *art. cit.*, p. 737.
13. *Ibid.*
14. *Ibid.*
15. Cf. *ibid.*, pp. 737, 740.
16. Cf. *ibid.*, pp. 740-41.
17. John L. McKenzie, *Authority in the Church* (New York: Sheed & Ward, 1966) p. 11.
18. New York: Herder and Herder, 1968.
19. *Ibid.*, p. 31.
20. John W. Glaser, "Authority, Connatural Knowledge, and the Spontaneous Judgment of the Faithful," *Theological Studies* 29 (1968) 745.
21. *Ibid.*, p. 751.
22. John J. Evoy, "Dialogue across the Gap," *America* 120 (1969) 356.

16

JOSEPH J. REIDY, M.D.

Doctor Leo Bartemeier has been a dear friend and has helped me in many ways, and I feel it is a privilege to join my colleagues in paying tribute to him. This paper is but one example of the ways in which Doctor Bartemeier has been an inspiration and a help. In the fall of 1968 he asked me my opinion of sensitivity training programs. I did not know then of any evaluation of these programs, and in the course of time this paper became the answer to his question.

Sensitivity Training for Religious

I HAVE OFTEN been asked for my opinion of sensitivity training programs. Many who have asked me are priests and religious sisters. Some have heard enthusiastic reports about these programs and hope that sensitivity training will help them. Some have misgivings because they have heard of persons who had emotional disturbances following sensitivity training. I have talked to persons who have returned from a sensitivity training week convinced that they were helped, feeling they were able to understand themselves and others. I know also of persons who have been admitted to mental hospitals following a sensitivity training experience. There have been very few evaluations of these programs, so that many important questions have not been answered. I have tried here to present ways to judge the goals and methods of sensitivity training.

Religious orders are using psychological knowledge and techniques to improve their community life, and they are interested in theories and techniques concerned with group living, especially those of the group dynamics and sensitivity training approaches. A recent issue of *Sisters Today* carried an article describing in an enthusiastic way the sensitivity training of religious sisters.[1] The religious have good reason for this interest. They know the importance of good relationships in community life and have recognized areas of ineffective group functioning which they had previously overlooked. The renewal of community life is leading to the abandonment of customs and rules which kept religious at a distance from one another, just as it is leading to a change of attitude about the "dangers" of being close to other people. The religious do not see intimacy as a hindrance to religious life, but believe that religious love is expressed in relation to others. There is more recognition of the value of feelings towards others and freer expression of these feelings.

The religious believe that the way to God is through love of others, and they have discovered that the secular sciences propose that a measure of the fullness of personality development is how well one loves others. But they often feel that they do not know how to relate to people. They want to learn what psychology and the other sciences say about love, openness, authenticity. What do these sciences say about how they can become loving, open, authentic? Improved communication, they find, can lessen loneliness; it can undo distortions and misunderstandings and projections. Getting to know a person is a necessary step to loving him. In their apostolate they want to know how they can change their relationship to the people they meet and work with. Some religious have lived isolated lives; and the experiments with religious dress, with small communities living away from the convent, with houses of study moving into the city, are examples of their attempts to undo this isolation.

But the apartness from the world which they once cherished was more than dress and dwelling place, because it came from ignorance of the values, beliefs, and ways of living of persons of different social backgrounds; and the apartness came from a fear that if they were open to the world they would become worldly. Now they want to relate to the world, to be involved in its problems. They wish honesty in their dealings with others; they know that often religious persons are dishonest, suspicious, and authoritarian. They see they have failed to reach people they work with, and know their approach to their apostolate is in need of change. The purpose of sensitivity training is to improve human relationships by making a person more perceptive of his own behavior and that of others, and by helping him remove hindrances to his relating to others. It is not surprising that religious persons are interested in these programs.

Here are the questions we need to ask and to answer. How does sensitivity training or any other "helping" program define its goals? Does it define them in vague terms, or does it specify what it can accomplish? Are the goals attainable? Does it promise lasting results in a short period of time, or does it have continuing, long-range program? Does it accept anyone who applies, or does it take only those applicants it has reasonable hope of helping? Does it refuse those who might be harmed? If it has criteria for accepting applicants, has it found by experience that the criteria are sound? Who conducts the programs? Is any professional background, any formal training required for those in charge? Can a person lead a program because he is a nice person, or because he has been a participant in a program, or has read about it? I know of an instance where a sister returned from a sensitivity program and convinced the community that she should run sensitivity training sessions for the other sisters. Another religious, not in any way connected with the training programs, received in a short time over a dozen requests from religious communities to lead sensitivity training groups.

What techniques are used in the programs? In evaluating these techniques I have drawn upon my experience and training as a psychiatrist and psychoanalyst. This does not mean that psychiatric treatment or psychoanalysis is the only way to help people, or that these treatments are suitable for everyone. There are many ways of helping people, but none of the methods which have proven beneficial disregard the essential requirements of the therapeutic relationship.

The structure and behavior of groups has been studied extensively by sociologists, anthropologists, social psychologists, psychiatrists, and psychoanalysts, and these studies have furnished some of the theoretical basis for the programs of the original training centers at the Tavistock Institute in London, and the Human Relations Laboratory at Bethel, Maine. In the years since their beginnings shortly after World War II, the theory and method of these organizations have been modified by various groups, so that it might be difficult to select any one as representative of the theory and practice. The program of one of these centers, the Esalen Institute in Big Sur, California, has had wide publicity and has been described by Clark Moustakas and William Schutz. Moustakas says:

> The purpose (of encounter groups) seems to be to face openly the forces of dissension, conflict, and general evil raging inside many people but rarely given opportunity for direct expression. The conviction is that straightforward, hostile tactics eventually lead to genuine, authentic transactions between persons, that direct attack and counter-attack, in a climate where the basic intention is honesty of self-expression, will result in compassion and intimacy. The ultimate aim is the development of a positive, loving, human relation. . . . From the depths of anger, rejection, and animosity, from

the revealing of personal guilt and torture, out of the combined forces of group life, individuals meet honestly and confront one another with conflict and resentment, as well as with tenderness and love.[2]

When individuals express their own convictions, beliefs, and feelings without defensiveness or facade, the usual, lengthy time arrangements are not required. Self-awareness, intimate contact with others, and trust are created suddenly and quickly rather than in a gradual, cautious way. . . . The alienated person is suffering; alone, he is unable to face his estrangement; but in a group, once the alienating thoughts, feelings, and mannerisms are out in the open, once they are met, recognized, and accepted or challenged, the individual begins to change; he moves in the direction of authentic presence, dialogue, and encounter. The established patterns and habits do not continue, because the alienated self has been honestly shared, and in sharing, an explosion occurs that dissipates the old connections and facilitates new relationships.[3]

Schutz describes the sensitivity training as removing the obstacles to realizing one's fullest potential: ". . . for feeling, for having inner freedom, and openness, for full expression of himself, for being able to do whatever he is capable of, and for having satisfying relations with others and with society."[4]

These authors state that the sensitivity training overcomes barriers to releasing feelings, barriers created by guilt, shame, embarrassment, fears of punishment, failure, success, or retribution. An encounter with another is a threat to many persons, and they handle the threat by various devices—withdrawal, aloofness, masks, roles. Their interpersonal relationships are not authentic; that is, they are not free from these defenses against closeness.

The sensitivity training groups are called T-groups ("training groups"), and a T-group numbers six to twelve people who are "normal" but wish to improve their relations with others. Although the stated purpose is to "train" and not to treat, and the method is not directed towards emotionally sick persons, there is usually no effort made to screen the participants. The participants meet for one or two weeks or a long weekend. The length and number of group sessions per day varies: there may be so-called marathon groups. Some groups exclude distractions such as television, radio, newspapers. There is no set agenda for a T-group; it takes as its agenda the interaction of the group and the feelings the members experience towards one another. It goes, so they say, in the direction in which its members take it. But the leader, called "trainer," is not necessarily passive; according to Schutz, he may be "silent, supportive, insightful. . . ." (p. 21). The T-groups use "free" association, dramatic techniques, elaboration of fantasies, dreams, and various types of exercises employing bodily motion and bodily contact.

They say that when the participants are able to express without reserve all of their thoughts and feelings about each other, a better relationship will result—that this change will occur during the short period of sensitivity training, it will be a lasting change, and it will give the person a new ability to make relationships. How the expression of feelings brings about change is not satisfactorily explained. The hodge-podge of explanations which Schutz culls from various sources shows no consistency, and when he uses psychoanalytic concepts to explain his methods, he shows a lack of understanding of these concepts. In one passage in his book Moustakas calls the change a miracle—". . . the miracle that happens when people are together—intimately, honestly—when they come to be sensitive and loving human beings" (p. 67).

Many of the things done in the T-groups bear a resemblance to the procedures of psychoanalysis. The writings of W. L. Bion, a psychoanalyst of the Tavistock Institute, on psychoanalytic groups have formed a basis for some of the sensitivity training programs.[5] However, Bion's theories of behavior have met with criticism.[6] A few psychiatrists and psychoanalysts have written favorably about these programs.[7,8] It may be that many persons have the idea that these programs are extensions of sound psychoanalytic theory and valid applications of psychoanalytic technique. As we will see, this is not the case.

You want to know: Is it sound? Is it safe? Does it work? What do religious hope to accomplish through sensitivity training? Are their hopes well founded?

Does it work? Something does happen. The seemingly unstructured setting provokes powerful feelings in the group members, and the trainer encourages the expression of these feelings. Participants are confronted with feelings others have about them, feelings which may never have been expressed before. They find themselves expressing feelings which they have never said, which they may not have been aware of. Others, they find, do not accept their feelings, attitudes, and motives. As a result of these interactions some change their feelings and attitudes.

Clinical experience is that it is unusual for a lasting personality change to occur this rapidly and under these circumstances. When Moustakas writes of not needing the "usual, lengthy time arrangements," I presume he refers to procedures which require long periods of time to produce permanent change. These procedures would include psychoanalysis and psychotherapy, education, and the cultural and political forces which produce change. Many are dissatisfied with the time and expense of treatment and educational methods, and wish for quicker means. But the repeated efforts of professionals from many fields have failed to produce quick results. The programs of sensitivity training offer no new information on how we can accomplish this.

The authors I have cited contend that the release of hostile feelings makes the person able to love. It seems to me that this view has its source in an "id psychology," that is, a psychology concerned only with the fate of impulses and not taking into account the ego, the part of the psychic apparatus which has among its many functions the control of impulse discharge and the mastery of conflicts. In every person there is the ambivalence of love and hate, an ambivalence which has its roots in unconscious conflicts. The release of feelings, or abreaction, which is the basis of the T-group encounters, does not affect these conflicts, and the unwanted feelings soon return. Because repression of feelings is often unhealthy, it does not follow that direct expression of those feelings is always healthy.

Total permissiveness regarding aggression is no more a solution of conflicts over aggression than is total permissiveness in sexual expression a solution to sexual conflicts. The manner of expressing, as well as the manner of repressing impulses has a great deal to do with determining what is healthy. Growth of a person is measured by his ability to control the discharge of his impulses in a fashion appropriate to his age and environment. Sometimes the most appropriate course is *not* to express feelings.

This naive idea—that repression is sick behavior whereas direct expression is healthy behavior—has taken root in some religious communities, and hostile incidents have occurred which would have been unthinkable in the past. A few years ago, for example, you would hardly have expected to find a community divided into two or three factions, where for weeks bitter denunciations and screaming insults were a daily occurrence. Some say that the religious has always had hostile and critical feelings, the only change is that she now says what she feels. She is open, and honest, and authentic. In the past she said things behind another's back; now she says them to her face. Or she expressed her hostile feelings in indirect and subtle ways; now she is more direct. Often a religious thought that she was a bad person if she had hostile thoughts. If her defense against these feelings was effective she would not admit the hostile thoughts into her consciousness and would have only kind thoughts about everyone. For some religious the new permissiveness has not really changed their attitudes, for they still feel the need to be rid of the evil, hostile thoughts, but now by expressing them directly. Then the good feelings will come. This is the message of the sensitivity programs, and it is no wonder it has a strong appeal for some persons. But does rudeness and crudeness mean honesty and sincerity? What does the discharge of hostile feelings do to the person who discharges them? One result can be a blunting of affects and a coarsening of the person. This seems to be the opposite of the sensitivity needed in community living, sensitivity to the other's weakness, respect for her defense. A loving relationship has tenderness and service and concern as part of it.

The release of hostile and aggressive feelings does make some of the T-group participants feel better. They have overcome barriers within themselves and the group has given them permission to say these forbidden thoughts. Not only has it given them this permission, but it has told them they are doing something healthy. This aspect of group functioning was noted by Freud in 1921 in his paper, "Group Psychology and the Analysis of the Ego."

> . . . in a group the individual is brought under conditions which allow him to throw off the repressions of his unconscious instinctual impulses. The apparently new characteristics which he then displays are in fact the manifestations of this unconscious, in which all that is evil in the human mind is contained as a predisposition. We can find no difficulty in understanding the disappearance of conscience or a sense of responsibility in these circumstances.[9]

The notion that the "joy" which comes after the release of pent-up feelings constitutes change is a sentimental, romantic, and superficial concept of change. Sentimental and romantic because it enthrones sentiment and ignores reality. "Let your feelings be your guide; do what your body says. If you do not, you cannot realize your potential for joy, openness, creativity." It is true that creativity, playfulness, and openness do involve elements of the irrational and the unconscious, but the use of these elements has to be disciplined, controlled.

A serious defect and danger of the method is that it directly attacks defenses which a person needs against anxiety. Schutz derives some of his ideas from Lowen, a follower of the early psychoanalyst Wilhelm Reich. When Reich published his *Character Analysis* in 1928 he made a notable contribution to the knowledge of psychopathology of character traits. Some character traits operate as defenses, so that they, like neurotic

symptoms, are ways of dealing with anxiety which comes from unconscious conflicts. A person with neurotic symptoms knows that they are
not normal. Yet he needs them in order to contain his anxiety. A person
who handles anxiety and guilt by formation of a character trait does not
experience this trait as something alien to his personality· or as irrational;
but he finds it useful. Examples are the traits of orderliness and thrift,
which even in excess can be put to practical use.

However, the inflexible nature of character traits makes a person less
free, less responsive, less creative. He may have difficulty getting close to
people, may keep feelings out of his awareness, and may lack spontaneity.
Reich called this state an "armoring" of character, and the sensitivity training advocates quite correctly point to this armor and to the masks people
assume as factors which prevent them from being open and responsive.

Since the character trait has served the person so well in controlling
his anxiety, and is often quite useful to him in his livelihood, he will see
little necessity for giving it up. He does not suffer, and he does not see
the personality distortions and limitations which may be apparent to his
friends. He does not seek treatment unless the character defenses break
down under stress. When he has treatment, change comes about quite
slowly. The psychoanalyst knows a good deal about treatment of the
person with this type of difficulty, for today he sees many more persons
with character disorders than the persons with acute neurotic disturbances
who were seen so frequently in the early days of psychoanalysis. And it is
possible that many who come to the T-groups do so because their character problems prevent them from becoming as involved with others as they
feel they should.

Reich's analysis of character was sound, but his technique of treatment was not. He advocated an assault on the character structure. His
approach was considered unsound many years ago, yet we find it reappearing in behavior therapy and in sensitivity training. People can be persuaded and intimidated and conditioned into giving up symptoms and
even character traits, but they gain no understanding of the conflicts
which led to the symptoms and traits. When the source of persuasion or
intimidation is removed, when the effect of conditioning weakens, the
symptom or trait may return, or the conflict may show itself in a new
symptom or trait. Or a person with a character disorder may reject these
approaches, even strengthen his defenses, when he fears that he might lose
them. But if his defenses are taken away and nothing replaces them, he
will become acutely disturbed.

Louis A. Gottschalk, a psychoanalyst, wrote about his experiences with sensitivity training, which included being part of a T-group in the Human Relations Laboratory in Bethel, Maine. In the T-group participants he saw psychotic and borderline psychotic reactions, depressions, severe emotional breakdowns with acute anxiety, sadistic and exhibitionistic behavior. He says:

> . . . the T-group sets up a powerful situation which is capable of evoking many kinds of dramatic reactions in individuals. Most of these reactions involve more than a mild exaggeration of the typical psychopathological traits of the participants.[10]

Redlich and Astrachan, both psychiatrists, have written:

> Such an experience usually is far from neutral. Quite frequently a number of participants become upset in this process; a few individuals whom we observed have become temporarily so upset that we had reason to call their behavior psychotic. Such responses in themselves testify to the powerful processes that occur in groups.[11]

Many persons who need to keep a tight control over their feelings have great fear of losing this control, and are threatened by sensitivity training. Gottschalk reports that persons who have good ego-strength and high self-esteem "survive the impact of unfolding and exposing their irrational and rational selves and getting stepped on or observing and participating in the harsh limit-setting of others."[12] Those who do not have good ego-strength and high self-esteem are frightened by their powerful unconscious feelings and they view loss of control as an explosive and destructive event. Further, loss of control diminishes the little self-esteem which they have. The directors of these programs seem to take little account of the dangers to emotional health. A number of the participants described by Schutz appeared disturbed: Rose who was phobic, Tom who had chronic stomach pains, Nora who had a "feeling of repulsion at her own body." In one place (p. 129) he describes some as "seriously disturbed people with identity problems, very rigid people. . . ."

Another source of the sensitivity training approach is the communications theory of interpersonal relations, which some have expressed as meaning that disturbed interpersonal relations are the result of faulty communication. This is an over-simplified view of the pathology of interpersonal relations. Aside from this, the claim that most persons in the T-groups have been able in a week or two to communicate, to understand the motivations and conflicts of one another, is completely misleading. The participants may talk readily, may say things about themselves and others which they have never said before. But they may be able to do so for many different reasons, one of which may be that they are playing a role. The role is that of a participant in a T-group and they are following the directions of the trainer and the cues given by other participants. Is this really communication? In psychoanalysis it takes a long time for revelation of any consequence to happen. This is so even though the psychoanalyst possesses skill in aiding the patient to reveal himself, the patient wants to communicate, and the technique and physical setting of psychoanalysis are carefully planned to provide the optimum conditions for this revealing.

It is important to know the qualifications of the trainer and the methods he uses. Gottschalk notes that the trainers come from many academic backgrounds, including education, psychology, philosophy, and psychiatry. He felt that "psychodynamic perceptiveness and comprehension" was wanting in the trainers he had observed. Trainers stress that the T-group experience is not treatment, but a learning experience. But in fact the results of the T-groups come about through techniques which are recognized elements of psychotherapy—discharge of feelings (abreaction), identifications with the group and the leader, persuasion, reassurance, and support. All of these techniques have very strong psychodynamic implications, especially the trainer's viewpoints on the expression of emotion and the pressure he exerts on the T-group participants to express their emotions and to change their attitudes and behavior.

Not only does the trainer expect the participants to express directly their emotions, but he points out emotions which he feels they are not expressing. For example, he may tell a participant that he is angry at the trainer or that he wants to dominate another participant. How reliable are these observations? How can the trainer or the participants be certain that they are due to the actual circumstances of the group and that they are not the product of the trainer's own imagination?

The pressure on the participants to change their behavior receives powerful reinforcement from the idealization of the trainer by the group, and by the reassurance that they can trust him. The laboratory at Bethel, Maine, has behind it the prestige of the National Education Association which sponsors it. Pressure also comes from the trainer's liberal use of techniques to belittle behavior and defenses which he does not consider appropriate. There are many examples of this in Schutz's and Moustakas' books.

The trainer misuses the most effective instrument that we possess for bringing about insight and true intrapsychic change. This is the interpretation of unconscious conflicts, and in particular those unconscious feelings which we call transference. Psychoanalysts define transference reactions as those unconscious feelings which the patient has toward his analyst, which do not in fact refer to the reality of the analyst, but to events and persons in the patient's life. Transference reactions occur in many other interpersonal situations besides psychoanalysis, and certainly occur in sensitivity training. The trainers regularly attempt to interpret these transference reactions. It takes the psychoanalyst years to master the technique of interpretation, and he himself needs a long and thorough personal analysis in order to understand his own conflicts which might interfere with his treatment of patients. None of this is required of the trainer. If it were, we might not see the clumsy, inexact and harmful use of interpretation which regularly occurs in T-groups. Not only does the trainer use this "wild" interpretation, but the group participants are encouraged to give their versions of the conflicts of other participants.

When the flow of words is slow, when the participants are unable to get to "honest confrontation," the trainer employs various devices to loosen up the participants. These sometimes involve bodily contact of both an affectionate and threatening nature. "Contact" is certainly made, but relating to another by means of bodily contact is a very over-determined way of relating, and it is often difficult to know just what the contact means to a particular person. For one thing it can be a very primitive and regressed way of relating. Bodily contact is the earliest way an infant relates, and it can be inappropriate for a group of adults. There is one technique, called the "crib" technique, in which an adult is cradled and rocked in the arms of several other adults, who may sing lullabies to him. Moustakas says:

> Discussions following this approach have often focused on maternal and paternal rejection and other experiences of rejection, both from the past and the present. Almost consistently, people emerge from this experience high, alive, feeling wonderful. The motion, the rhythm, the flow, the gentle rocking, all contribute to a sense of elation and peace.[13]

Other exercises are done to train the participants to trust one another, to break out of constricting habits and attitudes, and to express affection. It is difficult to believe that these can be seriously thought of as helpful, for they are caricatures of how people communicate and acquire important attitudes. One of the techniques is called "blind milling," and its purpose is to explore the nature of the other people. Here is how Schutz describes it:

> This can be done by having everyone stand up, shut his eyes, put out his hands and just start milling around the room. When people meet they explore each other in whatever way and for however long they wish. Slow accompanying music often enhances this experience. . . . Frequently its feeling is more general than individualized. That is, the experience is more significant for encountering the generalized other—the group—than it is in contacting individuals. For that reason, this method frequently enhances cohesive ties within a group. Moreover, it often sharpens awareness of the other people as human beings. If some individuals seemed of little interest before the blind milling, their identity and interest as people seem to be enhanced after it.[14]

Understanding an experience such as maternal rejection does not occur by playing these charades. When such understanding does come, it is because a person has experienced in a very personal fashion the many ways this maternal rejection has permeated his life. This working through, as it is called, takes time and an ability to judge one's self realistically. This is the very opposite of the naive viewpoint and methods of sensitivity training. The belief in the efficacy of these exercises must come from their having taken on a magic and ritualistic quality. Gottschalk remarks how similar to a religious experience he found the "confessing" that took place in T-groups; and we might add that the T-groups have other quasi-religious rituals. These encounters are nothing new. In 1832 Frances Milton Trollope, the mother of the English novelist Anthony Trollope, in her book *Domestic Manners of the Americans,* described a revival meeting in Cincinnati:

> When the room is full, the company, of whom a vast majority are always women, are invited, entreated, and coaxed to confess before their brothers and sisters all their thoughts, faults, and follies. These confessions are strange scenes: the more they confess, the more invariably are they encouraged and caressed.

Finally, these methods of verbal expression and bodily contact can provide occasion to gratify and to act out sexual and aggressive fantasies. I do not mean that this is necessarily the conscious intent of the trainer or the participants, but the descriptions of the group actions are filled with terms we usually use in describing impulse discharge. In a passage I quoted earlier in this paper, Moustakas described the "explosions" which occur. A few lines later he writes: "After the stormy explosions in a group, a glorious peace ensues, which brings with it a feeling of tenderness and communion."[15] In another place: "We were all exhausted (from the day-and-night struggle and exertion), but we were exhilarated."[16]

This is the language of the discharge of sexual and aggressive tensions, and of the effects which follow the release of these tensions. The group actions are an inducement to act out, and this is not therapeutic. Not only are they an inducement to act out, but the actions are rationalized so that persons who would not knowingly allow themselves direct gratification of these impulses feel assured that this is healthy and that it leads to better relationships. I think we should look beyond the rationalizations of the pushing, wrestling, massaging, embracing, and other forms of bodily explorations, and recognize what these experiences are.

Although participation in sensitivity training programs has helped some persons, the use of methods which do not take into account unconscious conflict and the defenses against anxiety, that misuse interpretation and provoke acting out, presents serious hazards. Many of the trainers have no more than a vague understanding of mental processes. In condemning overly rigid personality reactions, they have little appreciation of the importance of adequate structure and healthy defenses in psychic life. They are often not very clear on how one gains control of feelings and impulses, and seem to hold that simple discharge of feelings will lead to control.

According to Gottschalk, the persons who have high self-esteem and good ego strength benefit most from sensitivity training. These persons would probably benefit from almost any other kind of learning. Those who have told me that the T-groups were helpful were outgoing leaders who were always able to make good contact with others. The reasonable goals of sensitivity training—increased self-awareness and awareness of others, improved communication and empathy—are indeed worthwhile, and are not incompatible with the goals of dedicated religious. But we cannot say that emotional closeness, intimacy, and authentic encounters are necessary parts of religious love. These are concepts derived from the sciences which study human relationships, and not concepts of theology. Many persons are not psychologically capable of being open and authentic. Can we therefore say that they cannot possess genuine religious love?

Impulse gratification, release of feelings, intimacy, that come about through sensitivity training, may be exciting and perhaps meaningful for some, but they have no continuity with the reality of religious belief and love. Raymond Potvin, a sociologist, states that interpersonal relationship and communication on the affective plane are not the basis for a religious community except in a very limited sense.

> . . . On the one hand, there is the spiritual nature of the Mystical Body and its cultic dimensions which should help to create and express the Christian love binding all members. On the other, there is the sociological reality of limited, affective and communal relations. It would, however, be a fruitless task—not to say a theologically unsound one—to define this problem as one whereby supernatural charity must become translated into human emotion, or as one implying that the former is based exclusively on the latter. A person need not *feel* affection to have charity, nor need charity always express itself in a *social* relationship defined as affective. Christian love may impel a man to lend a helping hand to another, but this is a quite different phenomenon from "holding hands" for the sake of "holding hands." Though the temptation to unite the two expressions because of an appealing yet false idealism is great . . . this equation is frequently impossible. Again, as Harvey Cox insists, the good Samaritan did not form an I-Thou relationship with the man who fell among thieves. He bandaged his wounds, gave the innkeeper money to cover his expenses, and went on his way. Of such also is the unity of the people of God.[17]

Each religious who feels the need to change can be helped in ways that are best suited to her conflicts, her defenses, her goals, and her limitations. Some will be helped best by individual treatment, others by group therapy. Other methods may have to be worked out. Sherwyn M. Woods gives an example of the usefulness of a group process which recognized and respected the defenses of the participants, yet was sufficiently challenging that learning and change did occur. He worked with a small group of medical students to help them understand the psychology of sex, so that they could work more effectively with their patients. His aim was not only to give them knowledge of the attitudes and problems of their patients of various social classes, but to improve their communication and rapport with these patients, and to diminish their own anxieties which interfered with communication and rapport. Although the author did not consider these group sessions similar to T-groups, he felt they had elements in common with the T-groups and had achieved some of the results the T-groups try to obtain. Some of the students entered individual treatment (for which they had long recognized a need) because the experience in the group had helped them to overcome resistances to treatment.

. . . the experience was psychotherapeutic for some participants in that it resulted in a decrease in the anxiety, guilt, and shame they had experienced in their own sexual lives. This was an indirect effect of the group experience, which in no way attempted to focus upon any single individual or to directly assist him in exploring or working through a particular problem.[18]

Woods writes that the common personality pattern of the medical student is an obsessive compulsive one, and that they

rarely suffered from major psychiatric syndromes and in general struggled with characterological problems and conflicts that did not seriously interfere with their capacity to effect a successful general adjustment, achieve success in medical school, and maintain an outwardly poised and confident manner.[19]

But, he goes on to say, their capacity to establish an alliance with their patients and to be sufficiently flexible was limited.

The religious may be similar to the medical student in many respects, particularly regarding character structure. I have written about my own efforts in working with religious,[20] and found it close to the experience Woods describes. I met with a group of sister candidates every week for two years, and my goals were to help them to be aware of their attitudes towards their life and towards each other. I did not introduce topics, or force them to disregard their defenses, but I tried to help them understand the conflicts which resulted in the feelings they expressed. The discussions were not group psychotherapy, were not focused on any individual's emotional conflicts as such, yet they were helpful. Several sisters recognized their need for psychotherapy, and others decided that they should not continue in religious life. This way of looking at their attitudes was carried over to their other discussions and meetings.

There is a need for programs such as this and the one Woods describes, programs in which the group leader will not simply encourage the participants to discharge their feelings in the hope that something good will come of the discharge, but programs in which the leader is at the service of the ego of the participants. These should not be primarily didactic sessions, but there should be an affective interchange which challenges each, yet respects the defenses and the self-esteem of all. Perhaps in this way the religious can realize some of her very worthwhile aims and avoid the harm and disappointment which can result from unsuitable fads and methods.

230 *Hope: Psychiatry's Commitment*

REFERENCES

1. Sheehan, Frank X., "Sensitivity Training and Religious Life," *Sisters Today*, Vol. 40, April 1969, pp. 409-413.
2. Moustakas, Clark, *Individuality and Encounter*, Howard A. Doyle Publishing Co., Cambridge, Mass.: 1968, p. 45.
3. Moustakas, Clark, *ibid.*, p. 54.
4. Schutz, William, *Joy: Expanding Human Awareness*, New York, The Grove Press, 1967.
5. Bion, W. L., *Experiences in Groups*, London: Tavistock Publications, 1961.
6. Sherwood, Michael, "Bion's Experiences in Groups: A Critical Evaluation. *Human Relations*, Vol. 17, May 1964, pp. 113-130.
7. Frank, Jerome, "Training and Therapy," in *T-Group Theory and Laboratory Method*, L. P. Bradford, J. R. Gibbs, K. D. Benne, eds., New York, John Wiley & Sons, 1964.
8. Whitman, R. W., "Psychodynamic Principles Underlying T-Group Processes," in *T-Group Theory and Laboratory Method.*
9. Freud, S., *Group Psychology and the Analysis of the Ego*. The complete psychological works of S. Freud, Standard Edition, London, The Hogarth Press, 1955, p. 74.
10. Gottschalk, L. A., "Psychoanalytic Notes on T-Groups at the Human Relations Laboratory, Bethel, Maine," *Comprehensive Psychiatry*, Vol. 7, 1966, p. 475.
11. Redlich, F. C., and Astrachan, B., "Group Dynamics Training, *American Journal of Psychiatry*, Vol. 125, May 1969, p. 1056.
12. Gottschalk, *Op. Cit.*, p. 486.
13. Moustakas, *Op. Cit.*, pp. 87-88.
14. Schutz, *Op. Cit.*, p. 124.
15. Moustakas, *Op. Cit.*, p. 55.
16. Moustakas, *Ibid.*, p. 67.
17. Potvin, Rev. R. H., "The Liturgy and Community: A Sociological Approach," in *Experiments in Community*, The Liturgical Conference, Washington, D.C., 1967, pp. 91-92.
18. Woods, S. M., "A Course for Medical Students in the Psychology of Sex: Training in Sociocultural Sensitivity." *American Journal of Psychiatry*: Vol. 125, May 1969, p. 1517.
19. Woods, *Ibid.*, p. 1517.
20. Reidy, Joseph J., "The New Community and Personal Relationships," *Review for Religious*, Vol. 28, May 1969, pp. 383-392.

17

J. COTTER HIRSCHBERG, M.D.

It seems particularly appropriate that this paper on the factors which enter into the effective living of Sisters in a Community be part of a volume honoring Leo H. Bartemeier, M.D., since the ideas in it reflect two aspects of Doctor Bartemeier himself: his religious values and his psychoanalytic knowledge.

Doctor Bartemeier has been a friend and mentor over these many years, and I have learned from him and I hope I have also absorbed a part of his way of viewing life. He is a man of great warmth in his understanding, and of great understanding in his warmth. He combines a breadth and depth of knowledge with a sense of humanity and has the rare ability to share all this in his teaching. He is indeed "a man for all seasons."

Religious Communities: Psychological Factors

IT IS SIGNIFICANT that this paper originally evolved as part of a discussion on "Sister Formation" that occurred as part of an Institute for Mental Health given under the joint auspices of St. John's University and St. Benedict's College in Minnesota, since Doctor Bartemeier has for many years been a member of the Board of Directors of this Institute and an active participant in a great number of the sessions themselves. Novice Mistresses and Mother Superiors from all areas of this country worked diligently with a panel of priests, sisters, and psychiatrists to understand the psychological factors which come from a high sense of religious faith and spiritual motivation which is so basic to the group formation and the total task which a Community serves.

In thinking together about those elements which make for stable

231

and effective group living among women, one notes that there are several factors which contribute to a successful adjustment.

First, effective living within the group of Sisters means that each individual has a clear and unequivocal *sense of responsibility* toward the group as a whole. There can be *no* meaningful relationships without the acceptance of certain obligations, duties, and rules. Healthy relationships between people are built upon inescapable and necessary responsibilities. Group membership requires a participating experience and this does not mean freedom from responsibility; it means freedom within limits; it means an opportunity to conform as well as to differ; it means the gaining of a clearly marked group identity. Each member uses the group as a setting to search for and to find stable identification and ideals; as a place to ask what life is about, what she can receive from it, what she must contribute to it, and how to become a part of the Community and the world. Eventually such integration helps her to think not only of herself but of others, to be tolerant, and to be able to see herself as one of a group while still feeling that she has her own life to lead. To achieve this maturity, the conflict between her wishes and the reality of external and internal standards must be resolved without sacrificing completely either the satisfaction for wishes and needs, or the ethical ideals. The wishes of each member do *not* require that they be either directly gratified or repressed; they can be achieved indirectly through sublimations and accomplishments.

Toward this end the Order and each member are all working so that out of learning and working and loving and being loved, one becomes part of a Community. By experiencing frustration and by experiencing the satisfaction of independent activity, each member not only tests her own adequacy, but she learns to deal with a world of reality instead of one of imagination. The Community performs its function by not allowing an individual within it to impulsively test herself beyond her capacity instead of working toward achievable goals.

To take on inappropriate responsibility makes maturity not a stable achievement, but a tenuously accomplished and therefore easily lost and frightening fact. Appropriate responsibility leads to Community recognition of a capacity to work and brings about a healthy continuity between the inner conception of self and outside recognition. Out of this comes a feeling of being understood that enables her to understand herself better and to function on her own. One's work thus brings maturity and the eventual sense of adequacy as a woman, secure in herself, yet flexible within the group. It is out of this awareness of mutual responsibility that the group creates its security and that the group also serves to absorb the temporary periods of anxiety which an individual within the group may sustain. This sense of total purpose, this awareness of the *process* that enters into Community life is what maintains Community life during the inevitable periods of discord and disagreement.

This leads us to an immediate awareness of the second factor necessary for successful group living: namely, the capability of the group as a whole and of each of the Sisters *to allow and accept expressions of anger and hostility*. When one brings together necessarily a group of women having individual differences in backgrounds and in values, it is to be expected that conflict will occur and anger inevitably arise. One has to give up the illusion that there is such a thing as a perfect Sister, or a perfect Community. One also has to give up any tendency to suffer too much. Although the expression of anger needs to be allowed, this does not mean that the origin of it should not be actively explored. Too often anger is used as a psychological tool to manipulate one another, and this sort of "testing" needs to be examined for what it is. One does not allow anger to obscure examining the consequences of action.

An example which illustrates this point can be found in the Novice Mistress or the Mother Superior who "for the sake of peace and harmony" does not make the rules and the procedures of the Community crystal clear, and also does not establish clearly that violation of these rules will call for consequences that are equally fully known ahead of time by all. True freedom within a Community exists when each member knows that she is required to follow certain procedures consistently and that she must recognize those limits to her behavior which the function and the welfare of the total group require of each member. When one is uncertain about limits, one tends to test the extent of the behavior allowed. If when one unconsciously tests in this fashion, the limits are variable and inconsistent, then one becomes anxious and constricted. True freedom exists within limits; it is not anarchy.

Anger is not a reason to obscure facing each member of the group with what the reality is, since anger itself is only one aspect of a reality and not a threat to it. One does not allow any member of a group to use anger for the purpose of playing on the guilt of others or for playing the game of "who takes the blame this time." When one tries to ignore or escape from these inevitable differences of opinion, or of interest, one does so at the price of becoming submissive to others and at the price of ignoring or escaping from one's own sense of individuality and dignity. Without the expression of anger, without the expression of resentment, it is impossible for the Sisters really to know each other, and really to meet each other's important and realistic needs. When anger cannot be expressed, it too often means that there exist unresolved and unhealthy sustained dependency struggles rather than the mutual acceptance of realistic and shared needs and abilities.

The third of these factors is a *mutual fulfillment of normal dependency needs* that comes when Sisters living together strive to create the kind of climate where each member of the Order can feel relaxed and can experience within the group sufficient emotional security to be able to express honestly what her feelings and needs are. When this expression of her own feelings is accepted on a realistic level, each individual Sister is able to become a more effective adult.

One does not ask that each individual Sister repress and deny the feelings that she may have about any particular incident or about any particular behavior which she may or may not like. Rather, one hopes that each Sister will express whatever her feeling is so that the group as a whole not only allows the expression of the feeling, but is also able to absorb it. The group as a whole can also examine the situation fully and come to a consensus. In this way a Sister can realize when her own feeling is inappropriate to the occasion, or when the intensity of her feeling is beyond that which is warranted by the event. The group as a whole makes it clear how the rest of the Sisters feel as a Community, and thus provides a "base-line" for a sense of comfortable belongingness.

If the group members have an accurate awareness of the strengths and weaknesses of each other, the expectations which each has will be based on a realistic appraisal of what each Sister can do and be. There will be no magical expectations of perfect success and no fears of total failure. Adaptation to any situation is always a relative matter. Each of us succeeds to a certain degree and each of us fails in a certain measure. It is the achievement of more successes than failures which casts the balance on the side of good mental health.

Further, each person varies in his ability to cope with the tasks facing him. Each of us has our good days, and each of us has our poor days. One's adaptation must be evaluated over a span of time in order to express any judgment about succeeding or failing. Moreover, although each of us is able to be an effective adult most of the time, one must allow leeway for feelings of doubt and feelings of inadequacy about oneself, since each person must from time to time cope with such feelings.

Growth comes to each Sister as an individual when doubts and feelings of inadequacy are not cause for depression, but are seen as "signals" which say to the Sister that she is struggling with conflicts within herself and needs to explore the causes and the meanings of such internalized conflicts. Through this *use* of doubt and this *use* of feelings of uncertainty, the Sister gains a method for achieving personality growth. When such feelings say to the Sister: "Be aware that you have a struggle within yourself about this; examine what it is that troubles you, or that causes doubts, or that has resulted in feelings of inadequacy; use this moment to understand yourself more completely, not to berate yourself or to bemoan or to give yourself over to the luxury of depression."

There are occasions when it is necessary for an individual to feel temporarily helpless without feeling threatened and without feeling a loss of self-esteem because of it. Moreover, each of us has to be able to take a protective and even caring role for another when necessary. Sisters must know each other well enough to react to each other's needs, must allow for fluctuations of capacity without any sense of blame, while at the same time having realistic expectations of another's abilities.

All of this brings us to the fourth element essential to creating healthy Community life: the existence of a level of *self-sufficiency* within each of the Sisters. The Community itself can help the Sister achieve self-sufficiency by mapping out clear areas of specific responsibility for each Sister so that competition with each other is not built into the system itself. One wants to create a structure which makes rivalry inappropriate instead of allowing rivalry to become a part of a setting.

Too often when individuals live together in a group, they hope to gain esteem or to increase self-regard by unconsciously taking over the duties or the functions of another group member. The Community which makes the assignment of responsibility clear cut, and which respects the "territoriality" of the responsibilities of each Sister, is the Community in which succeeding by doing someone else's job becomes inappropriate rather than rewarding.

Competition should not be necessary to enhance relationships; yet one often can observe that a rivalry is created between two people in order to enhance the relationship of one of them with a third and usually superior authority figure. This kind of rivalry leads to childish dependency and not to the kind of normal effective reliance on each other that enhances the Sisterhood.

When one feels self-sufficient and has resolved childish dependency needs, then one is not caught in the bind of needing to idealize those in authority, as one in earlier childhood idealizes the mother. Self-sufficiency allows for objective appraisal and a realistic evaluation of those who exercise authority. One then needs neither to idealize nor to exclude an awareness of shortcomings. By this process a feeling of helplessness in group living is avoided. This permits the realization that no individual is absolutely necessary, that one is not helpless, and that one can indeed think and function on one's own. However, self-sufficiency should not be confused with a feeling of omnipotence.

Each member of the group, and particularly those in authority, need to avoid promising more than they can give or do, thinking they can handle more than they can, assuming more power than they really have, feeling that they can control too many variables, and allowing themselves to be spread too thin. What needs to be evaluated is the actual strength of each one in each particular situation since what is possible at one time may not be possible at another. Being self-sufficient does not require assuming that an individual can always function equally well, or can do the same level of functioning at all times. A self-sufficient person can expect each day to bring its own reward and she can avoid the need to dream that the next day will always be better.

And fifth, and last, healthy, effective group living among women requires *an acceptance of a sense of loneliness* and an awareness of the values that loneliness can bring. The experience of being a part of a group has to allow for the experience of feeling one's own individuality, and has to allow for moments in which the individual can be alone and use this apartness to deepen one's self-awareness. Loneliness helps one avoid the tendency to overintellectualize one's relationships and to obscure their emotional impact.

It is so easy to do that which is apparently the most comfortable and overlook the *relationship* meaning of the act itself. It is equally easy to be satisfied with one explanation of a problem in a situation that has multiple causes. Being alone gives one the opportunity to discover one's own small areas of intolerance rather than seeing them as "a natural opinion," the feelings of any "normal person." When one is alone one can ask the question: Is this difficulty or problem "bad," or is it just disturbing to me *personally?* Being alone with one's thoughts helps us to avoid hasty generalizations, to avoid seeing others as stereotypes, as "all good" or "all bad." It is out of the experience of *separation,* and the consequent experience of reunion, that further individuation and growth occur. One has to have time to one's self in order to commune with God, in order to know the nature of relationship with others, and in order to understand commitment to others and to one's self. A coherent and sustaining way of life is gained not only from one's group but also from the sense of faith which emerges in clarity from the experience of loneliness and from the need for increased communication and sharing which is the healthy result that an experience of loneliness brings.

Effective group living requires a simultaneous awareness of *stability* and *transition* and of the interconnection between these two elements which allows progress. Each member of the group has a responsibility for understanding the tested old truths and also the responsibility for seeking new truths in the emerging patterns of change.

A sense of responsibility toward the group must always be an *evolving achievement*. It has become vividly clear that we do not live in a stationary society, where the solutions of one generation are adequate to the problems of the next. Instead we face an open future, determined in part by our own knowledge and our own decision, but also in part by decisions still to be made which will commit us to new responsibilities not yet perceived. It is this very transition that requires of us a comfortable solidarity with the tradition to which we belong, a tradition that has itself been evolved by women who were able to welcome a higher level of human value and human functioning, even when this required the necessary changing of former values that could not continue unaltered.

However, changing one's values does not mean creating marginal people who try to stand clay-footed in both the old and the new, yearning vainly to accept both but ultimately believing in neither. The Community is not "on trial"; it is undergoing change and our best achievement as a member of an Order will come from a confidence in the worth of the Order and in our own worth as a member of a group in whose traditions and values we are intimately associated and confidently believe.

These are five of the elements which combine together to make for stable and effective group living among women. A group experience does not merely require maturity; a group experience in itself brings about important achievements in maturation and growth.

Part III

Section Two

SECULAR SOCIETY

We live in a time of revolution. Hope causes unrest—makes man dissatisfied with the gulf between present realities and future possibilities. Hope points to what has been called "the unfulfilled present."

In his article chronicling "Advances in Administration in Psychiatry," Dr. Walter Barton describes the ways in which psychiatry has attempted to "fulfill" the present—to come up with viable solutions to a succession of social problems. In "Civil Disobedience and Urban Revolt," Dr. Gene Usdin offers psychiatric insights on many of the crises besetting society today—especially those generated by the complex younger generation alternately operating as a force for renewal and an atavistic scourge. Dr. Eugene B. Brody, in "Project HOPE," records an enterprise which suggests that man, through his ability to symbolize, may achieve a modicum of peace and harmony. Doctors Kaufman, Romano, and Lemkau all concern themselves with the interrelationships between the physician, the medical school, the student, and the community as a whole—with Dr. Lemkau stressing the necessity for medicine to minister to the whole man, Dr. Romano discussing feasible interaction between the medical school and the community, and Dr. Kaufman pinpointing the obligation of the medical educator for instilling in his students the capacity for social criticism. Throughout the last three essays can be heard Chaucer's poor parson's sturdy avowal of moral and professional responsibility:

If gold rust,
What shall iron do?

18

WALTER E. BARTON, M.D.

To Leo Bartemeier who, as friend, and counselor, played such an important role in my own career development. Dr. Bartemeier made significant contributions to the history of administrative psychiatry and the form of psychiatry's organizations.

Advances in Administration in Psychiatry During the Past Fifty Years

THE GIANT STRIDES made in the administration of psychiatric hospitals have almost all been taken in the last fifty years. The genesis of many of these advances, however, may most often be discovered in the latter half of the nineteenth century. And—to any but the historian— these origins were not always salubrious. Rather they themselves were the short-range effects of tumultuous and temporarily adverse changes taking place in our society. Paradoxically, their ultimate consequences attest to man's equilibrium-seeking impulses, which, over the ages, have so richly justified students of human nature in their persistent hope for the human race.

BEFORE THE 1920'S

Fifty years ago, most psychiatrists were engaged in institutional practice. The pressures of immigration, industrialization, and urbanization had greatly changed mental hospitals. Gone were the small mental hospitals of the mid-nineteenth century that cared for 120 patients; they had given place to large institutions that housed more than 1,500 persons. Inevitably, the superintendent's personal concern with individual patients

241

had to give way to the problems of administering a complex social institution.[1]

Institutional psychiatrists, for the most part frustrated and pessimistic about what they could do for hospital patients, were, nevertheless, excited about the prospects the future offered. Neuropathologists like Alzheimer, Huntington, and Pick were increasing the understanding of organic brain disorders; microbiologist Noguchi had discovered the *treponema pallidum* in the brains of patients who had died from central nervous system syphilis. Sherrington, Pavlov, and Cannon were adding to the understanding of the physiological basis of emotions, and psychologists Binet and Thorndike were developing tools for measuring intelligence.[2] Adolf Meyer was expounding a unified theory of psychobiology that embraced all the new knowledge, and was teaching that nature could be altered to meet man's needs and that man could transform himself.[3] Psychiatrists were beginning their long struggle to emerge from the isolation of mental hospitals.

The Era of Social Rejection

The way the mentally ill are treated is largely determined by the way society reacts to them. The administrative policies of hospitals respond to social pressures. Early in this century, vast numbers of immigrants were pouring into the country. These immigrants, in addition to the normal stresses of life, had to bear the special stresses of unemployment, loneliness, and the difficulties of adjusting to a new culture, probably to a new language. A non-income producing sick member in a household could upset the delicate economic balance necessary for the survival of the immigrant family. Thus, a mentally unbalanced family member would be sent to the state hospital to give the rest of the family a better chance to succeed in the New World. The foreign-born, added to the other indigent mentally ill, filled and quickly overcrowded public mental hospitals. Society wished to care for those aliens as cheaply as possibly; as a result, the institutions were underfinanced.

With too many patients and not enough money and staff to care for them properly, it was not surprising that the belief spread that mental illness was incurable. Even professional psychiatrists subscribed to that idea, and their conviction, added to the public belief, led to diminished support for state mental hospitals. The optimism that had prevailed half a century earlier in the era of moral treatment and the extraordinary recoveries it produced gave way to pessimism and therapeutic nihilism.

To control disturbance, to prevent violence and self-destruction, and to reduce the annoyance to society became the mission of the hospitals, and those who threatened to disrupt the family and community were extruded from society and incarcerated in these hospitals. People increasingly relied on the state to accept total responsibility for the mentally ill and the retarded.

The hospitals controlled disturbance and violent behavior by the use of hydrotherapy, physical or chemical restraint, and isolation. The very disturbed were controlled by the use of wet-sheet packs; they were wrapped in a cocoon of sheets wrung out in cold water and insulated with blankets to retain the body heat that developed in response to the cold. The method induced somnolence. Others, not so truculent, were placed in a so-called continuous tub, a bath fitted with a canvas cover through which only the patient's head protruded; flowing warm water ran continuously through the tub and this, in a darkened room, was quieting and relaxing.

Whenever a patient became dangerous to others (interpreted loosely in practice to mean destructive or assaultive, and sometimes noisy or obnoxious behavior), a physician would sign an order for seclusion, and the patient would be confined alone in a "strong room" with a locked door. Physicians also prescribed restraint which consisted of putting a patient into a camisole—a canvas jacket that enclosed the folded arms and laced in the back. Alternatively, the patient would be spread-eagled on a bed and held down by sheets tied to his wrists, ankles, and around his chest. A patient who was suicidal or tried to injure himself would be restrained in his bed. It was not uncommon for depressed patients to be tied up for weeks or months. When a nurse was available, she would release them for bathing, massage, toileting, and meals.

Sometimes, restraining sheets would be tied around a patient seated in a chair, and today, in the American Psychiatric Museum in Washington, D.C., you can see a restraining chair that was used at McLean Hospital, Belmont, Massachusetts, before the turn of the century. Chair restraint was used for elderly or confused patients, or for those who were unsteady on their feet and might fall and injure themselves if they walked about without supervision.

Nurses prided themselves on the kindly, sympathetic care they gave patients. Anyone who abused patients was punished if it was discovered. Psychiatrists would prescribe periods of work and recreation for patients able to function at all. Most work assignments were designed to help the operation of the understaffed hospitals and included working in the farm, dairy, kitchen, scullery, laundry, or boiler room, shoveling coal, removing trash, or serving as household servants in staff quarters.

In 1919, the American Medico-Psychological Association, now the American Psychiatric Association, met in Philadelphia on its seventy-fifth anniversary. The April 1919 issue of the *American Journal of Insanity* (now the *American Journal of Psychiatry*) showed that the program of the meeting was devoted to administering hospitals and the problems of central state agency control. Because of the increasing reliance on state funds, it was becoming necessary to develop a system for managing state hospitals. Owen Copp, of Philadelphia, read a paper that detailed what the relationships of a mental hygiene division should be within a state department of public welfare.[5] James May, of Boston, explained the functions of a new type of facility called a psychopathic hospital.[6] E. A. Strecker, of Philadelphia, outlined the treatment of war neuroses as it existed at the end of World War I.[7]

Before 1920, most mental hospitals were located on the outskirts of town, where Kirkbride said they should be. In the 1850's Kirkbride had written detailed standards for the construction of mental hospitals.[8] Those standards had been institutionalized by the codes of the original Association of Medical Superintendents of American Institutions for the Insane. Those who believe that mental hospitals were originally built to keep patients out of sight and out of mind should read the early literature to understand the reasoning of these humane physicians.

Kirkbride recommended that mental hospitals be built about two miles out-of-town, but be easily accessible by turnpike or railroad so that labor and supplies could readily be brought in. A suitable site was chosen, about 200 acres for 200 patients, so that farm gardens and a viable farm could be created to supply nourishing food, fresh country air, and wholesome outdoor work for patients in the predominantly agricultural economy of that time.

Today, a Kirkbride building looks forbidding because of its iron-barred windows and heavy doors with strong locks.[9] The admission wards were in front of the building, close to the administrative services. Food and housekeeping services were in the central part of the building. From the administrative and admission core, the lateral wings of the buildings extended in either direction. The quiet patients were housed closest to the administrative center on "parole" or open wards. Noisy, untidy, and destructive patients were banished to the most remote or back wards of each wing.

In Kirkbride's day, a good hospital was shiningly clean. Its waxed floors had a high polish, burnished by patients who paced back and forth pushing a huge, heavy block of wood, called a swab, covered with carpet, and mounted on a long handle. Back wards had heavy wooden benches in the day halls and rows of seclusion rooms off wide central corridors. Those single-occupancy rooms were often unfurnished except for an "indestructible" mattress on the floor or sometimes on an iron cot.

But the winds of change kept blowing, and in 1905, Peoria (Illinois) State Hospital had opened its doors, removed all bars and gratings from windows and doors, and instituted the 8-hour day. For a time, women aides were allowed to work on all male wards, but for some reason that practice was abandoned in 1909.[10]

In 1906, the first psychopathic hospital was opened in Ann Arbor, Michigan; during the same year Goddard introduced the Binet-Simon Test into this country, J. H. Pratt began group therapy in Boston, and the Flexner Report on medical education called for higher standards in medical schools.[11] In 1908, the Toronto General Hospital established neuropathic wards.[8]

In 1909, Freud spoke at Clark University in Worcester, Massachusetts, and won the greatest support for his views given him anywhere in the world. In the same year, Clifford Beers established the National Association for Mental Hygiene, now known as the National Association for Mental Health.

In 1910 came Adolf Meyer's introduction of psychobiology, and in 1911, Noguchi discovered *treponema pallidum*, the cause of syphilis; also in 1911, Lashley and Liddell began experiments with animals which showed the importance of early mothering.

In 1912, Boston State Hospital opened a psychopathic division as a community facility for outpatient treatment, training, and research. In several years this division gained fame and became a separate institution known as the Boston Psychopathic Hospital, today called the Massachusetts Mental Health Center.

In 1913, the Phipps Psychiatric Institute in Baltimore and the Psychopathic Divison of the Boston State Hospital opened the first clinics for disturbed children, and Douglas Thom in Boston established a habit clinic for the "study and treatment of behavior problems of infancy and childhood." Earlier, however, in 1909, William Healy had founded the Juvenile Psychopathic Institute in connection with the juvenile court in Chicago.[12]

In 1916, Henry M. Hurd published a monumental description of psychiatric institutions in the United States and Canada. And in 1919, the beginning of our 50-year period, E. E. Southard advocated social psychiatry. Psychiatry had taken notice of the lessons World War I offered, lessons that were to have a tremendous impact over the next half-century. Not only was psychiatric screening necessary, it was also feasible for the armed forces; the emotionally unstable could not tolerate unusual stress; mental disorders in wartime were enormously costly, and psychiatric facilities should be a regular component of military medical care.

THE 1920's—SOME SCIENTIFIC DEVELOPMENTS

Early in the 1920's, the United States, reacting to the threat of an even greater flood of immigrants from the countries of war-ravaged Europe, passed a restrictive immigration law, establishing a quota of 2 per cent of the number of immigrants who arrived in 1890. That curb on immigration would reduce pressure on public hospitals.

The 1921 Washington Naval Disarmament Conference reflected society's determination to outlaw war by declaring a 10-year moratorium on naval construction, and in 1928, the United States joined with 62 other nations in signing the Kellogg-Briand Pact to outlaw war. During these years, the bootlegger, the prohibition agent, the speakeasy, and home brew appeared on the national scene as a result of the 18th Amendment which became effective in 1920. For the next 13 years, until its repeal in 1933, the slogan was "See America Thirst."

In 1928, thanks to the work of Goldfarb and Spies, it became possible to conquer an important mental illness, pellagra psychosis, that was characterized by the triad—diarrhea, dementia, and death. Primary prevention through proper diet also became possible. [13]

In 1924, St. Elizabeth's Hospital in Washington, D.C. applied malarial therapy for general paresis. In 1918, Wagner von Jauregg in Vienna had found that high fever was effective in destroying the *treponema pallidum* spirochetes which caused the illness. This was of great significance to hospital psychiatry because 12 per cent of all the patients they admitted at that time suffered from syphilis of the central nervous system.

In 1920, Freud's "Introduction to Psychoanalysis" elicited a comment from G. Stanley Hall on the growing impact in the United States of psychoanalysis on literature, history, biography, sociology, anthropology, education, and religion. Freud's contributions profoundly affected American psychiatry; they opened up the possibility of understanding dreams with their incoherent acts and symbolisms, and brought knowledge of the unconscious mind, of personality structure, of normal and abnormal mental mechanisms, and made it possible to interpret deviant sexuality.

In his Presidential Address to the American Psychiatric Association in 1921,[14] Owen Copp noted that standardization in hospital administration and construction and rigid adherence to the codes written in the 1850's had restricted initiative and creative experimentation. The number of public institutions had increased from 26 in 1844, when the Association was founded, to more than 500. The number of patients had increased, during the same period, from 3,000 to 235,000, and the cost of their care from $500,000 to $56 million a year. In New York and Massachusetts, Dr. Copp noted the cost amounted to one-eighth of the total cost of state government. He said that treatment initiated at the time of hospitalization was too late in the course of the illness to be effective, and called for better preparation of all physicians and nurses to work with the mentally ill. He called for more laboratories and diagnostic resources so that early recognition would result; finally, he called for the establishment of metropolitan and district psychopathic hospitals of 100-200 beds. He reminded the membership of about 1,000 that recoveries and discharge rates had declined below 10 per cent in many institutions, and commented that many psychiatrists believed that less than 5 per cent of schizophrenic patients could be expected to recover.[15]

Significant general events in the decade of the twenties included the 19th Amendment, which allowed women to vote, and became effective in 1920. By 1921, radio was beginning to develop as a mass communication medium. The Teapot Dome Scandal, which reached a boil in 1923 after the death of President Harding, was already brewing in 1922 when Harding's Secretary of the Interior leased the Teapot Dome oilfields in Wyoming without competitive bidding.

In 1923, Thomas W. Salmon became the first President of the American Psychiatric Association who was not a hospital superintendent.

In 1927, Lindbergh became the first man to fly across the Atlantic Ocean to Paris. In 1929, the Great Depression began with bank failures, foreclosures, and idle factories. Within a few months, 50 per cent of all voluntary hospital beds were empty. It was during this crisis that prepayment financing or hospital insurance by Blue Cross was born.

THE 1930's—NOT ALL WAS BLACK

As the new decade began, the United States and the rest of the world were still in the grip of the Great Depression. President Herbert Hoover declared a moratorium on war reparations and established the Reconstruction Financing Corporation. In 1933, under the new President, Franklin

D. Roosevelt, a multitude of government programs came into being in attempts to control the economy. They were known chiefly by their initials: FERA (Federal Emergency Relief Administration), NRA (National Recovery Act), CCC (Civilian Conservation Corps), PWA (Public Works Administration), and WPA (Works Progress Administration).

In 1932, drought in the southwest drove the Okies from their native Oklahoma to California. The one bright spot in the early 1930's was the repeal of Prohibition by the welcomed 20th Amendment.

It became easy for the mental hospitals to fill their staff vacancies, and for once, every authorized position was filled by physicians, nurses, and other mental health professionals. Under PWA, much needed new mental hospital buildings were erected, and the WPA supplied gangs of workers, financed by federal funds, to work on hospital projects.

Most of the knowledge available about mental illness concerned patients confined in institutions. Psychiatry was mainly based on Kraepelin's *Medical Psychology*. Treatment, in most institutions, consisted of control and restraint by physical and chemical means, although there were lively discussions about non-restraint. Important therapeutic modalities in some hospitals were habit-training, hydrotherapy, and occupational therapy.

Both the mental hygiene movement and psychoanalysis were gaining adherents. The social significance of mental illness was appreciated and public education programs began. Psychoanalytic therapy had but little impact on mental hospital administration; psychoanalysts felt they could not help patients with organic brain disorders, schizophrenia, and manic-depressive psychoses, the principal types of disorders found in hospitalized patients.

On the advice of my professor of psychiatry, H. Douglas Singer, I went to Worcester State Hospital in 1931 for my training in psychiatry. Under the leadership of William A. Bryan (1921-1940), Worcester was regaining the position of leadership it had held nearly a century earlier. Bryan's concept of administration emphasized patient treatment, staff education, research, and ties with the community. He surrounded himself with such men as R. G. Hoskins, Francis Sleeper, Clifton T. Perkins, D. Ewen Cameron, Andras Angyal, David Shakow, John Dollard, Geza Roheim, and many others. The aura of excitement, innovation, and change that resulted came at a time when most public hospitals were still stressing custodial care.[1]

At Worcester, we introduced group therapy, greatly extended occupational and industrial therapy, and established a child guidance clinic at a time when few existed. Dr. Bryan was the first to introduce the cafeteria system to improve hospital feeding practices. His classic book, *Administrative Psychiatry*,[16] was published in 1936, and captures the essence of the progressive program I had the good fortune to enter.

As a new resident, I was apprenticed to senior physicians and psychiatrists to learn-by-doing under their corrective and supportive guidance. My principal textbooks were Hart's *Psychology of Insanity*,[17] White's *Outlines of Psychiatry*,[18] Bleuler's *Textbook of Psychiatry*,[19] texts by Strecker and Ebaugh,[20] and Henderson and Gillespie,[21] Wechsler's *The Neuroses*,[22] Freud's *Psychopathology of Everyday Life*[23] and *General Introduction to Psychoanalysis*,[24] *The Happy Life*[25] by Levy and Munroe, *The Challenge of Adolescence*[26] by Wile, and *The Human Mind*[27] by Karl Menninger.

Every Monday morning, I gave injections of bismuth and arsenicals to 100 patients with syphilis and performed a dozen or so spinal punctures. After the busy syphilitic clinic, I did ward rounds on my service, treating injuries that resulted from accidents, administering tube feedings to patients who refused to eat, and prescribing continuous tubs and wet-sheet packs for the disturbed. We encouraged improvement by permitting better patients to go out on the grounds on so-called parole, and by assigning them to work and recreation. I also ran a sleep therapy unit and several therapy groups. I made my first research report on pericardial hemorrhage in scurvy.[28]

I was privileged to study neurology at the National Hospital in Queen's Square, London. I visited various mental hospitals in England and was amazed to find no disturbed wards resembling those I knew at home. The respect for human dignity and superior nursing care seemed to be responsible for the very different behavior of confined chronically ill patients. On my return to Worcester, I was permitted for a time to demonstrate the validity of my observations. We placed graduate nurses with experience in psychiatry on every ward. It was a sad day when the state ordered their dismissal because most of them had been recruited from outside the state. During the depression, we were obliged to fill vacancies from applicants who were residents of the state.

In 1933, William A. White, looking back over 40 years of experience, said that the most significant advances of the past were the establishment of psychopathic hospitals; the re-establishment of wards in general hospitals for psychiatric patients, which led among other benefits to a closer association between psychiatrists and others on the medical staff; the increased number of child guidance clinics; and the impact of the law. He referred in particular to the Briggs Law in Massachusetts, which called for psychiatrists to examine all recidivists and criminals charged with major offenses, and the contributions of psychiatry to the understanding of delinquency.[29]

Major advances in therapy for mental illness took place during the 1930's. In 1933, in Austria, Sakel introduced insulin, Moniz of Lisbon demonstrated prefrontal lobotomy in 1935 and von Meduna in Budapest introduced Metrazol. In 1938, Cerletti and Bini in Italy developed electric shock therapy, and its dramatic effect on agitated depressions is still, I believe, one of the great psychiatric advances of this century. The significant symptomatic relief produced by the new therapies made it possible to discharge hospital patients in a shorter time than had been possible before these treatments were available.[30] In 1939, Myerson in Boston introduced "total push" therapy to combat the harmful effects of prolonged institutionalization.[31]

Three most important methods of delivering care were also started in the 1930's although they did not reach their zenith for some years. Several general hospitals established special units for psychiatric patients.[32] Although the beginnings were laid in the 18th Century in Philadelphia, by the Toronto General Hospital in 1908, and the Henry Ford Hospital in 1924, it was the added impetus, at a time the field was ready to break out of the mental hospital, along with the discovery of new therapies, EST in particular, that stimulated the rapid growth of this care system.

The day hospital was created in Boston in 1935, the first one being Adams House, a private mental hospital that served mainly neurotic patients (from "The Annual Report, Adams Nervine," Boston, Massachusetts: 1935).[33] In Amsterdam, Querido devised a system of visits to patients' homes when a psychiatric emergency occurred. His original intent was to screen patients and assign priorities for scarce mental hospital beds, but the discovery that many of the mentally ill could be managed outside hospitals ultimately led to the community mental health program.[34]

Other important psychiatric events during the 1930's were studies on the impact of environmental stress; the classic work of Feris and Dunham on urban mental illness;[35] the increased number of outpatient psychiatric clinics; the development of mental hygiene programs in schools; and the establishment of psychiatric departments in industrial plants. Interest in forensic psychiatry increased, and so did awareness of the values religion and psychiatry had for one another. Family studies began to be made, and Skinner in 1930, Harlow in 1932, and Fulton in 1935 began experiments in the behavior of animals that added to our knowledge of operant conditioning and mothering, and the function of the frontal lobes of the brain.

Most important in the period, the American Board of Psychiatry and Neurology was formed in 1934.

The form of psychiatric practice was changing. In 1920, over three-quarters of APA members worked in institutions. By 1930, 29% were in private practice. This number was to grow to 38% in the decade ahead.[36]

THE 1940's—MILITARY PSYCHIATRY

Despite the war that enveloped Europe as the decade ended, there had been no effective preparation or plan by the U.S. military services to use psychiatry when the bombs fell on Pearl Harbor in 1941. The intensely valuable documentation of the experiences of World War I were gathering dust in books on library shelves.[37] Such experience had shown that for every four men wounded, there would be one psychiatric casualty. Yet, no preparation had been made to care for that fifth man.[36] The painful process of organizing an effective military psychiatric service has been well described by William Menninger and others.[36,38]

I was in the Neuropsychiatry Consultants Division in the Office of the Surgeon General of the Army, and I am tempted to dwell on the significance of that experience. I shall resist the temptation, however, and instead enumerate some of the lessons that we learned from World War II that were important to psychiatric administration, primarily in the services but also in general to civilian psychiatry.

The first was the importance of planning for psychiatric casualties within overall medical services. Between January 1, 1942 and December 31, 1945, a million patients with NP disorders were admitted to military hospitals. Psychiatric screening at the time of induction was not very effective, although it had been reported as effective in World War I in preventing psychiatric casualties. In World War II, a total of some 4,650,000 men were rejected for military service, 39% (1,825,000) for some type of personality disorder or mental disturbance.

A manpower pool of adequately trained and qualified psychiatrists and other mental health professionals was vital, of course. Ongoing training was needed to revise training to include instruction and supervised practice in dynamic psychiatry.

It was important to have psychiatrists in combat divisions in order to institute rapid screening of casualties and initiate immediate short-term psychiatric treatment while the individual was still in the combat zone. It proved possible to treat and to return to duty 65% of those who suffered psychiatric illness, compared with 60% for other illnesses or injuries.

Two-way channels of communication between the combat zone and the Office of the Surgeon General proved valuable. The attitude of military leaders toward psychiatric breakdowns was important. Military leaders began to recognize that every man has his breaking point under the disintegrating impact of continued stress. It was also necessary to understand that abstract patriotism and the willingness of a man to die for his country are less effective than the resolve to live up to his responsibility to his immediate group; hence the value of group replacement to a depleted combat unit. Also, leaders discovered that reconditioning for return to duty can be most effective.

Application of these experiences to civilian psychiatry includes a wider social application of psychiatric principles;[39] greater emphasis on the demonstrated value of mental health professionals working together to give treatment to the mentally disabled; the value of group therapy; the importance of rehabilitation; and the contributions psychiatry can make to patients suffering from the emotional aspects of blindness, deafness, paraplegia, and amputation.

The World War II experience led directly to the provision of psychiatric services to former servicemen in Veterans Administration hospitals. The VA made one colossal policy error that has seriously blocked psychiatric progress. A proposal was made to give each discharged veteran a comprehensive, prepaid insurance policy that would provide access to a common system of medical care that would serve all citizens. Instead, the VA adopted the policy of preferential treatment of veterans which led to the development of a competing system of health care at enormous public cost. A new chain of general and psychiatric hospitals was built which competed for scarce professional manpower, duplicated other expensive medical facilities, and were available only to veterans with service-connected disabilities. Sometimes the VA system has competed with community hospitals for patients—but not in psychiatry where there have always been enough patients to go around. VA hospitals are generally excluded in the planning of community mental health programs, making them an extravagant exception to regional medical planning.

Nevertheless, the VA originated many important contributions to administrative psychiatry under the progressive direction of Daniel Blain and later, Harvey J. Tompkins, in the VA Central Office. The formation of the Deans' Committees to oversee staff performance and procedures inspired excellent therapy. The newly established Department of Physical Medicine and Rehabilitation coordinated the efforts of occupational, physical, and industrial therapists with those of therapists in the new specialties of education, recreation, manual arts, and corrective therapy. The new hospitals were limited to 1,000 beds, and modern physical arrangements enhanced their efficiency. More patients recovered in the small, well-staffed hospitals. The VA also did much to help develop factory-type and community work programs for psychiatric patients.

The development of antibiotics changed the course of infectious diseases. Some toxic psychoses that were associated with them disappeared from admissions to the mental hospital. Knight's statistical study in 1941 of 600 patients treated by psychoanalysis aroused widespread discussion of the value of analytic psychotherapy. About 56% of the psychoneuroses in prolonged analysis were recovered or markedly improved.[40]

Shortly after the war, a number of science writers forcibly directed public attention to the pitiful state of decline that had characterized mental hospitals during the war years. A year or so later, Albert Deutsch documented those findings in his book, *The Shame of the States*.[41] The public response evoked a prompt professional response, and in 1945, the APA formed a committee, headed by Mesrop Tarumianz, to develop standards for mental hospitals. In 1947, a Central Inspection Board composed of ten psychiatrists was proposed to inspect mental hospitals and to suggest improvements. The APA Council approved its creation in May 1948, and in November of that year it began operation under Ralph M. Chambers. During its 12 years of operation, the CIB inspected 272 hospitals and its reports were used to help correct deficiencies. The board was discontinued in 1960 as the Joint Commission on Accreditation of Hospitals had instituted a program in 1958 of survey and approval of mental hospitals on request.

Meanwhile, in 1946, the newly established Group for the Advancement of Psychiatry pushed for the reorganization of the American Psychiatric Association. In 1948, for the first time in its history, the association employed a full-time paid Medical Director. Daniel Blain and his administrative associate, Robert L. Robinson, opened the Central Office in Washington, D.C. The following year, the APA Section on Mental Hospitals came into being and also the APA Mental Hospital Service.[42]

The most significant psychiatric event of the decade was the passage, in 1946, of the National Mental Health Act, under which the National

Institute of Mental Health was established. Under a great leader, Robert H. Felix, who surrounded himself with outstanding men, the NIMH got off to a flying start. Through grants to medical schools, it improved psychiatric teaching. Its stipends recruited men and women into solid training programs in various mental health professions. Grants stimulated sorely needed research. Funded demonstration projects encouraged innovations in mental hospitals.

There were many other important contributions during the 1940's that were to help in the management of psychiatric illness. One was Lindemann's 1944 study of grief reactions;[43] the brilliant work of Wolf and Wolff on the role of emotions in stomach ulcers was published during the same year;[44] in 1946, the Hill-Burton Construction Act enabled mental hospitals to be renovated and general hospitals to add psychiatric units. In 1945, Harry Stack Sullivan's work on interpersonal relationships was published;[45] in 1948, Wiener introduced cybernetics,[46] and in 1949, Barr and Bertram reported the first breakthrough in human cytogenetics that led to chromosome studies.[47]

THE 1950's—ERA OF NEW DIRECTIONS AND NEW HOPES

Society gets its daily work done through the power its organizations wield.[33] "An organization comes into being," says Bernard, "when persons are able to communicate with each other; are willing to contribute to action and to work toward a common purpose."[48] An organization is ". . . a system of consciously coordinated activities." Motivation is the means or inducement by which such coordination is effected. The group may compel acceptance of its goals; it may purchase acceptance, or the goals may be accepted through identification when the worker accepts the organization's goals as his own or hopes to make them accord more closely to his own. Decisions or policies, as well as matters relating to the common purpose, tend more and more to be formed by groups of experts rather than by single individuals. The shift in power and the understanding of systems within many types of organizations have led to the evolution of management theory.[49,50,51] The vast literature in this field has had a profound impact on all aspects of administration in the past two decades.

Other significant events that shaped the form and direction of psychiatry during the 1950's were improved teaching of psychiatry in medical schools; improved management of mental hospitals; advances in therapy, particularly through the introduction of new drugs; the extension of group therapy and crisis intervention; and the discovery of inborn errors of metabolism and the evolving science of cytogenetics.

Early in the decade, the APA joined with the Association of American Medical Colleges to hold three important conferences. The first, in 1951, concerned the teaching of psychiatry in medical schools. The aim, stated the report of the conference, was to prepare medical students to deal intelligently and skillfully with patients as people, and to provide students with some basic knowledge about psychological and social problems and resources in relation to health and disease.[52] The following year, a second conference focused on the training of psychiatric residents, and sought to formulate ways of improving the teaching of basic and clinical psychiatry and to advance the skills of the resident in recognizing and treating mental illness. The basic importance of a thorough grounding in psychodynamics was emphasized.[53] In 1956, a third conference dealt solely with the care and treatment of emotionally disturbed children in inpatient medical settings. The focus was on the treatment program and how children with mental disorders might be helped.[54]

The resurgence of the American Psychiatric Association into a leadership role was a principal factor in bringing about improved care of patients and the improvement of the institutions dedicated to that purpose. I believe the creation of the APA Mental Hospital Service (now the Hospital and Community Psychiatry Service) was enormously important in effecting the changes that occurred in this decade.[55]

Standards which were formulated in 1951 were revised in 1956, and again in 1958 as the hospital administrators on the committee hammered out guidelines to improve the quality of care.[56,57]

The annual Mental Hospital Institutes offered a forum at which to discuss common problems and to arrive at solutions that were usually quickly applied. The magazine, *Mental Hospitals,* now *Hospital and Community Psychiatry,* published by the Mental Hospital Service, presented practical articles on clinical and hospital management of patients— articles that stimulated change and improved practices.

As the result of a conference held early in 1952, the APA Architectural Project blossomed briefly as a mechanism for joint planning between architects and psychiatrists for the improvement of psychiatric facilities. Generous grants from the Division Fund and the Rockefeller Foundation made the project possible and financed the final report, *Psychiatric Architecture,* published in 1959.[58] The need for innovation and joint architectural and medical planning, however, continued long after the money for this ambitious project had run out.

At about the same time, Stanton and Schwartz carefully studied a small group of patients on a ward at Chestnut Lodge, a private psychiatric hospital in Maryland. They concluded that the social situation in a mental hospital is closely related to and strongly affects the illness of patients, and is an area directly accessible to psychiatric administration. When the hospital organization works smoothly and the morale of personnel is high, patients usually tend to improve. When disagreement occurs among the staff about how to manage patients, that disagreement is reflected in disturbance among the patients. Patients who are subjected to loss of self-esteem or feel devalued by the attitudes of those around them become incontinent. But administrators who are sensitive and alert can offer satisfying activities to patients often before the patients themselves have become aware of their need for attention or stimulation.[59]

During these years, I was the superintendent of the Boston State Hospital. We had developed a competent medical and professional staff and employed many consultants. Thus we had become able to treat newly admitted patients intensively. Screening procedures brought into therapy many others from the intermediate and long-stay wards. Even before the use of the new drugs became widespread in 1954 and 1955, the hospital census began to decline. This experience convinced me that an adequate number of qualified staff, dedicated to giving individual patient care, is the one essential to having a good program.

In 1954, the unit plan was introduced in Clarinda, Iowa. It was essentially an administrative mechanism that provided for one section of a mental hospital to be responsible for the care of all patients from one geographical area. The large institution was decentralized into smaller, more manageable units that made individual care possible.[60] There were other advantages too: many facilities were used by both sexes; intermediate and long-stay patients were in the same wards as the short-term, acutely ill; staff roles were clearly defined and personnel from other units were not moved in to cover for absentees. The most important result was that continuity of therapeutic personnel was provided at all stages of treatment.

In 1958, Harry Solomon, in his Presidential Address to the American Psychiatric Association, made an admirable summary of the achievements of the preceding ten years. One paragraph of that address, however, exploded the complacency of mental hospital administrators for many years to come. Said Dr. Solomon: "The large mental hospital is antiquated, outmoded, and rapidly becoming obsolete. . . . I do not see how any reasonably objective view of our mental hospitals today can fail to conclude that they are bankrupt beyond remedy. I believe, therefore, that our large mental hospitals should be liquidated as rapidly as can be done in an orderly and progressive fashion."[61]

In any period of great change, the major barrier to progress is the difficulty of creating awareness of the need for change. The old ways of doing things are familiar and comfortable. The accumulated experience of years weighs the balance in favor of proven responses. Yet, today's problems cannot be successfully managed with yesterday's solutions. The large mental hospitals had so many defects that others besides Dr. Solomon said they should be abandoned and new facilities built where they were needed. Legislatures, sensitive to the high cost of caring for the mentally ill, were eager to stop spending large sums of money on ineffective public hospitals. But there was little eagerness to support new facilities until they demonstrated their usefulness.[62]

The most dramatic psychiatric event of the 1950's was, of course, the introduction of drugs that could profoundly change the symptoms of mental illness. The event that triggered the development of a series of successful tranquilizers was the discovery of chlorpromazine by Deniker and Delay in Paris in 1951.[63] Chlorpromazine controlled the symptoms of excitement, overactivity, and violence in mental patients, and made it possible to care for many with serious mental disorders in general hospitals and in the community. The anti-depressant drugs were foreshadowed by the introduction of isoniazid for the treatment of tuberculosis, and the discovery that it was accompanied by mood elevation, to the point of euphoria.

During the decade, group psychotherapy was widely used to modify behavior, and it was extended to embrace the concept of the therapeutic community[64] and the milieu of the whole institution. Patient government was developed at about the same time, not only to give patients a voice in policy decisions that affected their welfare, but also to increase their sense of dignity and responsibility. In the 1960's, it took riots for the poor to gain the right to participate in the government of their cities.

Although operant conditioning was not a new idea, its applications were extended into clinical settings, both for the mentally ill and the mentally retarded. The time-tested method of giving rewards was applied by rewarding patients for demonstrating socially acceptable behavior.

Among the other significant events of the decade was the Durham Decision handed down in 1954 by Judge David Bazelon of the U.S. Court of Appeals of D.C. The decision made the old M'Naghten test of "knowledge of right and wrong" inadequate, and adopted what is essentially the

New Hampshire Rule: "An accused is not criminally responsible if his unlawful act was the product of mental disease or mental defect."[65]

In 1953, Kenneth E. Appel, then President of the American Psychiatric Association, called for a "Flexner Report" on mental hospitals, which ultimately led to the establishment of the Joint Commission on Mental Illness and Health.

Social scientists were becoming actively involved in studying mental hospitals and social psychiatry.[66,67,68,69]

A new classification of mental disorders was adopted by the APA (DSM-I), and the association also established a commission to develop professional manpower, long before this topic became popular.

Crisis intervention was introduced,[70] family therapy extended,[71] inborn errors of metabolism were discovered, and extensive studies in communication made.[72] Studies of sensory deprivation contributed significantly to understanding the effects of isolation,[73] and several missions of psychiatrists toured psychiatric facilities in Europe, in particular England and Holland, to study rehabilitation programs involving factory-type employment in hospitals, a practice that was subsequently widely adopted in the United States.[74]

THE 1960's—SOCIAL CHANGE, PSYCHIATRIC CONTRIBUTION

The present weighs too heavily upon us to permit us to make truly objective evaluations of contributions in this decade that ultimately will prove to have historical significance.

A new America is emerging in response to challenges to nearly all social institutions. Protests in troubled inner cities are as common as robberies. Nudity and sexual practices are shown by the entertainment media. Few books are as widely read as those that describe copulation and sexually deviant acts. The government manipulates taxes and interest rates, and deficit spending is standard procedure. It promises equal rights and equal opportunities to everyone, but places little emphasis on service to one's country and on social responsibility as an obligation of citizenship.

Alcohol and drugs are taken as soporifics to blur the anxieties of a society that has not yet determined what its new directions should be.

In the 1960's, the government increased its support of research and manpower development. The right of all to receive high quality health care was proclaimed. Billions were poured into financing health care, but our ability to provide the service promised still fell far short of public expectations. One remedy suggested was a national health service involving complete governmental control of medicine. A better solution would be adequate financing for the development of medical manpower. In a world with too many people, it is shortsighted of society not to prepare the bright ones to fill top-level jobs. Equally important is to develop a health care delivery system that will conserve manpower and put services where they will be the most effective. In this decade, we are just beginning to study unification and coordination of services.

In 1961, *Action for Mental Health,* the final report of the Joint Commission on Mental Illness and Health, stirred citizens to support improvements in the care of the mentally ill.[75]

In 1963, President John F. Kennedy delivered to Congress his now famous Message on Mental Health. Probably no single administrative statement has had so profound an effect on the direction of psychiatry in the United States.

The expectation of President Kennedy and his advisors was that the establishment of comprehensive community mental health centers would diminish the need for public mental hospitals. Accordingly, that program proceeded at an accelerated rate, and as I write this, more than 300 community mental health centers have started operating under federal support. Many more have been started with state and private funds. Today, too, nearly 600 general hospital psychiatric sections admit more patients each year than all our public mental hospitals.

The Joint Information Service, jointly sponsored by the American Psychiatric Association and the National Association for Mental Health, based at the APA Central Office in Washington, D.C., has carried out a series of studies that constitute a principal resource for a national overview of community efforts in psychiatry. These studies incorporate the findings of national questionnaire-surveys together with field studies of prototype facilities. The site visits are made by a team of multidisciplinary experts, after which the site visit team and the directors of the prototype facilities hold a conference to discuss issues and problems of the particular subject under study. The monographs that have resulted from this technique provide a meaningful assessment of major aspects of community-based psychiatric services.[76,77,78,79]

Dr. William A. White spoke out boldly in his Presidential Address to the APA in 1925 in support of the new ideas about mental disease based on psychoanalytic principles. In 1952, Dr. Leo H. Bartemeier traced the development of psychoanalytic theory and its applications to psychotherapy in his Presidential Address. He cautioned against uncritical enthusiasm and what he called "wild analysis." He deemed it important for the therapist to take a complete anamnesis, interview relatives and maintain good relationships with family physicians; he deplored ignoring the importance of the patient's life environment. He deplored the tendency to embrace ". . . an illusory psychoanalytic respectability," saying that psychiatry had responsibilities beyond treating only patients ". . . whose prognosis appeared favorable under psychoanalytic theory."[80]

In the 1960's, psychoanalytic psychotherapy was coming under heavy attack as the pressure increased to give high quality treatment to all mentally ill patients. An hour spent in individual psychotherapy was only useful to the few who could afford to pay the analyst's fee. But who would care for the medically indigent equally effectively? There was talk of abandoning the medical approach in favor of the unproven social systems approach. In a recent paper, I commented as follows: "From one point of view, instant therapy for the masses seems called for. If we respond and spread ourselves tissue-paper thin, we may be faced with re- nouncing the 50-minute hour for the 15-minute exhortation, with closing the hospital ward in favor of life at home with a neurotic spouse and group therapy membership, with viewing an exclusively private practitioner of psychiatry as irresponsible, if not immoral. An obvious rejoinder to the accusation of *second-rate* as to what is evolving in medicine is that some help is better than none at all. First aid can stop the bleeding, splint the broken leg, and counteract shock. This truth does not reassure those engaged in the pursuit of excellence, nor should it. The community mental health movement is at present handicapped by over-enthusiasm, partly because of childishly gullible fascination with the new and adolescent rejection of the old. We have been through these phases many times be- fore. In the beginning, two-thirds of schizophrenic patients were said to be cured by insulin coma; sixty per cent of paranoid schizophrenics were allegedly improved by convulsive therapy; and similarly rosy results were initially attributed to psychoanalysis, lobotomy, tranquilizers, and the therapeutic community. This enthusiasm is not necessarily all bad: the new must be tested, applied with considered indiscrimination, and evalu- ated after a period of time in order to find the truth. This is the obligation of science."[81]

Social therapists, concerned about living space, decent housing, educa- tion, equal access to jobs, poverty, and family problems, began experi- menting with neighborhood and storefront psychiatric facilities and com- munity health centers.[82,83] "Indigenous non-professional" was the awk- ward label devised for non-professional mental health workers. Such assist- ants are often the first workers a person meets when he comes to a center,

They may be assigned to take his history and to gather information from other agencies. With this information in hand, the assistant makes a preliminary judgment about whether the program available is suitable for the individual. He will probably have a professionally trained mental health worker as a supervisor, and it is usually the latter who reports to the psychiatrist. The indigenous nonprofessionals may well be the principal therapists under this tenuous psychiatric surveillance.

Developing knowledge about the effects of bio-chemistry on perception, behavior, and feelings is bringing psychiatry closer to other medical practice. As new drugs are introduced and new biochemical knowledge about their action becomes available, psychiatrists are better able to relieve the symptoms of mental illness and to restore the victims to a functioning role in society.

It is more urgent than ever to demonstrate the value of various forms of therapy through controlled studies. Two recent works of importance have particular value. Pasamanick, Scarpetti, and Dinitz showed that many schizophrenic patients need not be hospitalized and for some, drug therapy is effective in preventing hospitalization; indeed, for some, home treatment may actually be better.[84]

May compared controlled groups of mental hospital patients receiving drugs, electroconvulsive therapy, psychotherapy, and drugs combined with psychotherapy. This study showed that drugs and drugs plus psychotherapy were the most effective modalities. Patients receiving EST were in the middle, and those on psychotherapy or milieu therapy alone showed the poorest results.[85]

Perhaps the most important of the new trends in administration is the national effort to plan for regional and local mental health care. Such planning must be a cooperative enterprise between professional mental health workers, and the citizens of the community that is to be served. The focus of the planning must be on the resources needed to create a total plan for health services.

Books by Barton, Ewalt, Clark, and a GAP Report on administration in psychiatry all offer valuable assistance to hospital administrators.[33,86,87,88]

Standards for all psychiatric facilities have been revised.[89] The Joint Commission on Accreditation of Hospitals has assumed responsibility for inspection of psychiatric facilities of all types and is planning a reorganization that will provide for a categorical council on psychiatric facilities, an organizational component that will take the responsibility for inspecting and developing standards.

The new classification of mental disorders (DSM-II) has brought the United States' nosology into harmony with the international classification.[90] A study of the current state of nosology demonstrated, however, that we have a long way yet to travel before the classification system can be said to really meet the needs of modern practice.[91]

Contributions to recruiting psychiatric manpower and studies on the use of existing manpower have been helpful in defining the extent of the problem that we must solve in order to develop adequate psychiatric services for all who need them.[92,93]

Psychiatry, like the rest of medicine, is exploring the many uses of various types of automation, and of the computer in particular. Automated laboratory procedures and electroencephalogram analyses, scanning devices that read X-rays, automated ways of monitoring patients' vital signs and observing their behavior are some examples of systems being developed. Needless to say, computers speed up bookkeeping and billing operations. They can also store medical records, and retrieve them immediately upon demand. Networks of computers combine the resources of several centers to solve specific problems.

Perhaps the most dramatic achievement in the stormy 60's has been the reduction in the number of persons in state mental hospitals—from 536,000 in 1960 to 426,000 in 1967—a decrease of 21 per cent. It is the more dramatic because of the expanding general population and the increasing number of admissions to public mental hospitals. Patients stay a shorter time in the hospital and complete their treatment in the community.

The financial problems of treatment are also receiving attention. The extension of insurance plans to cover mental illness is a most important mechanism for financing mental health care, by providing for many access to treatment that would not otherwise be available in our free enterprise system. The APA is taking an active part, together with the National Association for Mental Health and the National Institute of Mental Health, to demonstrate the feasibility of insurance plans to cover mental disorders.[94] The association is currently involved in a study of health insurance that offers both inpatient and outpatient psychiatric care to more than 700,000 blue collar workers; the study will be completed in 1971. Meanwhile, the APA has published guidelines for insurance plans and a summary of the present insurance coverage available for mental illnesses.[95,96] The association has been in the forefront of the campaign to include mental disorders in Medicare and Medicaid programs.

There is a ferment in medicine as it accommodates to the pressures of rapid social change.[97] Society has agreed that treatment must be available to all, regardless of their financial situation. The worker and his family now are able to pay for health care through insurance. The elderly have Medicare; the unemployed and the medically indigent are increasingly cared for by state or federal governments. Nevertheless, the delivery systems for health care are still inadequate. They function badly for the poor, for children, and for special groups like those with alcoholism and elderly people with chronic disorders.

The role of government in delivering health services leads to greater concern with health legislation. American medicine and medical institutions are diverse and heterogeneous. That diversity serves as a protection against abrupt, sweeping change. But we must abandon the image of the old family doctor, standing by his dying patient through the long night in support of the grieving family. This is but a nostalgic wish for a bygone day in a simpler time, in an unstructured society. The doctor of today has at his command resources for treatment that are increasingly effective in the management of illness. Advances in medical practice undreamed of today will be tomorrow's reality.

REFERENCES

1. Grob, G. N., *The State and the Mentally Ill: A History of the Worcester State Hospital in Massachusetts, 1830-1920*. University of North Carolina Press, Chapel Hill: 1966.
2. Lebensohn, Z. M., "American Psychiatry: Retrospect and Prospect," *Medical Annals of the District of Columbia*, 31:379-392, July 1962.
3. Lidz, T., "Adolf Meyer and the Development of American Psychiatry," *American Journal of Psychiatry*, 123:320-332, September 1966.
4. Dane, N., *Concepts of Insanity in the United States, 1789-1865*. Rutgers University Press, New Brunswick, New Jersey: 1966.
5. Copp, O., "An Administrative Ideal in Public Welfare Work," *American Journal of Insanity*, 76:1-14, July 1919.
6. May, J. V., "The Functions of the Psychopathic Hospital," *American Journal of Insanity*, 76:21034, July 1919.
7. Strecker, E. A., "Experiences in the Immediate Treatment of War Neuroses," *American Journal of Insanity*, 76:45-69, July 1919.
8. Meyers, D. C., "Neuropathic Wards in General Hospitals," *American Journal of Insanity*, 65:533-540, January 1908.
9. Kirkbride, T. S., *On the Construction, Organization, and General Arrangement of Hospitals for the Insane*. Second Edition. J. B. Lippincott Co., Philadelphia: 1880.
10. Zeller, G. A., *7th Biennial Report, Illinois General Hospital for the Insane*. Peoria, Illinois: June 30, 1908.
11. ————, *100 Years of American Psychiatry*. Collmbia University Press, New York: 1944. *American Journal of Psychiatry* Centennial Anniversary Issue Supplement: 1944.

264 *Hope: Psychiatry's Commitment*

12. Kanner, L., *Child Psychiatry.* Third Edition. Charles C. Thomas Co., Springfield, Illinois: 1957.
13. Spies, T., in Kelly, E. C., *Encyclopedia of Medical Sources.* p. 384; William and Wilkins Co., Baltimore: 1948.
14. Copp, O., "Some Problems Confronting the Association," *American Journal of Psychiatry,* 78:1-13, July 1921.
15. Tourney, G., "A History of Therapeutic Fashions in Psychiatry, 1800-1966," *American Journal of Psychiatry,* 124:784-796, December 1967.
16. Bryan, W. A., *Administrative Psychiatry.* W. W. Norton Co., New York: 1936.
17. Hart, B., *The Psychology of Insanity.* Fourth Edition. Macmillan Co., New York:1931.
18. White, W. A., *Outlines of Psychiatry.* Nervous and Mental Disease Publishing Co., Washington, D.C.:1929.
19. Bleuler, E., *Textbook of Psychiatry.* Macmillan Co., New York:1930.
20. Strecker, E. A., Ebaugh, F. G., *Practical Clinical Psychiatry for Students and Practitioners.* P. Blakiston Co., Philadelphia:1931.
21. Henderson, D. K., Gillespie, R. D., *A Textbook of Psychiatry.* Second Edition. Oxford University Press, London:1937.
22. Wechsler, I. S., *The Neuroses.* W. B. Saunders Co., Philadelphia:1929.
23. Freud, S., *Psychopathology of Everyday Life.* Macmillan Co., New York:1930.
24. Freud, S., *A General Introduction to Psychoanalysis.* Horace Liveright, New York:1920.
25. Levy, J., Munroe, R., *The Happy Family.* Alfred A. Knopf, New York: 1938.
26. Wile, I. S., *The Challenge of Adolescence.* Greenberg Publisher, New York:1939.
27. Menninger, K. A., *The Human Mind.* Garden City Publishing Co., New York:1930.
28. Barton, W. E., "Pericardial Hemorrhage Complicating Scurvy," *New England Journal of Medicine,* 210:529-531, March 1934.
29. White, W. A., *Forty Years of Psychiatry.* Nervous and Mental Disease Publishing Co., New York:1933.
30. Cameron, D. E., Hoskins, R. G., "Some Observations on Sakel's Insulin Hypoglycemia Treatment of Schizophrenia," *American Journal of Psychiatry,* 94:265-269, Supplement, May 1938.
31. Myerson, A., "Theory and Principle of the *Total Push* Method in the Treatment of Chronic Schizophrenia," *American Journal of Psychiatry,* 95:1197-1204, March 1939.
32. Bennett, A. E., "Problems in Establishing and Maintaining Psychiatric Units in General Hospitals," *American Journal of Psychiatry,* 115:974-979, May 1959.
33. Barton, W. E., *Administration in Psychiatry.* C. C. Thomas Co., Springfield:1962.
34. Querido, A., "Home Treatment of Mental Illness," JAMA, 157:73-74, January 1, 1955.
35. Feris, R. E., Dunham, H. W., *Mental Disorders in Urban Areas.* University of Chicago Press, Chicago:1939.
36. Menninger, W. C., *Psychiatry in a Troubled World.* Macmillan Co., New York:1948.

37. ————, *The Medical Department of the United States Army in the World War. Neuropsychiatry.* Volume X. U.S. Government Printing Office, Washington:1929.
38. Anderson, R. S., Glass, A. J., Bernucci, R. J. (editors), *Medical Department of the United States Army. Neuropsychiatry in World War II.* Volume I. U.S. Government Printing Office, Washington:1966.
39. Rees, J. R., *The Shaping of Psychiatry by War.* W. W. Norton Co., New York:1945.
40. Knight, R. P., "Evaluation of the Results of Psychoanalytic Therapy," *American Journal of Psychiatry,* 98:434-446.
41. Deutsch, A., *The Shame of the States.* Harcourt, Brace and Co., New York:1948.
42. Blain, D., "Better Care in Mental Hospitals," Proceedings of the 1st Mental Hospital Institute, American Psychiatric Association, Washington:1949.
43. Lindemann, E., "Symptomatology and Management of Acute Grief," *American Journal of Psychiatry,* 101:141-148, July 1944.
44. Wolf, S., Wolff, H. G., *Human Gastric Function.* Oxford University Press, New York:1943.
45. Sullivan, H. S., *The Interpersonal Theory of Psychiatry.* W. W. Norton Co., New York:1953.
46. Wiener, N., *Cybernetics.* John Wiley and Sons, New York:1948.
47. Barr, M. L., Bertram, E. G., "A Morphological Distinction between Neurons of Male and Female and the Behavior of the Nuclear Satellite During Accelerated Nuclear Protein Synthesis," *Nature,* 163:676-677, April 30, 1949.
48. Barnard, C. I., *The Functions of the Executive.* Harvard University Press, Cambridge:1938.
49. Dubin, E., *Human Relations in Organization.* Prentice-Hall, New York: 1954.
50. Petrecello, L., Bass, B. M., *Leadership and Interpersonal Behavior.* Holt, Rinehart and Winston, Inc., New York:1961.
51. Galbraith, J. K., *The New Industrial State.* Houghton Mifflin Co., Boston:1967.
52. Whitehorn, J. C. et al. (editors), *Psychiatry and Medical Education.* Report of the 1951 Cornell Conference, Ithaca, New York. American Psychiatric Association Washington:1952.
53. Whitehorn, J. C. et al. (editors), *The Psychiatrist, His Training and Development.* Report of the 1952 Cornell Conference, Ithaca, New York. American Psychiatric Association, Washington:1953.
54. Robinson, J. F. et al. (editors), *Psychiatric Inpatient Treatment of Children.* Report of a 1956 Conference, Washington, D.C. American Psychiatric Association:1957.
55. ————, Mental Hospital Service Bulletin, January 1950. (evolved to *Mental Hospitals* in 1951 and to *Hospital and Community Psychiatry* in 1966) American Psychiatric Association, Washington, D.C.
56. Duval, A., "Formulation of Standards," *Mental Hospitals,* 2:3, September 1951.
57. ————, *Standards for Hospitals and Clinics.* American Psychiatric Association, Washington:1956.
58. Goshen, C. E. (editor), *Psychiatric Architecture.* American Psychiatric Association, Washington:1959.

266 *Hope: Psychiatry's Commitment*

59. Stanton, A. H., Schwartz, M. D., *The Mental Hospital.* Basic Books, New York:1954.
60. Garcia, L., "The Clarinda Plan: An Ecological Approach to Hospital Organization," *Mental Hospitals*, 11:9-31, November 1960.
61. Solomon, H. C., "The American Psychiatric Association in Relation to American Psychiatry," *American Journal of Psychiatry*, 115:1-9, July 1958.
62. Barton, W. E., "The Care and Treatment of the Hospitalized Mentally Ill," *Mental Hygiene*, 44:281-289, April 1960.
63. Delay, J., Deniker, P., "38 Cases of Psychoses Under Prolonged and Continuous RP 4560 Treatment," Compt. Rend. Cong. Med. Alien. Neurol,. July 21, 1952; p. 7.
64. Jones, M., *Social Psychiatry: A Study of Therapeutic Communities.* Tavistock Publications Ltd., London:1952.
65. Fortas, Abe, "Implications of Durham's Case," *American Journal of Psychiatry*, 113:577-582, January 1957.
66. Caudill, W., *The Hospital as a Small Society.* Harvard University Press, Cambridge:1958.
67. Greenblatt, M., Levinson, D. J., Williams, R. H., *The Patient and the Mental Hospital.* The Free Press, Glencoe, Illinois:1957.
68. Leighton, A., Clauson, J. A., Wilson, R.N., *Explorations in Social Psychiatry.* Basic Books, New York:1954.
69. Belknap, I., *Human Problems of a State Mental Hospital.* McGraw-Hill Book Co., New York:1956.
70. Caplan, G., Four Crises Studies, unpublished. See *Principles of Preventive Psychiatry.* Basic Books, New York:1964.
71. Ackerman, N. W., *The Psychodynamics of Family Life.* Basic Books, New York:1958.
72. Ruesch, J., "Psychiatry and the Challenge of Communication," *Psychiatry*, 17:1-18, February 1954.
73. Solomon, P., Leiderman, P. H., Mendleson, J., Wexler, D., "Sensory Deprivation: A Review," *American Journal of Psychiatry*, 114:357-363, October 1957.
74. Barton, W. E., Farrell, M. F., Lenehan, F. T., McLaughlin, W. F., *Impressions of European Psychiatry.* American Psychiatric Association, Washington:1961.
75. ———, *Action for Mental Health.* Basic Books, New York:1961.
76. Glasscote, R., Sanders, D., Forstenzer, H. M., Foley, A. R., *The Community Mental Health Center.* Joint Information Service, American Psychiatric Association, Washington:1964.
77. Glasscote, R., Cumming, E., Hammersley, D., Ozarin, L. C., Smith, L. H., *The Psychiatric Emergency.* Joint Information Service, American Psychiatric Association, Washington:1966.
78. Glasscote, R. M., Kraft, A., Glassman, S., Jepson, W., *Partial Hospitalization for the Mentally Ill: A Study of Programs and Problems.* Joint Information Service, American Psychiatric Association, Washington:1969.
79. Glasscote, R., Sussex, J. N., Cumming, E., Smith, L. H., *The Community Mental Health Center: An Interim Appraisal.* Joint Information Service, American Psychiatric Association, Washington:1968.
80. Bartemeier, L. H., "Presidential Address," *American Journal of Psychiatry*, 109:1-7, July 1952.

81. Barton, W. E., "Prospects and Perspectives: Implications of Social Change for Psychiatry," *American Journal of Psychiatry*, 125:147-150, August 1968.
82. Duhl, L. J., *The Urban Condition*. Basic Books, New York:1963.
83. Srole, L., Langer, T. S., Michael, S. T., Opler, M. K., Rennie, T. A. C., *Mental Health in the Metropolis*. Blakiston Division, McGraw-Hill Book Co., New York:1962.
84. Pasamanick, B., Scarpetti, F. R., Dinitz, S., *Schizophrenics in the Community*. Appleton-Century-Crofts, New York:1967.
85. May, P. R. A., *Treatment of Schizophrenia: A Comparative Study of Five Treatment Methods*. Science House, New York:1968.
86. Ewalt, J. R., *Mental Health Administration*. C. C. Thomas Company, Springfield, Illinois:1956.
87. Clark, D. H., *Administrative Therapy*. Tavistock Publications, London: 1964.
88. ―――, *Administration of the Public Psychiatric Hospital*. Report #46. Group for the Advancement of Psychiatry, New York:1960.
89. ―――, *Standards for Psychiatric Facilities*. American Psychiatric Association, Washington:1969.
90. ―――, *Diagnostic and Statistical Manual of Mental Disorders (DSM-II)*. American Psychiatric Association, Washington:1968.
91. Katz, M. M., Cole, J. O., Barton, W. E., *The Role and Methodology of Classification in Psychiatry and Psychopathology*. USPHS #1584, U.S. Government Printing Office, Washington:1968.
92. Burch, C., Van Atta, W., Blain, D. (editors), *Careers in Psychiatry*. The Macmillan Company, New York:1968.
93. Whiting, J. F., *Psychiatric Services and Manpower Utilization*. American Psychiatric Association, Washington:1969.
94. Avnet, H. H., *Psychiatric Insurance*. Group Health Insurance, New York:1962.
95. ―――, *APA Guidelines for Psychiatric Services Covered Under Health Insurance Plans*. American Psychiatric Association, Washington:1968.
96. Scheidemandel, P., Kanno, C., Glasscote, R., *Health Insurance for Mental Illness*. Joint Information Service, Washington:1968.
97. Magraw, R. M., *Ferment in Medicine: A Study of the Essence of Medical Practice and Its New Dilemmas*. W. B. Saunders & Co., Philadelphia: 1968.

19

GENE L. USDIN, M.D.

It is a compliment to be invited to participate in this anthology honoring Dr. Bartemeier on his 75th birthday. Dr. Bartemeier exemplifies the finest traditions of a physician and of an ethical human being. His impact on psychiatry and religion as well as on young physicians is equaled by few and exceeded by none. His friendship is valued by so many of us.

Civil Disobedience and Urban Revolt

WHILE THE DOCTRINE of civil disobedience had much earlier origins, it became more clearly defined in the mid-summer of 1846, when Thoreau spent a night in jail in conscientious disobedience to what he considered an unjust law; it was tested by the successful overthrow of British arms by an unarmed nation led by a wizened old man named Gandhi dressed in a loin cloth and humbly preaching passive disobedience to a tax on salt and obedience to all laws but those that he considered immoral; it matured in the peaceful strike against the bus lines and businesses in Montgomery, Alabama, led by a then little-known preacher named King. It has developed both as philosophical doctrine and tactical strategy in a struggle to change society.

In essence, this doctrine advocates the willful and open violation of any law deemed so immoral or unjust that the violator cannot in conscience obey it. The violation is itself a form of appeal to society to change the law. At the same time the violator willingly undergoes the penalty for its violation in order that his punishment may itself serve as a further appeal to the conscience of society.

This chapter is a revision of an article published in the *American Journal of Psychiatry* vol. 125, pages 1537-1543, 1969. Copyright 1969, The American Psychiatric Association.

Such disobedience may occur in situations seemingly far from those we usually think of. Consider, for example, physicians who, in a non-clandestine way, perform abortions or provide birth control advice in states where the law prohibits these acts and who thus seek to bring the issues to the public attention in the hope of effecting statutory changes. The goal of civil disobedience today is to change the law tomorrow.

The dissenter who engages in civil disobedience recognizes that he is a lawbreaker. As Solicitor General Edwin Griswold stated in a recent address:

> It is of the essence of law that it is equally applied to all, that it binds all alike, irrespective of personal motive. For this reason, one who contemplates civil disobedience out of moral conviction should not be surprised and must not be bitter if a criminal conviction ensues. And he must accept the fact that organized society cannot endure on any other basis. His hope is that he may aid in getting the law changed. But if he does not succeed in that, he cannot complain if the law is applied to him.[2]

The fact is that those guilty of civil disobedience should object if the law were waived in their favor, since such waiver would subvert the basic purpose of drawing attention to a law or system considered unjust.

The Confusion of Disobedience with Disorder

Both the passive public and the law violator often confuse this doctrine of conscience with a twentieth-century American phenomenon—civil disorder. But this is a mistake, because civil disobedience, which is neither irrational nor anarchistic, is in the best democratic tradition. Practiced wisely, it has often been a great force for good. In civil disorder, on the other hand, the lawbreaker is in revolt against the social system, including the institutions of the law, and he breaks the law as an expression of defiance; in addition, he may seek to secure immediate materialistic gains. Although the act of defiance may be overt, the lawbreaker who engages in civil disorder seeks to avoid punishment, usually by acting anonymously or as part of a mob. Destruction of property, looting, and personal violence characterize civil disorders.

The use of the term *civil disorder*—so misleadingly similar to the phrase *civil disobedience*—is a reflection of the confusion the public suffers in distinguishing these phenomena. Let us turn aside from the interesting psychodynamic problems in civil disobedience and direct our attention only to the area of civil disorder. In fact, it is incumbent upon us as psychiatrists to do so, for it is only by analyzing the phenomenon and parceling out pathological attitudes and consequences that we will derive the insight necessary to psychiatry's functioning as a responsible element of society.

In order to identify more accurately the phenomenon we are discussing, let us call civil disorder what it primarily is: *urban revolt*. The term "urban revolt" is used, at least in part, because the phenomenon we are observing is not only one of violent protest, as summed up in the word "revolt." It is also peculiarly "urban"—a pattern of group action in metropolitan areas.

Urban revolt may occur in a variety of contexts: as an outgrowth of civil rights activities, as a means of student action, as a protest against society's economic institutions. But even when urban revolt is fomented in the name of a moral cause, such as the civil rights movement, many of those who answer the call to action have no moral conviction and their involvement is to satisfy personal psychodynamic frustrations. Their needs may be to destroy, to rebel, to get caught and punished, to be one of the group, to secure attention, or to be martyred by injury or imprisonment. The psychologic equilibrium of many persons is maintained by compulsive action in this context, just as it may be maintained for some by other forms of acting out, such as hippiedom, compulsive involvement with civil rights actions, intolerance, or fanatical patriotism. However, to the extent that all behavior is motivated by personal conscious, preconscious, or unconscious factors, the social value or merit of various behaviors and attitudes cannot be judged solely by the psychodynamics producing the behavior. Many right deeds can be done for wrong reasons, and many injustices are perpetuated despite good intentions.

When civil disobedience was invoked by the Reverend Martin Luther King in 1956, it was a method to be used in the struggle to obtain equal civil rights (for example, the right to vote, the use of public property and privileges, equal treatment by local and state officials, and protection of civil rights advocates against harassment and murder). But in today's urban revolt those who profess to seek equal rights are often in the vanguard of violent action, many times using techniques of looting, property destruction, and violence at the expense of someone else's rights.

The urban revolt itself denies civil rights to thousands of persons caught in the disturbed cities. The citizen is denied his right to walk in public areas; his life is endangered by violent individuals; his property is violated by burning, looting, and pilfering. At times the urban revolt deprives others of the opportunity to disagree, to pursue gainful occupations, to own property, to operate businesses unmolested, and to maintain basic rights to life itself. In this sense the urban revolt is regressive and atavistic; at best, it is only an exchange of roles in a most extreme degree.

The Nature of Urban Revolt

Recognition of the contradictory nature of urban revolt does not, of course, imply condonation of the social wrongs that American society has committed in the past, nor of those that it allows to flourish today. Instead it merely implies the necessity of analyzing such debacles as the Detroit riots of 1967 and the student revolts of 1968-69 for the factors contributing to irrational excesses and the actual postponement of those improvements in society most of us sincerely desire. Actually, success in achieving certain benefits in individual situations may be often at a loss to the overall cause.

Urban revolt destroys at least temporarily the institutions of orderly living. It is for this reason that the legal profession has become increasingly concerned. Justice Frankfurter said, "Violent resistance to law cannot be made a legal reason for its suspension without loosening the fabric of our society."[1] Adherence to orderly methods of changing the law is especially important in a democracy, where legal and social institutions should be susceptible to change by peaceful majority action. In addition, and apart from basic principle, the violence of urban revolt may marshal resistance of the other extreme and bring about opposition from political moderates.

In the past (and despite such sporadic outbreaks as the 1830 anti-Catholic riots, the Civil War draft riots, the widespread 1877 labor uprisings, and the 1943 Detroit race riots), American society has viewed itself as one of law and order, its orientation influenced by the innate conservatism of rural areas and small communities.

Recent years have seen a marked change in our living patterns as well as in public attitudes toward law. As our society has become increasingly educated, urban, and anonymous, it has become more tolerant of purposeful violations of the law in furtherance of what the violators proclaim to be a just and moral cause. As peaceful protest has spilled over into revolt, violence has been widely publicized, often glamorized, and virtually legitimized. Individuals have been permitted to make their own choice about the binding nature of law. Protest too often sits high on the throne of emotional reactions, which may serve as a substitute for reasoning.

Dissenters have a right to express opposition—this no one denies—but by what means and to what extent? There are some people who consider violence undesirable but say that there are situations in which it is justifiable.

The Adolescent as a Model for Understanding Rebellion

Our American society has been oppressive to many minority groups: it has oppressed blacks in some ways; it has oppressed the youthful in others; it has disturbed college students in yet different ways. It is interesting to compare the modus operandi and dynamics of the militant Negro and the activist student groups. They have expressed a communality of interests. Despite their differences in background and goals, the leaders of the black revolt and of student action groups certainly feel a bond for each other and have much in common.

A model for understanding both groups may be an understanding of the adolescent. Emancipation is a necessary developmental phase of a mature personality as well as of a mature culture. As part of his emancipation, the adolescent needs the means to rebel against parents or parent surrogates. The wise parent, or authority figure, will afford the opportunity to express this emotional rebellion, while setting appropriate and clearly-defined limits upon the degree and type of rebellion of his child or subject. Many of those involved in civil disorders have no parents, and the closest they may come to rebelling against a parent is to rebel against a parent surrogate. For them this can be a society or some form of the establishment.

Adolescents are especially attuned to the approval of their peers. For years, blacks considered themselves "subjects" subservient to the pleasure of the "master white race." Now, they are ready subjects for mob action. Indeed, such action is attended by so many seeming gains that participants may find it to be an effective technique not only for the present but also for the future.

But we must remember that one of the crucial developmental phases of the ego is the development of personal courage. Such personal courage involves the ability to take a stand regardless of peer group opinion. Mob action substitutes the group standard for the individual standard. For many, the exhilaration found in the mob may prevent the development of personal courage. Will the young man who participates in mob action always need the screaming mob, the group glamour, and the spectacle of the power of the group in order to be brave? Will group intoxication result in the abdication of individual responsibility? Healthy rebellion should be accompanied by constructive ingredients. But many of those involved in urban revolt are caught up by the thrill of being part of the mob, of being enthralled by a dynamic leader, or seduced to a destructive violence by the desire to be effective—at any cost.

Another adolescent feature that lies behind the resort to mob action is the feeling of alienation from the mainstream of so-called "law-abiding" society. The revolters are convinced that society—a parent surrogate—does not understand them or take them sufficiently into account as individuals. Blacks feel they are not sharing in the mutual benefits "the others" have and that this stems from society's rejection of them as individuals. College students feel "lost in the crowd" and neglected by adult members of the university community, especially the administration. When these blacks and students join a mob, they experience a sense of power. It is ironical that for some the only emotionally creative thing they have achieved is to destroy something. By an act of violence, they have ceased to be a minuscule part of the universe and become factors to contend with.

We should differentiate between the constructive activist student and the student rebel. The anti-Establishment nature of the students' revolt and the need to throw off any restraint has resulted, for many, in a type of destructiveness that may be considered an immature exaltation of aimlessness—eroticized or libidinized. The infantile nature of some is apparent in the sadistic behavior whereby pure joy is found in destruction for its own sake. For some, extreme anti-Establishment activity may be a type of substitute hippiedom in which students proclaim that they don't *have* to do anything. Their dress and personal habits are the initial proclamation of nonconformity.

Their second proclamation—overt defiance of and belligerence toward authority—represents their adolescent need to rebel, but *not,* in many instances, legitimate protest. Few classes in history have been permitted as much freedom as has the American student. The average student has been raised in comparative affluence by permissive parents. He has grown up in a country governed since its birth by men who generally subscribe to Edmund Burke's dictum, "Freedom and not servitude is the cure of anarchy; as religion, and not atheism, is the true remedy for superstition." Some may argue that our system of government has been democratic enough to allow a change with access to dissent to the law and, because of this, radicals have had to create artificial tyrants.

The Myth of the Violent Hero

We must also consider the American tendency to covertly admire violence. Our national heroes have included the Indian fighter and the western gunslinger, who have been idealized in the fantasy that they kill only the evil men in black hats for good cause. This American idealization of violence adds fuel to a dangerous field. We admire the hunter, the warrior, the air ace, the killer. This is the myth of the violent hero, exploited by our entertainment media. Adolescents see themselves merely as extending the limits and type of violence.

Violence is a symptom, not a cause. It is an integral part of human nature. We cannot stamp it out, but we may be able to channel it into less harmful and more constructive outlets. Violence is coupled with violation of human dignity. As a result of slavery, oppression, and subjection to indignity, the black accepted the status of an inferior being and turned violence inward, striving to escape his black identity. One result has been extensive black intraracial violence.

It was not until the historic Supreme Court school desegregation decision in 1954 that blacks began to assert self-respect and, as a concomitant, to turn their violence outward. This was a moment of decision. The decision? To assert self-respect or fall back. Civil disobedience was a means of securing self-respect.

But the progress of the black has been disappointing to him. It has been sufficient to enable him to buy a TV set, insufficient to enable him to participate in the more meaningful social, intellectual, and material benefits of the culture he sees televised. Hence, he has experienced bitter frustration of earlier hopes. Revolutions start among rising classes, especially among those who have experienced a rise in living conditions or in feelings of potency, then suffer a setback.

Adolescents are enjoying a precocious maturation—not only the physiological advantages accruing from advances in medicine and research in nutrition, but also the sophistication and general awareness resulting from a lifetime of exposure to television, newspapers, and other information media. Furthermore, the ubiquity of these media enhances the position of student dissenters, according them an attention commensurate with that which was formerly directed to adults only.

With the competition for "newsworthy" events have come increased efforts by the media to cover happenings that are dramatic, violent, or unusual to the degree that they will attract readers or viewers—and the media's ability to spread emotions brings with it responsibility yet unmet.

We cannot expect an underplay of events, but are the media yet responsible enough to report and portray events in the proper perspective? Perhaps only a widespread campaign to educate people in healthful mental attitudes will eventually counteract journalistic tendencies toward sensationalism—and the public's appetite for it.

A New Rate of Social Change

The affluence of our society enables virtually our entire population to have access to the various communications media. Events are vividly presented while they are still "hot." The audience is nationwide. At the same time, rapid transportation permits an effective rabble-rouser to assume prominence and to use his unique talents in one city in the morning and in a distant city in the afternoon. The same rapid mass transportation permits vast numbers of people to converge and assemble, with weapons of destruction ready in hand.

Technology has thrust upon us problems which indeed are threatening and anxiety-producing. The population explosion, the explosion in knowledge (making relatively recent knowledge obsolete), the possibility of nuclear destruction, and the erosion of boundaries of race, time, and geography—all of these are productive of anxiety that may be discharged in a diffuse nature seemingly unrelated to the issues.

Adolescents have been caught up in the rapid change of our culture. Like adults, they are frightened by the rate of social change. The adult culture has demonstrated a rapid evolution of its social system and a capacity for swift change (unfortunately many of these are but superficial cultural changes). This raises the question of the need for an adolescence which may be considered a transitional phase or moratorium in personality development, for adolescents can exist only in societies in which the adult population represents solidified beliefs. In emerging societies, adolescents are required to combat the ossification of the society.

Adult society is undergoing so many changes that the adolescents are deprived of their normal avenues of rebellion. At the same time, adults express an air of permissiveness that encourages the development of adolescent revolt without setting definable bounds. Blacks may be leapfrogging the adolescence of their cultural and societal development. Add to this the fact that the period of infantile dependency on which so much of our psychological development depends is being shortened and we have a serious strain on the family structure.

It is significant that the more advanced the development of the animal, the longer is the period of infantile dependency. Is "adolescence" disappearing and are we reverting to a form of young adulthood beginning right after puberty such as existed in earlier centuries when youths went to work as soon as they could guide a plow?

Urban violence must have a psychological effect on the teen-ager, either as a participant in the disorder or as an observer of the actions of the revolters and of his elders in the disorder. Many psychiatrists, by their training, have been individual-oriented. Yet we should not ignore the possible effects of group interaction. We cannot and must not overlook some of the basic concepts of personality formation such as the mimicking of actions and need for identification, the advisability of having appropriate and clear limits set, and the necessity for the maintenance of a relative consistency within the societal fabric. Again consider the similarity between adolescents on the one hand and the black or student revolt group on the other. Adolescents must find confirmation of inner needs in existing society. So it is also with the black and the college student.

The Air of Permissiveness

It is interesting to examine the permissive attitude that so much of the public has toward urban revolt. The surprise has been not in the white backlash but in the relative tolerance of the majority. One reason for the acceptance of urban violence lies in the sad but realistic commentary that such action often abruptly accomplishes what legal and other means have been unable to. If our society is to end the use of violence as a technique of social change, it must afford the means to accomplish what is moral and appropriate by other means.

Another factor contributing to indulgence may involve the guilt toward adolescents and minorities that fosters masochism in many of us who form the dominant group in society. Our own trouble may be that we take seriously such allegations as "You haven't handled the world. You haven't solved these problems." Perhaps, in taking to heart such comments, we are projecting our own omnipotent thoughts and frustrations onto the critics. We may handle our own anxieties by projecting them onto the adolescent or the substitute adolescent—the black and the college student—and then by letting them express our emotion for us. But this is an unrealistic and mentally unhealthy tactic. Why should we be so grandiose as to accept blame for the world? What makes us think that, within one or two generations, we should be able to build a society without pain, frustration, and turbulence?

Another hypothesis for our permissiveness is the guilt attributable to the injustices that we have perpetrated on the underprivileged and on many minorities. Each of us carries a cultural identification and, with it, guilt feelings for many of the sins and actions not only of our forebears but also of our present classes or groups. As behavioral scientists, we are aware that overprotection or overpermissiveness is a response to guilt feelings, and that reaction formation is a response to ambivalence and ineffectiveness, which in themselves are a response to insecurity and indecision. White America, almost in a masochistic fashion, seems to be encouraging the violence of the black culture by its very inconsistent, ambivalent, double-standard, self-punitive role.

In this context, consider the situation a decade or so ago when enlightened black leaders deplored the "too fair" justice meted out for over a century by white courts to Negroes convicted of crimes against other blacks. Minimal sentences were imposed in these circumstances. It was as if the white society were saying that blacks were an inferior lot and white man's justice should not apply so long as a white person was not involved. May a similar pattern be perceived in the nominal punishment imposed on a person who burns a store during an urban revolt? Should the person who destroys property be given the normal punishment for arson? Or are we doing something similar to what we imposed as "Negro justice" when we assume a more lenient attitude toward those involved in acts of violence during an urban revolt?

The Urgency of Time

Most importantly in considering the possibility of a change in patterns of violence—and here the outlook is devastatingly depressing—what chance does a child of poverty beginning life with emotional and nutritional deficiencies in a crowded home, dominated by a working mother, and without even the physical presence of a man—let alone a father figure—have of avoiding the development of psychic and physical defects with severe, indelible scars? Children reared in such homes must be grossly affected. May not destructive violence be an understandable outcome in later years?

Regardless of how much and how ably society theorizes, its educated conjectures will not help unless it keeps its pledges of equal opportunity, equal rights, and genuine respect. In Nikos Kazantzakis' powerful (and surprisingly popular) book about a modern, non-violent hero, Zorba says to his idealistic young comrade:

"Let people be, boss; don't open their eyes. And supposing you did, what'd they see? Their misery! Leave their eyes closed, and let them go on dreaming!"

He was silent a moment and scratched his head. He was thinking.

"Unless," he said at last, "unless . . ."

"Unless what? Let's have it!"

"Unless when they open their eyes, you can show them a better world than the darkness in which they're gallivanting at present. . . . Can you?"[4]

Zorba, out of his practicality and also his great compassion for humanity, was constrained to put his finger on the weakness of many men of intellect (philosophers, scientists, even psychiatrists)—i.e., the tendency to observe rather than assess, the willingness to let time and the process of happenstance evolution alter the status quo. The remark attributed to Marshal Lyautey when he was French Governor-General of Morocco might appropriately serve as a precept for those inclined to too much observation and too little action. Having seen a particularly beautiful tree, the marshal asked his gardener about the possibility of planting the species in his own garden.

"But, General," said the gardener, "that tree takes 200 years to reach maturity."

"In that case," said Marshal Lyautey, "we have no time to lose. Plant them this afternoon."

In an age of rapid transportation, instant communication, and automated manufacture, goods—including the ethical as well as the material variety—must be delivered fast, not *because* we are pressed or *when* we are pressed but because certain rights—adequate housing, education, economic opportunity, and cultural identity—are just and moral, and morality should not have to wait upon pressure or expediency. We must preserve the societal fabric, but this can and must be done while preserving hope for the young and poor.

Those who are preaching violence argue that the wheels of change in our democratic society move too slowly and that almost any means justify the ends. It is uncomfortable for so many of us to recognize the basis behind so many of their claims.

Psychiatrists have essentially been liberals, striving for the dignity of man and the rights and needs of the individual. We recognize the destructive effects of poverty and discrimination. But in our liberal, intellectual zeal, have we shown personal courage by refusing to accept the glib diagnosis, the cliché of the moment as the explanation or putative solution of society's ills? We might do well to reevaluate the individual ingredients in our society's present dilemma and become action-oriented in our consideration of both the good and the bad. We have an obligation to put our creativity at the service of society.

William Hazlitt, in describing the process of creativity, compared it to the muscular state of a man standing upright and motionless in a moving coach. It was not the *fait accompli*, he contended, that signified creativity. Rather it was the process—the striving and contending with the exigencies of time and place.[3] So it is with social progress. To be viable, it must be the result of a dynamic equilibrium maintained in the face of opposing forces. Man was designed to be perfect*ible*, not perfect. Only in our awareness of this humanly incomplete state—and the resolve and never-ending effort to improve it—rests hope for the future.

REFERENCES

1. Cooper v. Aaron, 358 U.S. 1, 22, 1958.
2. Griswold, E. N.: Dissent—1968, Tulane Law Review 42:726-739, 1968.
3. Hazlitt, William (The Complete Works of), ed. by P. P. Howe (London: J. M. Dent and Sons, Ltd., 1930-34) Vol. XVIII, p. 161: "On the Elgin Marbles."
4. Kazantzakis, Nikos, *Zorba the Greek* (New York: Simon and Schuster, 1952), pp. 61-62.

20

EUGENE B. BRODY, M.D.

Most of us are living examples of Meyerson's concept of homo ambivalens. Leo Bartemeier has resolved as well as any man I know the inherent contradictions that pull us in different directions. He is, thus, a fitting recipient for the gift of an essay on hope.

Project HOPE — A Pragmatic Endeavor

HOPE IS AN ACRONYM for Home Ownership Plan Endeavor. Supported by private as well as federal funds it buys, renovates and sells homes at cost to low-income families. In 1969 it is the most biracial of Baltimore organizations and has been referred to by one of its associates as "a classic example of how people of different races can work together." Started in 1965 by a white woman who had been associated with the Archdiocesan Women's Committee for Civil Rights, its goals by 1968 had moved beyond the supplying of adequate low-cost individual-owned housing. It now looks forward to the development of an educational complex in the inner city. With these goals there has been increasing emphasis on the development of black leadership, and the active involvement of an order of black nuns. There has also been injected the element of activism; a key person in the project, Sister Mary Paraclete, principal of a private Catholic high school for Negro girls, has declared that "inner city Negroes have grown tired of promises by white officials and 'no longer believe in them.' "[1]

It is not my purpose to devote this essay to a description of HOPE Inc.—but rather to the motives which instigated it. *Hope* as a human attribute may be considered at a variety of philosophical, abstract or concrete levels. This paper approaches it from the viewpoint of the pragmatic clinician, concerned with the adaptation of individual human beings to their environment, and of the social biologist interested in the future of the species. If man wants a future on the planet Earth, he should understand that he can assure it only through perceiving himself as a member of a single biological and cultural species. One world means one race, the human race. The organization HOPE—like the virtue for which it is named—is at base a unifying mechanism. Despite the new note of militancy (which may simply supply necessary fuel during an era of confrontation), the organization is aimed at undoing the division of our society effected by biases against color and class. Concretely it is a counterforce to the "blockbusters" who, breeding on fear and greed, buy cheaply from the racially frightened whites and sell dearly to the home-hungry blacks. Man is a nest-builder, a home-based animal. Perhaps through such endeavors as HOPE, it will be possible for him to extend his view of home and family from his own microscopic piece of earth territory to the entirety of his microscopic floating-dot-in-space while it can still foster survival.

The gradual division of the United States into black and white cultural subspecies and antagonists represents not a national but a worldwide phenomenon. Human beings are prone to antithetical polarization on non-genetic bases in a manner not observed among other living creatures. Polarization is made easier and reinforced by social visibility on the basis of color. But it also occurs between people of similar color, physiognomy and socioeconomic status on the basis of religion, politics or whatever other symbolic system has the greatest drawing power of the time and region.

Perhaps there is cause for hope as well as despair in man's symbolic ability. His capacity for complex symbolization, including concept formation, and his capacity to create and maintain a socially transmitted culture are, after all, basic to his ability to engage in sustained collaborative behavior. Without them there could be no HOPE. Nor would there be a city, or a church, or a community in which such schemes could originate. Much of human adaptability and survival depends upon behavior called collaborative, cooperative, collective or even altruistic. Individual survival throughout man's existence as a species has depended upon his capacity for collective action.[2]

This is part of the puzzle. Ideologies, involving symbols as motivating forces (rather than food, water or sex), lead man both to his most remarkable achievements and his most destructive acts. Wars, which are organized attempts by one society to destroy another, require shifting allegiance to a variety of ideologies. This is in sharp contrast to the relatively fixed patterns of intro-species aggression which lead members of one rat family, for example, to automatically attack members of another differentiated from them on the basis of scent rather than of beliefs.[3]

Symbolization also allows man to look forward into the future and backward to the past. Without it he would have neither his quality of self-awareness nor the existential anxiety associated with it. He could not conceive of himself as a time-limited entity suspended in a void; he might also be less plagued by some of the horrors called "mental illness." He would not have developed the moral and ethical systems which regulate his individual and group behavior; yet he would not be in a condition of perpetual inner conflict primarily *because* his self-awareness and value systems, combined with the technical mastery of his environment, permit such a perplexing array of behavioral alternatives. Abraham Meyerson has observed the paradox of man's condition, aptly contrasting his cruelty and rationally justified war-making with his tenderness and conscious love. He describes man as *"Homo Ambivalens,* a creature who builds up contradictory, hostile and opposite patterns of life and attempts to live them simultaneously."[4]

HOPE and other organizations like it reflect the rudimentary process of resolving the contradictory tendencies within man. Most agencies of this kind, while their conception may have been motivated in part by a concern for the underprivileged—or fear of their eventual rebellion, are the creations of detached, reasoning, symbol-manipulating intellects. A man can intensely dislike another of different color and subculture, but at the same time know that his own survival will ultimately depend upon the relative well-being of the other. With that knowledge he can devise a mechanism to ensure the well-being of the other, even though he harbors hatred for or, at best, indifference toward him.

The reiteration of these mechanisms over the short period of recorded human history appears to reflect the gradual and uneven move through cultural evolution toward the development of a system of social homeostasis, of "social wisdom"; this is as necessary for the survival of humans as is the physiological homeostatic system constituting the "wisdom of the body" and ensuring the relative constancy and survival of an individual organism in the face of physical environmental vicissitudes.[5] The great philosophers and religious leaders have underscored this theme as a central aspect of their moral codes. Confucius said, "What you do not want done to yourself, do not do unto others." Plato wrote, "It is worse to inflict wrong than to suffer it." Jesus said, "All things ye would that men should do unto you, even so do ye also do unto them." And Rabbi Hillel, Jesus' contemporary said, "What is hateful unto thee do not do unto thy fellow,"

HOPE represents positive social action, and it is perhaps encouraging to see it as a reflection of rational, secular, rather than religious thought— even though it sprang from a lay religious group. Its existence implies the recognition of its founders that, for man to have hope, he must have a place to live. And it attests the powerful potential in man's ability to transform abstract concepts into collaborative efforts. It may also augur the survival of the human race through the transmission of acquired, as well as inherited (or genetic), intelligence.

Yet each consideration of man's capacity to transcend genetic evolutionary forces and to rescue himself through the conscious creation of social mechanisms leads back to the classic dilemmas.

The unlocking of nature's storehouse of energy for peaceful purposes, leading at the same time to the building of engines of total destruction, is one.

The conquest of communicable disease and the application of public health knowledge, leading to explosive overpopulation in regions without adequate food resources or educational facilities, is another.

The development of new tranquilizing drugs which permit the early discharge of schizophrenics into the community—and a consequent rise in their rates of reproduction and ability to perpetuate distorted child-rearing environments—is yet another.

The survival of mental defectives, resulting in an increased need for caretakers, represents an ironic "good."

The development of cheap, efficient transportation enables migrants to move from undesirable rural living areas to the cities in such numbers that municipal services are totally overwhelmed.

The growth of industry, while promoting national fiscal "health," is also responsible for the biological assassination of our rivers and lakes.

The development of computers which free man from the slavery of interminable calculations and open unforeseen research horizons may make real the old specter of loss of personal privacy as one's social security number becomes the key to a magnetic-tape record of his life history.

And without the rise in living standards and a concomitant increase in the dissemination of information leading to ever-greater expectations, there would probably not have been as yet a black-white confrontation in the United States' inner cities. For example the deprived masses of Latin America, where the difference between haves and have-nots is far greater than it is in the United States, continue to be so weak and powerless, so excluded from the informational and participatory system, that they have neither the attitudes nor the strength to strive aggressively toward a new identity.

There seems, however, to be no growth possible without a period of upheaval. A move from one status to another requires a transitional period, and it is during this period, when people are no longer what they were nor yet what they will be, that tension rises. Given his history of slavery and emancipation in America, the black man could not achieve socio-economically adult status *without* a phase of stormy adolescence.

Most national societies have not yet progressed to the point where confrontations of the varieties occurring in the United States—between black and white, rich and poor, powerful and powerless—are possible. Our very confrontations, with all their tension and casualties, reflect the distance we have travelled toward honest self-perception and a view of ourselves as members of a single species—in other words, as inhabitants of one world. We may look upon the Home Ownership Plan Endeavor as heartening proof that man is capable of learning to control his own technology and even of developing ethical systems to accommodate it. We may see in such organizations as HOPE the promise of sufficient strength to bridge the transition period and, ultimately, the gulf between societies.

REFERENCES

1. The *Sun*, November 18, 1968, p. C14.
2. Brody, E. B. Culture, Symbol and Value in the Social Etiology of Behavioral Deviance. In *Social Psychiatry* (J. Zubin, ed.) New York, Grune & Stratton, Inc., 1968, pp. 8-33.
3. Lorenz, K. On Aggression, 1963. English translation. New York, Harcourt, Brace and World, 1966.
4. Meyerson, A. Speaking of Man. New York, A. A. Knopf, 1958.
5. Brody, S. Science and Social Wisdom. The Scientific Monthly, 59:203-214, 1944.

21

M. RALPH KAUFMAN, M.D.

Leo Bartemeier: "A man for all seasons." He practices what he preaches.

The Physician's Role in Social Issues

THE RESPONSIBILITY of a medical school, particularly a new one, is to relate itself to the state of medicine not only in 1969 but in 1975, 1980, and even the year 2000. The physician to be graduated within the next ten years will become a member of a profession whose practice may bear little resemblance to that of today. What are these changes that are taking place and predictably will take place? Who are the students who are entering medical school today? What are their attitudes and expectations? How should and can one relate these attitudes and expectations to the realities of twenty-five years from now?

One of the oldest and most fundamental canons of the physician stems from that part of the Hippocratic Oath which enjoins physicians to impart their knowledge to others aspiring to be doctors—"to teach them this art if they so desire without fee or written promise; to impart to my sons and the sons of the master who taught me and the disciples who have enrolled themselves and have agreed to the rules of the profession, but to these alone, the precepts and the instruction." The Oath further states, "I will prescribe regimen for the good of my patients according to my ability and my judgment and never do harm to anyone. To please no one will I prescribe a deadly drug, nor give advices which may cause his death. Nor will I give a woman a pessary to procure abortion. But I will preserve the purity of my life and my heart."

Ancient as it is, the Oath contains the essence of many of the problems that still confront physicians and that will become even more pressing in the days to come.

285

There seems to be, if not a new, at least a more active type of student today. This is true not only in medicine but in all areas of student life. The phenomenon does not seem to be limited to our country or even to our socioeconomic point of view. Red China, Soviet Russia, DeGaulle's France, Wilson's England, as well as Nixon's America—all are filled with the sound and fury of activists, whose style must be taken into account for any program of education and training—more particularly in the field of medicine.

The first student-edited issue of *The New Physician* carried an editorial which expresses the viewpoint of the young physician as activist. Its initial statement is a confrontation:

> Student activism is only one facet of the spectre of revolution which haunts the Establishment. Yet the fact that it is beginning to touch upon the Medical Establishment in a significant way is perhaps most surprising and important. The physician, says Martin Gross in his well-documented book [sic], *The Doctors,* has changed "from a societal leader, intellectually and humanly . . . to a man of mediocre intellect, trade-school mentality, limited interests, and incomplete personality—the contemporary Non-Renaissance Man. . . . Student activism in medicine reaches its highest potential when it is effectively organized. It was easy for the Medical Establishment to dismiss, in fact destroy, the first responsible, but weakly organized, group of activist medical students, the old Association of Interns and Medical Students.

The editor goes on to claim, "It is clear that our older professional colleagues are listening. They are listening partly because the voice which they hear reflects their best teachings, and partly because they must realize that it is the voice of the future."[1]

In a similar vein and of major interest is the preamble of the Free University of the Mid-Peninsula, Palo Alto, California, printed in the same student-edited edition of *The New Physician* quoted above. This emphasizes that the American educational establishment has not met the needs of our society and that students are neither encouraged to think critically nor provided training which helps them understand the crucial issues of today. American education, the preamble asserts, is too bound to the existing power structure and modes of thought to consider freely and objectively the cultural, economic and political forces rapidly transforming the modern world. In capital letters the preamble proclaims:

> THAT EDUCATION WHICH HAS NO CONSEQUENCES FOR
> SOCIAL ACTION OR PERSONAL GROWTH IS EMPTY. THAT
> ACTION WHICH DOES NOT RAISE OUR LEVEL OF CON-
> SCIOUSNESS IS FUTILE.

The significance of such attitudes for the future of medicine cannot be underestimated, whether the premises on which they are based are altogether true or mostly false. Contrast the attitude of the student of today with his fantasy of the passive student of yesteryear—browbeaten, spoonfed, didacticized, lectured at and stuffed with what passed for knowledge with a complete irrelevance to the task at hand.

Looked at from one point of view, the new medical student and his activist philosophy can be passed off as a pain-in-the-neck. But glibly to dismiss him would be to overlook the significance of his protest: he is bringing to the field of medicine his ideal of what the role of the physician should be in society; he desires a new and more humane approach to the problems of the world; he recognizes that the right to health and medical care should be more than a political slogan or shibboleth, and he wants to convert that hypothetical right into a palpable reality. He also recognizes that the right to become a physician should not be restricted to an economic class or related primarily to the color of one's skin. He questions some of our basic assumptions about how one qualifies to become a medical student. (There is a good deal of talk about the "disadvantaged" and what change in the Establishment System is necessary to obliterate inequities and limits.)

The challenges implicit in both the preamble and the editorial confirm the impressions that the activist is a young man in a hurry—that he is unwilling to wait for tomorrow since he feels that everything should have been done yesterday. (And even when something *was* done yesterday, he regards the accomplishment dubiously, since he is convinced that yesterday's techniques are almost by definition today's museum-pieces.) They corroborate many an administrator's opinion that, immediately upon admission to medical school, the average student wants to become a member of the Admissions Committee and revamp the standards for qualification. They also tend to support the uneasy suspicion that, if the student had his way, all aspects of medical education would be turned over to him with the faculty playing a purely secondary role—inasmuch as wisdom is no longer regarded as a factor of age but its inverse. In the extreme, it seems to medical educators, today's student does not even want a dialogue. Many of his terms are underlined as non-negotiable, and the younger the protester, the more certain he is that things should be done his way or not at all.

Since these attitudes and points of view are reflections of what has been called the generation gap and its conflicts, there is a danger that, in faculty-student confrontation, the solution demanded by the medical student may become the overriding basis for Faculty action. It seems as if a series of complex psychological phenomena results in a kind of leaning-over-backwards which may give the faculty members the illusion that they are not, as the students imply, really "old fogies" but that they are as "with it" as their young tormentors. Such uncritical surrender may proceed from the desire for peace, a hankering after popularity, or the guilty conviction that the older generation is indeed culpable and a consequent tendency to over-compensate.

Evidence that leaders in medical education have not been as oblivious to changing conditions as the activists may believe is found in the recommendations of the Association of the American Medical Colleges based on a study supported by the Commonwealth Fund. The AAMC recommended that:

1. Medical schools must increase their output of physicians;
2. Increased numbers of students should be admitted from geographic areas and from economic and ethnic groups that are inadequately represented today;
3. The medical student's training must be individualized to fit varied rates of achievement, educational backgrounds and career goals;
4. Medical school curricula should be developed by interdepartmental groups that include students;
5. The medical schools must now assume a responsibility for education and research in the organization and delivery of health services, with the total span of the physician's education revised so that his professional competence will be most relevant to meeting the changing health needs of the people.[2]

The Commonwealth study gives various examples of the way these goals have been accomplished in different medical schools as they do more to implement the recommended changes.

Additional facts to be martialed in defense of the Old Order are those relating to the backgrounds of many entering students, the non-traditional roles coveted by today's aspiring physicians, and the extent of the information and skill that must now be communicated to the medical student. Increasingly the beginning medical student brings with him a highly specialized education. Ever since Sputnik, secondary schools throughout our country have laid a heavy emphasis on science, and today's students often find themselves, upon graduating from high school, better posted on modern concepts of physics, and chemistry, and mathematics than were their professors at the conclusion of *their* pre-medical years in college. As a result, many medical students appear to identify more with the scientist-physician or the graduate student in the sciences than with the practitioner. They have little in common with older clinicians practicing in the community and, because of a failure in communication, often misjudge the motives and intentions of older doctors. Furthermore, the speed with which new knowledge is accreting and making obsolete the old axioms produces an almost unavoidable lag between discovery and teaching, thereby eroding confidence in educators as up-to-date dispensers of vital information and techniques. It is unfortunately true that awareness and understanding of the new cannot be superimposed upon anything but a firm grasp of the old, and that, ultimately, only the incentive to continue study throughout his career will keep the physician abreast of the latest developments in his field.

There can, however, be no counter-argument to the contention that schools of medicine should take the lead in studying the ways medical care is delivered. Their concern should be not only with acute care but also with prevention and rehabilitation, with comprehensive family care as well as with specialization. The university-sponsored medical school is in an unequalled position to bring the resources of many disciplines—including the behavioral and social sciences—to bear on a wide range of medical responsibilities.

As Cecil Sheps has observed:

> There are few countries in the world today which do not find themselves coping with the tide of rising expectations in the field of health services on the part of citizens. In the less well-developed, less industrialized, and poorer portions of the world, where the mass of the people themselves are not fully aware of the benefits to be gained from the availability of modern health services, political forces are at work which are aware of these opportunities.[4]

Edmund Pellegrino, Dean of the Medical School of the State University of New York at Stony Brook, wrote:

> Medical care in our country is undergoing a profound transformation induced by two potent ideas long nascent in our society. The first of these is the awakening of our universities to the potential of their role in public service and community action. The second is the public decision to establish health as a major goal and to take the means to define that goal and achieve it optimally . . . the fact is that an informed public has already decided to devote a significant part of its material resources to the purposes of better health and has expressed its will in legislation and appropriation. It promises to go much further in this direction in the future. In so doing, it regards

the physician and the university as instruments of social purpose. While the initiative has not been theirs, the university and the community of practicing physicians are now impelled toward a confrontation for which they have had little time to prepare and for which there is little precedent . . . this confrontation will surely complicate the interrelationships of medical schools and practitioners.[5]

Those who are physicians and students of medicine should be particularly sensitive to the signs and symptoms of inequality and injustice. The health status of our Negro, Mexican-American, Puerto Rican, and Indian citizens is stark evidence of the disastrous consequences of discrimination. We find among these groups shorter life expectancy; malnutrition; higher infant and maternal mortality rates; and more than their share of mental illness, chronic disease, mental retardation and orthopedic and visual handicaps. It is not only this pattern of disease and disability; it is even more the lack of dignity and decency with which health services often are provided that is a shame on all the health professions.[6]

In the words of John Gardner, the distinguished former Secretary of Health, Education and Welfare:

There has been significant progress in recent years in removing the barriers to health services for the poor of the country—Medicare; Medicaid; migrant health programs; maternal and infant projects; neighborhood health centers. All are important steps forward. Yet, few can seriously question that we still have a long, hard road to travel before we can say that access to high-quality health services is not only a right but a reality for all Americans.[6]

Wilbur reminds us that medicine has been considered primarily a personal thing between a physician and his patient, but today, and even more tomorrow, medicine and health are matters of total public concern.[7]

The population explosion confronts medicine with perhaps its greatest challenge. Few doubt that the rapid application of modern science and engineering skills to the problems of sanitation and the control of infectious diseases has contributed significantly to rapid rates of population growth—far more, undoubtedly, than medical studies of human reproduction and fertility control have contributed to a decline in the birth rate.[8]

Scientific advances also lead us into perhaps one of the most controversial areas, embedded as it is in religion, philosophy, ethical and taboo situations—namely, that of abortion and sterilization. Relatively few medical schools even today enter into a discussion in depth of these problems. Too often the medical student is given an attitude he must adopt rather than an opportunity to examine, to think about and to take the position in terms of his own individual makeup and his role as a physician.

A recent spate of papers deals with various aspects of medical ethics and morals brought to urgency through technical advances. Current technical advances in biomedical endeavor, such as organ transplantation and fertility control, challenge our understanding of moral problems associated with medical practice. No longer are there solid and immutable absolutes for our comfort.[9]

Many ethical issues which are raised anew with the advances in organ transplants have been aired repeatedly throughout the centuries whenever medical advances were made. Anesthesia, surgical asepsis, and blood transfusion in their turn were each criticized on ethical grounds. In their day, these procedures were considered by some critics to violate 'natural law.'[10]

There is currently a good deal of concern with the area of transplant. Many of the technical advances in the operative procedures have been overcome though problems still remain, particularly in the area of immunology. Hopefully, most of these will be solved. The discussions are no longer primarily in terms of the technical advances but rather center in ethical, religious and psychological aspects. Medicine is being forced to look into its basic assumptions in regard to time of death. Within the medical profession itself such terms as "vultures" and "grave snatchers" have again come to the fore.

And, at the same time, the opposite ethical position on transplants is expressed by Christian Barnard who said, "The question is, whether it is moral to bury that organ which could save somebody else."[11]

Keith Reemtsma, in his article in the new book, *Ethical Issues in Medicine*, writes, "Taking a kidney from one individual for use in another violates a fundamental precept: *primum non nocere* (first of all, do not harm)."

Use of organs from cadavers raises the question of the definition of death. Classically and legally, death is defined as cessation of heartbeat and respiration. Biologically, death is a complex and prolonged process, not an instantaneous event. Organs die at varying rates, and cells and subcellular systems cease functioning before or after circulatory and respiratory systems have failed.[12]

Artificial insemination raises still other ethical problems. As Feingold noted:

Officially, artificial insemination does not exist. No court in the United States, Great Britain or Canada has any statutory law aimed at A.I.D.* Countries boasting prolific legislation and complexities of laws have made no effort to recognize the procedure. This is surprising when one is apprised that five individuals are concerned in each insemination in which a donor is used. A patient, her husband, the donor, the doctor and the child are involved. Each requires a measure of legal protection. . . . The American Medical Association is aware that, in spite of a serious void in the law, doctors are practicing and will continue artificial insemination. The director of the legal and socioeconomic division of this organization stated that he doubted that the AMA had the authorty to say to the physicians of America that they can or cannot properly engage in this practice.[13]

In search of enlightenment and guidance in order to be able to fulfill in part the obligations of a teacher and mentor to the student who is to become a physician, I reread the Opinions and Reports of the AMA Judicial Council, Section 10 on Principles and Medical Ethics. The introduction tells me that: "The honored ideals of the medical profession imply that the responsibilities of the physician extend not only to the individual, but also to society where these responsibilities deserve his interest and participation in activities which have the purpose of improving both the health and the well-being of the individual and the community."

I eagerly read this section which I found dealt with 1. Physicians as Citizens; 2. Public Health; 3. The Relationship of the Physician to Media of Public Information; 4. Advertising and the Daily Press; 5. Medical Public Relations; 6. Physicians Writing Health Columns; 7. Release of Medical Information to the Press; 8. Use of the Physician's Name in Connection with Civil Enterprises; 9. Disclosure of Information to Insurance Company Representative; 10. Discussion of Medical Facts with Patient's Lawyer.[14]

Information under this section, valuable as it is, offers very little to discuss with my students about the burning social issues of the times. It affords no response to some of their most urgent questions and demands.

There has been an explosive recognition that the patterns of the delivery of health services are defective at almost every level. The changing concepts of health involve a recognition that "health is a basic human right and is no longer a matter for professional and public debate. It is a fact, and we must plan within its context and act to fulfill its content. A sound mind, in a sound body, in a sound family, in a sound environment is the goal for every individual and no less will do."[15]

---

* Artificial Insemination Donor

This concept leads to re-examination of one aspect of practice, namely that of group practice. It also raises the necessity for re-evaluation and emphasis on the education, training and up-grading of paramedical personnel.

The shortage of physician manpower is so serious that, even if the planned increases in medical school enrollment are achieved, the schools will barely be able to keep pace with population growth, much less increase the availability of physician services.

Teaching and learning in the entire spectrum of medical education, from paramedical education through residency training, is still too rigidly structured and compartmentalized and too stifling to intellectual initiative. It is also not sufficiently adaptable to provide the diverse range of physician manpower demanded for the future.

It becomes increasingly evident that no medical problem should be solved purely in terms of technology. Indeed, technological advance can introduce new problems or increase the magnitude of old ones. Cultural, sociological and psychological factors relating to illness and health seem to be as important today as they always were and the physician must be prepared to understand them if he is to function as a healer.

The traditional fee for service in terms of direct payment of such a fee on a personal basis plays a lesser role in the practice of medicine today and it will play an even smaller role in the future. Government involvement, Medicare, Medicaid, third-party-payment through insurance, and medical care through fringe benefits all make it necessary to re-examine medicine's traditional attitudes towards the payment of fees. Medical care in many instances—particularly as it relates to hospitalization and certain kinds of ambulatory care—may too often be determined by the payment pattern and regulations rather than by medical determination of the patient's need. For example, 90-day limitation for hospitalization in general hospital departments of psychiatry in New York City creates the necessity for a treatment program that must be limited on this account. The ideal of continuity of medical care may be impossible to carry out under certain circumstances. Also, these third-party payment plans seem to have altered even the traditional professional courtesy that for so long has been part and parcel of the etiquette of the practice of medicine.

The education of medical students and house staff members also has felt the impact of third-party payment. As more hospital and other medical costs are paid for by governmental and other third-party sources, the ranks of the non-paying ward patient—the "teaching patient"—are reduced. New relationships between the patient and his doctor need to be established if we are to carry on a viable education in these areas.

Technological advances continue to expand the medical center concept. Utilization of special instrumentation and technics for the care of patients has resulted in an increasing use of the team in which each individual becomes more highly specialized in a specific aspect of patient care. In most instances this has made it impossible for any one physician to function without the aid of a complex manpower group. This will require a physician who is accustomed to, and can work comfortably with, a greater number of specially trained teammates. It will also enlist the leadership skills of the physician who has to coordinate several different functions and the work of others on behalf of his patient.

These are but some of the highlights of the current and future trends that constitute the generic field of medicine. Our problem therefore as educators is how to create a climate for the medical student which will enable him to make the necessary commitment and to obtain the necessary skills—which will enable him to be a member of the medical profession in all its aspects in the year 2000.

One thing is certain: that this change cannot evolve by precept alone. The future physician's attitudes towards the dignity of his patient will be molded by the example of the physicians who teach him. Attitudes and relationships fostered in current outpatient departments would seem to indicate that certain current operational procedures in the practice of medicine must change.

The basic model for identification should be the teacher who practices what he preaches.

REFERENCES

1. *The New Physician*, Vol. 17, No. 9, September 1968.
2. Harold M. Schmeck, Jr., "Medical School Survey Urges Drastic Changes in Universities and Medical School for the Education of Future Physicians," *Journal of Medical Education*, Vol. 43, 1968, p. 436.
3. Daniel H. Funkenstein, "Implications of the Rapid Social Changes in Universities and Medical Schools for the Education of Future Physicians," *Journal of Medical Education*, Vol. 43, 1968, p. 436.
4. Cecil G. Sheps, "The Medical School—Community Expectations," *Trends in New Medical Schools*, in Hans Popper (ed.) New York: Grune & Stratton 1967.
5. Edmund D. Pellegrino, "Regionalization: An Integrated Effort of Medical School, Community, and Practicing Physician," *Bulletin of the New York Academy of Medicine*, Vol. 42 (1966), p. 1193.
6. Philip R. Lee, M. D., "Medicine and the Four Revolutions," *Pharos of Alpha Omega Alpha, Honor Medical Society*, October 1968.

7. Dwight L. Wilbur, M.A.C.P., "Medicine as the Leader of Change," *The Bulletin of the American College of Physicians*, Vol. 9, No. 10, October 1968.
8. Lee, *Op. Cit.*, p. 131.
9. Chauncey D. Leake, Ph.D., "Theories of Ethics and Medical Practice," presented at the Second National Congress on Medical Ethics, October 5-6, 1968, Chicago, Illinois.
10. Paul S. Rhoads, M.D., "Medical Ethics and Morals in a New Age," *Journal of The American Medical Association*, Vol. 205, Aug. 12, 1968.
11. "Dr. Barnard Discusses Transplant Moral Issue," New York *Times*, December 7, 1968.
12. Keith Reemtsma, "Ethical Problems with Artificial and Transplanted Organs: An Approach by Experimental Ethics," E. Fuller Torrey (ed.), *Ethical Issues in Medicine*, Boston: Little Brown and Co., 1968.
13. Wilfred J. Feingold, "Artificial Insemination," in E. Fuller Torrey (ed.), *Ethical Issues in Medicine*, Boston: Little Brown and Co., 1968.
14. Judicial Council, Section 10, *Opinions and Reports*, 1966. American Medical Association.
15. L. E. Burney, M.D., et al, "Planning for Comprehensive Health Care at Temple University Hospital," *Public Health Reports*, Vol. 83, No. 6, June 1968.

22

JOHN ROMANO, M.D.

It is a pleasant assignment and an honor to share with others the privilege of paying tribute to a colleague and friend of many years. A European journey many years ago during the war with Leo Bartemeier, Karl Menninger, Lawrence Kubie and John Whitehorn has given vivid and fond memories of Leo's clinical wisdom and kindness. As can be said of only a few men, one can say of Leo, only the strong can be gentle.

Engagement Versus Detachment

PROGRESS IN THE MEDICAL SCIENCES and the education of the public to its benefits have led to the assumption that health, no longer a privilege, must be considered a basic human right. Modern scientific discoveries and the methods to apply them have affected how we are born and live and die. The intent of federal legislation and the tax authorization to support it is to improve medical care not only for the privileged but for the many. This movement is an expected extension of federal tax support to the health services. In the past two decades support was restricted to project and programmatic medical researches and to selected training programs.

All this leads quite directly to issues of significant increases in trained personnel, to provisions for the availability and continuity of care, to the distribution of services, to community planning and organization, and to public education in preventive, curative, and rehabilitative services. The central and urgent relevance of this movement to the university medical

---

* Abridged from paper initially presented on the occasion of the dedication of the Connecticut Mental Health Center, Oct. 1, 1966, New Haven, Conn. Published in "The University and Community Mental Health" pp. 25-39. Reprinted by permission from Yale University Press, 1968.

centers is clearly apparent. There are now, and there will be many more, serious and significant requests and demands made of the university medical centers for extension of health services to citizens in their communities and beyond to regional areas.

There is need for the medical school, its constituent departments and teaching hospitals, like all social organizations, to examine their internal systems and their constant exchange with their environment. Since the publication of Abraham Flexner's "Bulletin No. 4 of the Carnegie Institute for the Advancement of Teaching" (1910), there is evidence of an increasing and mutually profitable exchange between the medical school and its parent university. More recently there are attempts to examine with greater care the exchanges between the university medical school, together with its teaching hospitals, and the community or region in which it exists and which it serves.

What must not be lost sight of is the fact that the environmental context in which we exist—beyond the parochial boundaries of local town and gown—the national, political, economic, and social scene, is changing at an increasing rate. Its rate of change may outdistance by far the changes within our systems and will doubtedly influence our destinies for many years to come. The powerful impact of government aid and influence is not restricted to the medical school. It is felt, too, by the university-at-large. And if you listen to America, you will hear a persistent chorus—sometimes plaintive, often eloquent, and always literate. It is made up in great part by the voices and writings of university presidents and faculties, of government administrators and commentators on the social scene.

It says that the American university is facing an identity crisis of major production, often spoken of as "the time for decision."

The themes are multiple and often intimately interwoven: quality versus quantity; teaching versus research; isolation versus regionalization and commitments to area study programs throughout the world; science versus humanities; the freedom or restriction attached to funds solicited and received, with particular reference to the matter of secrecy. But there is another, not born of the moment. While it has existed from the beginnings of the establishment of the university in society, it has special significance for us today. Let me quote from President Goheen, of Princeton:

> Behind all these other tensions is a larger one which has troubled men and institutions for centuries: how to strike the proper balance between detachment and involvement. This tension is felt in myriad

ways in the modern American university. How we treat it, how we can best utilize its potential forward thrust, should be a matter of the gravest moment not only within universities but to men outside concerned about the contributions universities can make. . . . The university must not surrender its position as a place of relative detachment where cool reflection, objective study, and the long view can flourish. At the same time, men in the university must be alert and sensitive to the pressing needs of our times; they must be prepared to respond to important calls for service from outside the university; in doing so they must seek to bring to current issues the force of that kind of intellectual competence and candor which is most peculiarly the product of the university.[2]

And Barnaby C. Keeney, recently retired as president of Brown University, and appointed by President Johnson to head the National Endowment for the Humanities, issued a warning against both extremes, activism and detachment:

A college or a university traditionally requires a certain detachment, a physical or symbolic separation from the daily business of society. Such separation is rapidly diminishing, particularly in the case of universities, which are perhaps the largest reservoirs of expertise available to society. We have, therefore, locally and nationally and now internationally been utilized by society to find and teach information necessary for its purposes. The demands upon these institutions will grow as knowledge constantly becomes more important to modern life.

However, he clearly dissociated himself from the position of extreme detachment:

On the other hand, the academic institution cannot and should not turn its back on these problems. It should, in the first place, if it properly can and has the resources to do so, attempt to produce studies which make a problem clearer and which may lead to a solution. It should, if it is capable of doing so, teach the background of the situation involved and the foreground as well. It should permit and indeed encourage members, both students and faculty, to participate as individuals in efforts to solve the problems. This, I believe, is the proper contribution of colleges and universities to contemporary society—to produce information, to interpret it, to teach it, and to disseminate it in other ways, to accumulate data and then to free people capable of assisting society. It is not the proper function of a college or a university to commit itself to a particular solution.[3]

The relevance of this matter to the medical school must be apparent. As a professional school of the university, medicine (particularly, but not exclusively, in its clinical departments), like its sister schools of education, music, engineering, business, theology, and law, has been less of a spectator and more of a participant observer of the human comedy than are other divisions of the college or the university.

Obviously the teaching of clinical medicine in all of its divisions is not —nor should it be—a spectator sport. It can take place only with the significant engagement of the medical student, under the supervision of his teacher, with his patient, and his patient's family—in the setting of the community in which they live and work.

While there appears to be concern that the modern physician has become too impersonal, too scientific, or insufficiently informed or skilled in understanding his patients' psychological and social problems, there is general acknowledgment and appreciation of the contributions made to medical science, as well as the successful application of new knowledge and skills on the part of our medical school graduates. The critics of our modern university medical centers accuse us of two severe and serious shortcomings. The first relates to the doctor shortage; the second alleges that we have not participated fully in community health planning and services.

We are a deficit nation in medical education. We import many more physicians than we export. The need for more physicians and for other trained paramedical professions and ancillary persons is now generally accepted. The faculties of our medical schools, accused of resisting increases in the size of student bodies, have been called snobbish, unimaginative, timid, and insensitive to urgent, if not imperative, social needs. Greer Williams recently concluded a critique by saying, "The Flexner concept of excellence has served American medical education well, but have we not learned enough about large group organization and management in the 55 years since publication of his report to produce excellence in larger number? Perhaps it is time to say farewell to Flexner and move ahead."[4]

Equally critical are the comments about the relations between the teaching hospital and the community:

> The potential of the teaching hospital for leadership in achieving the new synthesis of scientific medicine and community health programs is almost limitless. As it stands midway between the medical school and the research laboratory on the one hand, and community hospitals, physicians, and other community health resources on the other, its historic role has been to translate progress in medical research and education into new and improved technics of patient care.

Despite their brilliant history, however, many—perhaps most—teaching hospitals now appear uncertain and defensive as to their appropriate role. Some turn their backs on the community altogether, concentrating all their resources on teaching and research, and accepting only enough patients to provide the required amount of "teaching material." A few attempt to open their doors to all who wish to enter and sometimes find themselves overwhelmed, especially in their outpatient departments, by the flood of social, as well as organic, pathology. If the care is provided in an atmosphere that attracts paying patients, the hospital may find itself locked in combat with the local medical society.

Much has been written and said in recent years about the harmful effects of such town-and-gown schisms. Much of the responsibility for the frequent breakdown in communications between academic medicine and community physicians and hospitals does not belong to academic medicine. But it is hard not to suspect that at least part of the difficulty is due to the intellectual snobbishness of some academic institutions and lack of adequate concern for general community needs and willingness to work with other community resources. In any case, in such situations society is less likely to seek a precise allocation of blame than to proclaim, "A plague on both your houses!"[5]

Within the limits of personal experience with the faculties of five American medical schools, I have not noticed a selfish or consciously insensitive lack of concern on their part with these issues. Some appear to believe that these matters should be solved by persons other than themselves, but in general, there has been a persistent and pervasive concern with quality, even though Coggeshall may have been correct when he said, "There has not been an objective, thorough study that has shown any clear relationship between the size of a medical school and the educational results achieved."[6] Our defense is based in great part upon impressions of the graduates of the diploma mills of yesterday, and upon more recent experiences with the graduates of the monstrously large medical schools in many continental and asiatic countries. While I am aware of the multiple determining factors, such as age of student, curricular pattern, teaching facilities, there is little question that there are significant differences between our graduates and theirs in information and knowledge, and, particularly, in clinical experience. Unlike our students, few of theirs have been seriously and continually engaged and supervised in events of human interaction which constitute the basic method of the clinician.

In our schools there have been serious and persistent attempts to keep abreast of the information explosion and to select consciously and wisely the information and knowledge basic and essential to the preparation of tomorrow's physicians. Furthermore, this has been taking place in a setting hardly contemplative, but in one characterized by urgent human needs, and with serious limits of experienced teachers, of funds, and of space. Almost everyone agrees that we need more physicians, and that it will be necessary not only to establish new schools but also to expand the size of the classes of existing schools. Additional funds, of course, will be necessary and probably forthcoming. It seems unlikely, however, that funds, however sufficient, will answer all of our problems. It is going to be necessary for us to examine closely and clearly our basic concepts and our current methods of medical education, and to learn how better to adapt to the tremendous changes in our society.

Similarly, in terms of community planning, even our harshest critic recognizes the difference between the functions and operations of the teaching or academic hospital and the community hospital. The challenge, it is stated, is not to repudiate scientific medicine, the high standards of medical education, the remarkable technological achievements, or the high levels of patient care, but, rather, to seek to extend them into the community-at-large.

As academic departments of psychiatry, what have we done, what are we doing, what is it we plan to do in the future to improve medical care for the many and not the few? I believe I am correct in stating that many, if not most, university departments of psychiatry have traditionally been more involved and engaged in community services—in schools, courts, public and private social, legal, and medical agencies—than have most of their fellow clinical departments.

Perhaps this circumstance is due to implicit, as well as explicit, concern for the human condition. Much of the biology of modern medicine can be understood and studied in infra-human terms, but this is hardly sufficient for our task. Furthermore, we constantly remind ourselves and our colleagues that man is a social animal. We are, I believe, the most personal, the most human, of the clinical disciplines.

Unlike our fellow department of medicine, psychiatry did not have a Rockefeller Research Institute to play its germinal part in grooming and selecting future professors and chairmen of academic departments. While the present recruitment of academic psychiatric faculty comes in great part from our university settings and to some degree from the NIMH, we must not forget how recent is this development. For example, eighty per cent of the psychiatric units in general hospitals, including academic hospitals, have been established since 1947. Earlier, those who were recruited as faculty to serve in the university departments of psychiatry (in themselves, these departments were limited in number and even more limited in scope) came in great part from extramural community service assignments in child guidance, social agency, public school, and court clinics, and from the government hospitals, state more than county or federal. Many psychiatric departments survived their early years principally through funds provided by community chest and public tax sources for the continuing services of the department members to the community. This was the case in Cincinnati, when I went there in 1942, and in Rochester in 1946. My personal experience of thirty years, I believe, is quite representative. It provided me with both obligatory and elective assignments to community health agencies, particularly in Denver and Cincinnati, and in Rochester; less so for various and different reasons in Milwaukee, New Haven, and Boston. These engagements have been with both private and public social, health, welfare, and legal agencies in these communities and include direct service to patients and clients, supervision of professional staff, membership on and consultation to lay agency boards, participation in clinical and social researches and in whatever overall community planning was being formulated. We have also been seriously engaged in national planning for health services in our field, including assignments to the NIMH, from its beginnings in 1946, and later with the Ford Foundation.

This has been our experience, our commitment, our tradition. Much of this has "growed like Topsy." Much of it, too, has been community crisis-oriented, unrelated or isolated from other health services, and subject to the whims and vagaries of personal interests and disinterests and short-lived budgetary commitments. Only recently is there a clearer awareness of the need for more systematic knowledge of the community in terms of extant health facilities and plans for the extension and coordination of services to all citizens in the community or region. Today in Rochester after many years of effort, and with the immense support of Marion Folsom, there has been established a planning group of lay and professional persons responsible for community and regional planning in all aspects of health services, including mental health.

Obviously, many factors will determine the form and substance of health service planning in communities. Consideration will be paid, of course, to basic demographic data, but planning will be determined in great part by the nature of the mosaic of relations between the university medical center (should there be one or more), its affiliated hospitals, local and regional community hospitals, relevantly concerned public and private health agencies, and the practicing medical profession with its professional bodies. Successful planning will also require the realignment and reorientation of existing traditional patterns of service. Many of these have been supported by local citizenry, with special dedication to ad hoc goals of the agency or clinic concerned. We have learned that it is not an easy matter for such persons to relinquish, or even to modify, existing patterns for which they have been responsible, at times have initiated, and have supported generously with funds and with personal services. It requires, too, compassionate understanding and clear exposition on the part of community planners in outlining the needs and advantages of realignment of such services to the community-at-large.

As an academic department of psychiatry, is our contribution essential to the task? Are there unique or idiosyncratic aspects of our contribution to contemporary society? How prepared are we to undertake new and different assignments? Earlier I drew attention to the remarkable changes which have taken place in the growth and development of academic departments of psychiatry in our nation. I pointed out that this has taken place principally in the past twenty years; further, that the increases in faculty and staff, the establishment of educational programs at graduate and undergraduate levels in clinical psychiatry, the broad scope of research activities of both student and faculty, have been made possible by the support of the NIMH extramural programs. There is little question that the single, most important determinant of change in the departments of psychiatry in the United States resulted from the enactment of the National Mental Health Law, passed by the 79th Congress, in 1946.

The scope of our intellectual concerns has been broadened. After a century of neglect there is a renascence in neurochemistry; psychologists, psychophysiologists, and psychopharmacologists are approaching with increasing sophistication their studies of cognitive functions, affective states, and human growth and development. The useful contributions of psychoanalytic psychology have been woven into the fabric of clinical psychiatry as well as into general psychology. There is increasing dissatisfaction with the dichotomy of individual-society, as there has been about mind-body, and unified theories of behavior have been introduced. This has led to renewed studies of the group, the family, and the community. We are even becoming more familiar and comfortable with the numerical method and the use of statistical means to assay intervention, and in undertaking epidemiologic studies.

Moreover, in addition to our research and educational functions, many of us in the academic teaching hospitals have stimulated, nourished, and pursued studies relating to patient care, that is, in systematic studies of the nature of the care of all patients. This, too, has brought with it concern for the patient and the patient's family. It has led us to examine more closely the basic tasks of the clinician and the need for him to understand the relevant events of human interaction, and the nature of the disciplining of his capacity for human intimacy. It has led us, too, to reevaluate and examine carefully our concepts of health and disease and to distinguish between the concept of disease in traditional, biological terms, and sickness as a state of social dysfunction, which affects the individual's relations with others.

All of these I believe to be relevant to the movement concerned with what is variously called social psychiatry, preventive psychiatry, community psychiatry, and public health psychiatry. At the moment this matter is certainly confusing, if not controversial. Careful reading of selected definitions of community, social, preventive, public health, administrative, and other adjectival forms of psychiatry, thoughtfully submitted by our peers and published as an addendum to the NIMH publication, *Concepts of Community Psychiatry*,[7] regretfully did not help me to discriminate between the fields defined.

Daniels quoted those who consider "Community Psychiatry is the psychiatry of the future . . . [that] we are in the midst of a third psychiatric revolution, which will result in new patterns of psychiatric practice." He quoted, too, from the opponents, who said, "Community Psychiatry is nothing more than good psychiatry. We have been practicing in this way for 15 years. . . . There is no basis of knowledge or experience for community psychiatric practice. . . . We will raise the public's hopes for help with their myriad social problems and then we will disappoint them."[8]

We owe Bell and Spiegel special gratitude for their thoughtful and scholarly review of the usages and connotations of the term, "social psychiatry," from its initial use in 1917 by Ernest Southard. They indicate that the central elements in the concept have recurred cyclically a number of times in the past fifty years, with varying engagements with social work and with sociology, and more recently by a combination of psychiatry and the social sciences. They conclude: "Apart from its usefulness as a label for a certain type of cross-disciplinary research training and research procedure, the term 'social psychiatry' would appear to have no logical meaning. There is little merit in applying it to the many and heterogeneous methods of practice and prevention in the area of community mental health, now being elaborated in an experimental fashion."[9] I have been impressed by the lucidity of the operational criteria for a community mental health program as outlined by Swerling.[10]

Less controversial appears to be the evidence of movement toward the following objectives:

1. Reducing the size of public mental hospital services.
2. Increasing general hospital services.
3. Promoting greater community participation by psychiatrists and others in preventive, first aid, and rehabilitative measures for patients and their families.

Among the multiple, complex, often intimately related and derived determinants of this movement are the following:

1. Major changes in federal legislation to improve medical care for all peoples.
2. Intent to return responsibility for the care of the mentally sick to local communities, from which it had been taken a century ago by state governments.
3. The development of community mental health centers.
4. Realization of obligatory, no longer elective, basis for planning of health services in order to avoid unnecessary duplication and proper availability, continuity, and distribution.
5. Liberalization of health insurance programs, both public tax, and voluntary, to cover psychiatric care, intra- and extramural.
6. Increase in the number and broadening of the scope of psychiatric units in general hospitals, providing diagnostic, therapeutic, consultative, first aid, and emergency services, with day and night care facilities.
7. The successful use of the psychotropic drugs and of electroconvulsive therapy in reducing materially the length of individual patient hospital stay.
8. The increased number of psychiatrists available to be associated with clinics, hospitals, and community social agencies, as well as in extramural practice.
9. Search for better ways to coordinate traditionally trained helping persons, like nurses, social workers, child care, etc., and the preparation of new types of paramedical personnel.
10. Liberalization of patient care practiced in psychiatric hospitals, both short and long stay, as to admissions, trial visits, readmissions, discharges, and aftercare.

11. Introduction of public health measures with the assistance of social scientists, statisticians, data processing personnel, and more sophisticated register studies, incidence, prevalence studies, transcultural epidemiological surveys.

12. After a period of neglect, a period in which there has been a major emphasis on biological and intrapsychic psychological phenomena. (There is general awareness of the rediscovery not only of the human family, but of the human community, with the increasing participation of social and behavioral scientists in studies of the family, other groups, and the community.)

In my teaching about the concepts and practices of what are called social, or community, or preventive, or public health psychiatry, I have found it useful, with the obvious risk of oversimplification, to distinguish between two basic components.

The first is fundamentally conceptual. It holds that the field of clinical psychiatry is concerned with the human condition in conflict; further, that this concern must include within it, knowledge of relevant biological, psychological, and social issues. In my view the most concise and penetrating exposition of this point, with particular relevance to the education of all physicians, including psychiatrists, is that of Norman Cameron in his presentation of "Human Ecology and Personality," which he gave at the First Ithaca Conference, fifteen years ago. He defined human ecology as the interaction of human organism with human environment, and personality as the characteristics of human organisms resulting from this interaction. You will learn that he considers perception and learning; emotion and motivation; language and thought; the genesis and decline of complex human activities in infancy, childhood, adolescence, maturity, senescence, and senility; the nature and development of personality; society and culture; the family; social organization and disorganization.[11]

So far as I can determine, within the past two decades comprehensive models for viewing human behavior have developed. In general these models point toward unified theories of behavior, with assumptions of the intimate interrelatedness and interdependence between physical, biological, psychological, social, and cultural phenomena. I have looked upon this material, as have most of the members of our department, not in terms of a special discipline, nor as an addendum, but, rather, as the basic matrix of clinical psychiatry. This does not mean that we have been able in our teaching or in our practice to be as fully informed about all of these matters as we would one day wish to be. But we will continue to pursue our own studies and also hope to continue to be enriched by the contributions of our colleagues in biology, psychology, and the social and behavioral sciences.

The second component, perhaps less conceptual, is more operational, and I believe it refers more to those areas which are usually subsumed under the term, *community psychiatry*. In great part, this deals with logistical problems, with management, and with the introduction of public health methods. At the moment it is given great impetus by the federal legislation to which we have referred.

It is concerned with attempts to improve medical care, to coordinate heretofore isolated or unrelated elements of health services. Attempts are being made to increase the availability and continuity of health services, to reach those who are reluctant to ask for help and those who become more confused by multiple, fragmented attention. It also intends to provide proper distribution of services locally and regionally and to make discriminate selection of appropriate services for children, adolescents, and the aged, for first-aid in crisis intervention, as well as for traditional intramural and outpatient care.

It is also involved in the preparation of new types of paramedical personnel and is searching for better ways to coordinate traditionally trained helping persons, like nurses, social workers, teachers, psychologists, parole and probation officers, child care workers, and youth and group workers. It is also calling upon epidemiologists, statisticians, social scientists, and community planners to assist in the designation of population catchment areas, public health education, and in epidemiological studies.

In my view, academic departments must become engaged with both components. Our involvement in the first is perhaps more familiar. This is the traditional role of the university department: to examine critically its current knowledge, skills, and belief systems, to pursue new knowledge, to disseminate this knowledge, and to take part in the formation of the minds of our students. In turn we hope that this may enable them to maintain high standards of practice and, hopefully, in some instances to generate that restlessness which may lead to discovery. And, as we are clinical departments, in pursuing our traditional objectives we will be intimately involved with our patients, their families, and our community. The fortunate introduction and acceptance into departments of psychiatry of psychologists, social and behavioral scientists, and statisticians will undoubtedly contribute further to the conceptual revolution taking place in considering the interrelatedness and interdependence within a field of behavior of physical, biological, psychological, social and cultural phenomena.

What is to be our responsibility in terms of the second component, in terms of the operational area of community psychiatry? Within our abilities to do so, and with adequate resources available to us, we have, we should, and we will participate in this movement toward the coordination and expansion of health services. As a department, or as a medical school, we know that our usefulness would be seriously impaired and our survival in danger should we become exclusively a community clinical service station. At the other extreme, if we were to become exclusively a research institute, detached from our environment, we would fail in our principal obligation—education.

In some way, we shall have to strike the proper balance. We must care for the sick, not only because of the obvious social need but also because in caring for the sick we educate the student, since he cannot learn without assuming responsibility for such care. But we must also have the privilege and opportunity to pursue new knowledge, whether it be useless or useful at the moment. Within a department faculty, there will be those capable of and interested in assuming certain public responsibilities in planning, and there will be others less interested or capable. Our needs are such that we need both.

We have serious problems of manpower, of fulfilling current clinical services and educational assignments, of providing time and facility for investigative work, and of financial support. I believe it is in the New Testament, in Matthew, where one learns that "For where your treasure is, there will your heart be also." At times our needs are so great and so urgent that we are apt to accept public monies from local or federal sources, even when the grants made available are conditioned by terms not necessarily favorable to the furtherance of basic objectives. Urgent and necessary as increased or expanded services to our communities may be, I believe the university departments must make clear to our fellow citizens their multiple duties, their responsibilities and, particularly, their primary obligations to education. If this task if evaded, the potential manpower for service needs will obviously be reduced.

Does this mean that our posture will be that of detachment, of lack of engagement in participation in community planning? I do not think so. There is little question that the academic hospitals may have to define not only what they way be able to do now and later (populations to be served, nature of services), but also how this is to be woven into the fabric of comprehensive medical care for the defined population groups. I believe the academic hospitals will have to take the initiative in the creation and establishment of new types of paramedical workers. The problems posed make more relevant the basic questions of the organization of the university medical center. Should there be established a new department of preventive health services, encompassing much of what is done now in preventive medicine, epidemiology, community psychiatry, pediatric family practice, well-baby clinics, planned parenthood, and well-woman clinics? Has the traditional departmental organization outlived its usefulness? Or, should we more boldly consider the establishment of a school of psychological medicine, as proposed by Kubie[12] and others in the past?

Should the department of psychiatry be established as a university department transcending the medical school and hospital, and relating directly to the parent university, in this way facilitating working relations with many departments in the university-at-large and with the community? Should universities establish schools or divisions for applied social studies in order to eliminate the unnecessary duplication of personnel engaged in survey research or in ad hoc responses to emergency inquiries and studies based upon community needs? There is little question that, as participant observers of the human comedy and clinical activists, we must continue to be engaged in service to our communities. However, we must in some manner or other learn to identify the contributions which the academic department, alone, may make to this venture and to adapt the health services we offer to the new needs.

REFERENCES

1. Pusey, Nathan M., "The American University Today," *School and Society*, 89:47-51, Feb. 11, 1961.
2. Goheen, R. F., "The University in the World Today," *Vital Speeches*, 27:281-283, February 15, 1961.
3. Keeney, B. C., "The Dilemmas of Relevance and Commitment," *Liberal Education*, 52:21-26, March, 1966.
4. Williams, Greer, "Quality Versus Quantity in American Medical Education," *Science*, 153:956-961, August 26, 1966.
5. Somers, Anne R., "Role of the Teaching Hospital in Community Health Planning," *Hospital Topics*, 43:53-58, June, 1965.
6. Coggeshall, Lowell T., Planning for Medical Progress Through Education, Association of American Medical Colleges, Evanston, Illinois, 1965, p. 35.
7. *Concepts of Community Psychiatry*, U. S. Department of Health, Education & Welfare, Washington, D.C., Public Health Service Publication #1319.
8. Daniels, Robert S., "Community Psychiatry—A New Profession, a Developing Subspecialty, or Effective Clinical Psychiatry," *Community Mental Health Journal*, 2:47-54, Spring, 1966.

9. Bell, Norman W., and Spiegel, John P., "Social Psychiatry," *Archives of General Psychiatry*, 14:337-345, April, 1966.
10. Zwerling, I., "Program of Community and Social Psychiatry in a Health Center," *Health News*, 40:14-191 August, 1963.
11. Cameron, Norman, "Human Ecology and Personality in the Training of Physicians in Psychiatry and Medical Education," 1951 Conference, American Psychiatric Assoc. 1952, pp. 63-96.
12. Kubie, L. S., "A School of Psychological Medicine within a Framework of a Medical School and University," *Journal of Medical Education*, 39:476-480, 1964.

23

PAUL V. LEMKAU, M.D.

This paper begins with a quotation from Adolf Meyer with whom both Leo Bartemeier and I had the privilege of training, though he knew the "Old Man" a few years before I came along. I suppose I learned Leo's name first at the Phipps—we had a way in the late night conversations, after completing the "Formulation for Staff" for the next morning, of remarking those who had survived the training and had made it in the psychiatric world outside. His first professional influence on me I recall vividly. I had already committed myself to the field of Mental Hygiene and was learning all I could about it when I found the literature put out by the Cornelian Corner. It was clear, had a sound clinical base, built on the experience of laymen as well as patients and psychiatrists. It had great appeal and usefulness for a beginning teacher and could be, and was, enriched by conversations with one of its sponsors, Dr. Bartemeier.

It was my privilege to be serving on the Medical Advisory Board of the Seton Institute in 1954 and to help in the decision to invite Leo back to Baltimore. It has been a wonderful thing to have him around. One gets security from his being in the same town—the assurance that with him around there will be no serious errors and that there is an anchor of wisdom at hand. I do not mean to underestimate his scientific productivity or his leadership, but it does seem to me that his most valued traits are his wisdom and his lovableness.

It is a pleasure and an honor to have this part in honoring Leo Bartemeier as an old and valued friend and leader.

Mental Hygiene and the Public Health

However much of a dreamer I may be, I pride myself on having seen a good many of my dreams come true. Can you see the ward or district organization—with a district building instead of the police station? With policemen as constructive workers rather than as the watchdogs of their beats? A district center with reasonably accurate records of the facts needed for orderly work? Among the officers a district health officer and a district school committee, a district tax committee, a district charity or civic work committee, a tangible expression of what the district stands for.

With a system of helpfulness and fairness and true democracy, avoiding bureaucracy as well as militarism and its primitive residual, the boss system, this country can safely go on developing methods tolerant of individuality and yet effective in its essential purposes.

There is not a solitary line of prevention and constructive work in which we do not sooner or later run up against insufficiency of community work, of registration, of collaboration, and even of acquaintance of those who should work together.

ADOLPH MEYER, 1915[1]

THE TWIN GOALS of continuity and comprehensiveness of health services have emerged with increasing clarity in the last few decades. Continuity of care became apparent as a need largely through investigations that revealed the so-called multiproblem families:[2] those in the population which absorbed disproportionate amounts of the available community health, welfare and consultative services. The studies showed that in most cases the services were applied in a seriatim fashion in the attempt to rescue the family and its members, but that rarely could all reparative or altering forces be brought to bear simultaneously or in a rational, successive pattern as they were needed. The needs of the patient in cardiac decompensation were met but the housekeeper necessary to prevent relapse after recovery was not supplied. The acute schizophrenic breakdown could be reversed, but the supply of drugs and the motivation to take them after discharge from the hospital were neglected items. Continuity of care, implying the coordination and collaboration of services, both in timing and in availability, became clear issues in furnishing more effective medical care and in the restoration of optimal function.

These investigations revealed the need for greater attention to the tertiary phase of prevention rehabilitation, and resulted in the development of the extensive programs in that area. As large and effective as they have been, they have suffered from organizational separation from health services, being in most cases administratively lodged in Departments of Education. This location evidenced the primacy of vocational and economic goals at their inception; broader goals more geared to personality function and personal satisfactions have gradually emerged and programs have been altered to meet them. But the coordination of acute therapeutic and rehabilitation programs remains a challenge in many areas, and for many types of illnesses.[3]

Continuity of care implies that various types of services will be organized in a temporal pattern of continuity. The extent and variety of services are the subject of the comprehensiveness of care. The range of services considered to operate in support of health has been broadly expanded since the recognition of the fact, first positively stated by the World Health Organization in 1948 as a definition, that health is "not merely the absence of disease, but complete physical, mental and social well-being." This definition brings into the health area all etiological factors which are sources of discomfort and dysfunction in man, whether of primary or contributory nature. It prescribes an inescapably multifactorial concept of etiology which operates not only in the initiation of a disease process but also takes into consideration the symptoms of the disease itself as additional factors of importance in the understanding of the illness episode—from its first symptom until the individual is restored to a new kind of adjustment. It is recognized that the individual emerging from an illness episode cannot be the same person as he was when he entered. A whole new block of experiences has been added and, to some extent at least, integrated into his personality structure.[4]

In a particular illness episode the etiological factors are often of bewildering complexity. The primary one, both in time and importance, may be an infectious, oncological, metabolic or hormonal one, but by the time the episode is finished, psychodynamic, sociodynamic, receptive, toxic and other factors may well become effective in altering the course of the episode. For example, diabetes is discovered in a middle-aged man. His "physical" needs are relatively easily met. But there may be other needs. He is frightened by this evidence of his aging, his failing physique. He fears his wife may now underrate him, and the role he assumes as a sick man may invite her to respond in this way. Her response drives him to test his physical and sexual prowess with others, further complicating his psycho- and sociodynamic situation. At work, he may employ the mechanism of over-compensation and change from a motivating but tolerant boss to a tyrannical one, calling forth reactions from his fellow workers to further complicate things. His religious security may be undermined, leading to anxious consultations with his minister. Merely letting the imagination run through the range of primary and secondary etiologies occurring in the course of a disease episode makes the goal of comprehensive treatment formidable. One factor not included in the illustration above is the economic—certainly a most important one which brings in its train many psychodynamic and sociological considerations, whether it appears in the highly productive years or after retirement.

This paper aims to make two points. The first is that the twin goals of continuity and comprehensiveness of care are appropriate to the whole field of health care—that no class of illnesses may be excluded. Once the goals of comprehensiveness and continuity are stated and accepted, the classification of illnesses into mental and physical will no longer be justified for every illness will involve both aspects in its etiological complex. In general, the concept of sociodynamics in etiology is less clearly formulated, but what is known would lead one to include rather than exclude it, particularly when the distribution of mental retardation by social class and cultural pattern is considered.

The second point of the paper is that in striving toward the twin goals of continuity and comprehensiveness of health care, identical problems of communication and coordination will be encountered. Hence, my conclusion is that the mental health field should become more influential in the area of general health services. Those patients for whom mental health workers traditionally are responsible are entitled to profit from the learning taking place in the management of general health problems, and the mental health worker can contribute his specialized knowledge of psychodynamics and his more limited grasp of sociodynamics to enrich the whole health effort. Conversely, mental health workers have much to gain in broadening the range of other etiological thinking as well as to see new avenues of service that do not now come to attention.

To return to the first point: that the goals of continuity and comprehensiveness of health care imply an all-inclusive concept of health in which the identifiable mental diseases meld indistinguishably with all other illnesses.

The term "mental illness" has many connotations. It implies that there is something special and distinguishable about diseases which have behavior deviation as their common symptom. I much prefer the term "mental illness*es*" (the plural), if we must make the separation at all. "Mental illness" as a term also implies, at least to me, that such illnesses have some common factor in etiology. If we speak of "infectious disease," it is implied that the sickness is the result of competition between the host and some invading organism—two competing biological systems, one of which is a human being. When one looks to the prevention of an infectious disease, the strategy is to list the places where the man may be strengthened and the invader weakened so that the man may survive. The grouping itself carries the implication of the strategy of the medical attack on the problem. Similarly, strategies are implied by such terms as metabolic, hormonal, oncological, degenerative and other classes of diseases. The names indicate a particular type of strategy to be used in conquering the primary etiology of the illness.

The term "mental illness" cannot carry such strategic implications. The word "mental" refers exclusively to the results, a particular kind of symptom of illness, and says nothing whatever about its cause or causes. Were it used as are other types of groupings, we would have to assume that the strategy for the prevention and the treatment of mongolism, phenylketonuria, oligophrenia, schizophrenia, depression, senile psychosis and neuroses all have something in common. We quickly recognize that this is quite preposterous. Of the list, schizophrenia, depression, and neuroses may be primarily of psychogenic origin; in all the others in this list of "mental" diseases, the primary cause lies elsewhere and only the symptoms justify their being included in the mental group at all.[5]

Certain grades and types of mental retardation appear to be culturally induced; their primary etiology lies in inadequate experience early in life. Although such cases are included as "mental" because of their behavioral inadequacy, the term refers again only to late symptoms and implies nothing as to the strategy of prevention and treatment.[6]

Such statements are often interpreted as tending to restrict the field of psychiatry and of mental health concern—to rather traitorously "turn it over to" some other specialty or group within or without medicine. In some instances, this does happen—and rightly. The type of mental retardation last discussed has properly become a responsibility of educational systems. After having been the very paradigm of a psychiatric illness for a century or two, central nervous system syphilis is now detectable before behavior disorder is severe, and venereologists prevent the illness or cure the patients so that psychiatrists rarely see such cases at the present time.

On the other hand, there has been great advance by psychiatrists in the management and understanding of diseases which have behavior disorder as their most disturbing symptom. The late Clifton Perkins, formerly Maryland's Commissioner of Mental Hygiene, used to say that the most rewarding efforts for the care of behavior disorders in state hospitals were to be found on the wards for senile patients. Treatment aimed at the underlying primary pathological process cleared the behavior symptoms more rapidly than anywhere else in the hospital. The development of drugs capable of altering more or less specific parts of behavior patterns has contributed to easing management problems which occupied much of psychiatrists' time and skill only a decade ago. The expertise of the clinical psychiatrist in the control of behavior symptoms, ranging from convulsions to moods, and from tremor to delusions, has greatly expanded. One can hope that in the relatively near future he will be able to perform this treatment task as successfully as the endocrinologist controls diabetes. This will allow the psychiatrist to deal with the more fundamental problems of primary etiology and with the thorny issues of motivation which surround the secondary prevention of all illnesses controlled only by the continuous taking of medicine. The better management of these problems will, in turn, perhaps, allow researchers to give more thought to primary etiologies; the gerontologist may concentrate on degenerative senile processes; the internist on arteriosclerosis, the oncologist on tumors, and the psychiatrist on those illnesses in which the primary etiology is known or suspected to lie in the psychodynamic and personal relationship areas —the schizophrenic reactions, the psychopathies, the mood disorders, the neuroses, and some types of mental retardation.

Under this scheme, mental illnesses are of two general sorts—those which demand psychiatrists' skills for the control of disordered symptomatic behavior and those which are of concern because their primary etiology may be in the areas of psychodynamics and social relationships but which also show symptomatic behavior which requires management. This is no new distinction; it was expressed in the American Psychiatric Association's nomenclature until it was recently superseded by a new one, but the defense of the old position was not, for me at least, as clear as it has become more recently.[7]

Mental health work, like all medicine, has as its goal controlling disordered behavior. Its special status rests in the fact that it struggles with a unique area of etiologic agents, those related to psycho- and sociodynamic forces. Psychiatric specialization stands in the same position as does cardiology, for example. The cardiologist is concerned with the etiological agents which disturb heart function but particularly with physiological agents related to arteriosclerosis. He looks to the psychiatrist for help, however, in managing the cardiac delirium and cardiac neuroses as well as exploration of particular types of functional disorder. The psychiatrist, on the other hand, sees the management of behavior disorder as his area of concern and looks to the cardiologist to deal with the agents acting to cause the symptoms insofar as they lie outside the psychodynamic area. Both specialists are a part of the profession dealing with human malfunction—the loss of well-being—whatever its causes.

The second point concerns the fact that mental health work must use the same agencies in comprehensive care as does the rest of medicine. Poverty is a threat to family stability whether it be caused by the hospitalization of the wage earner for tuberculosis, schizophrenia, operation for the removal of a lung for tumor, or for an acute pneumonia. The need for rehabilitative effort will be dependent on two issues—the length of the disability and the residual left by the illness, whether this be the status of an amputee or the presence of apathy. The need for supplying mother-love and maternal care to children is the same whether the mother is away from home undergoing surgery, treatment of an infectious disease, or psychiatric hospitalization. Marital counseling will be demanded in some cases, whether the complaints are of sterility or of incompatibility. Family planning services may be needed, whether the reason is to avert cardiac decompensation, economic decompensation, decompensation in personality function or respiratory decompensation. Services to maintain motivation to insure the regular taking of medication are very similar whether the medicine be insulin, phenothiazine or dilantin.

The problem of providing continuity of care is one of making available various specialized agencies offering various types of services, at the proper time and in proper sequence so that maximal therapeutic effect is experienced by the patient and those dependent upon him during the episode of illness. It is a problem that has long been recognized but has only recently become a matter to be considered for action. It is a part of what is perhaps the most important issue in health planning.[8]

Action for health planning at the national level came first from the mental health field. Under the mental health planning act of 1962, each state was induced to prepare a plan for the future of its mental health services.[9] The planning process was somewhat confused by the interjection of new programs while it was underway, but the plans were completed. For the first time planning included a rather large range of community services which are often associated with health efforts. The plans included the newly conceived social institution, the mental health center, but, in general, did not concern themselves with the integration of mental health with other health programs in the community.[10]

Meanwhile, the overall health field had also become concerned about whether services fit the needs as completely as possible. One result of a large commission study was the conclusion that planning would make it possible to clarify the direction future programs should take.[11] This found eventual expression in Public Law 88-749, the comprehensive Health Planning Act. Mental health was specifically included in the proposed planning, even to the extent of designating 15% of the federal funds supplied to be spent in this part of the effort. The large area to be covered, the interposition of the new medicare and medicaid operations, the heart, cancer and stroke program, and the politics involved have thus far made progress in comprehensive planning rather slow in most areas of the country. In many instances it has not included mental health personnel very actively, probably because some of the notions included in this paper are not recognized by leaders either in psychiatry or in general health. It is hoped that this exposition may suggest bases for more complete realization of the need of each group for the other. Genuine continuity of care will be fostered when it is realized that the services required for the symptomatic control of pathological functions are, for the most part, the same, regardless of which particular group of specialists may be concerned in the primary etiology of the illness episode.

Except for the occasional examples introduced, much of the discussion in this paper is abstract—far removed from the clinical situation. There are, however, powerful factors tending to unify all specialties at this level of conceptualization also. Health care, even in the most radical schemes proposed for its future development, is always assumed to involve a more or less personal relationship between the complainant, the patient, and a person whose goal is to help him.[12] The qualities of this relationship are conceded to be part of the *sine qua non* of active preventive or therapeutic programs. They include reasonable insurance of confidentiality and confidence that the helping interest is genuine.

The helping functions to be dispensed in this relationship are of two sorts, first, diagnosis and treatment planning, and second, the motivation of the patient to carry out the plan. In almost all situations the first is a specialist's function—that of a physician, a social worker, or a nurse, depending on the case and the setting. The second function is a more general one. When the case is one involving acute discomfort, physical or psychic, a physician is likely to be involved. If, however, the case is chronic, with relatively slow movement in the pathological process, the person carrying on the dyadic relationship is likely to be a generalist, carrying responsibility for a wide range of health problems in the community. The art of creating and using the relationship to persuade the patient and those about him to follow a health-promoting regimen usually lies not in the hands of a specialist, but in the generalized public health nurse, the first-level staff social worker, the physician's office nurse, or the nurse who works in a clinic or an industrial setting.

In some parts of the world, the concept of the generalist at this level is rejected. In Europe it is my impression that most psychiatrists have come to the conclusion that generalized personnel cannot successfully care for chronic psychiatric patients. In this country, on the other hand, there are many successful demonstrations of the fact that they can.[13] The same argument has appeared in other specialty fields from time to time. New Jersey once had specialized public health nurses to work in maternal and child health; many agencies once had specialized nurses to serve the needs of ambulatory tuberculosis patients and in many areas home nursing care of patients is separated from the other services of public health nurses. In general, and in the United States, the trend appears to be toward greater confidence in the capacity of the "front-line" person to carry the fundamental type of relationships needed in all these various situations. The special knowledge needed to make the contacts maximally effective can be supplied by consultative back-up to deal with technical matters and mental health consultative service to deal with the problems inherent in the relationship itself.[14] The issues of this basic, health-protecting relationship are, of course, very apparent in the psychiatric interview in which psychodynamic issues are dealt with as etiological and not management matters.

In summary, the twin goals of continuity and comprehensiveness of care are incompatible with a medical care system which separates mental health from other health endeavors. Comprehensive care almost always involves mental health experts, because behavior disorder is symptomatic of illnesses which have a variety of primary etiologies, and because episodes of illness have effects which are not necessarily dictated by the primary etiology. Psychiatry has its own special concern in primary etiology, psychodynamics, but it serves to help manage symptomatic pathological behavior, regardless of its cause.

The achievement of continuity of care through an illness episode involves the use of many community services which are essentially the same, whatever the primary etiology of the illness may be. Because of this fact, genuine planning for continuity of care will perforce include the care of psychiatric patients.

The purpose of most health service is first, to achieve a diagnosis and treatment plan, and second, to ensure that the patient will be motivated to follow that plan. The latter function is usually assigned to generalized "front line" personnel who are found capable, with adequate consultative backing, of implementing the treatment plan.

REFERENCES

1. Meyer, Adolf. *Where Should We Attack the Problem of the Prevention of Mental Defect and Mental Disease?* National Conference of Charities and Correction, Proceedings XLII (1915) 298-307. (Reprinted in the Collected Papers of Adolf Meyer Vol. IV, pp. 190-197). Baltimore: The Johns Hopkins Press, 1952.

2. Buell, B., *et al. "Community Planning for Human Services."* N. Y.: Columbia University Press, 1952.

3. Sussman, M. B. (ed.) *"Sociology and Rehabilitation,"* Washington, D.C.: Am. Soc. Assn. and Vocational Rehabilitation Administration, 1965.

4. Usterman, L. *"Psychological Aspects of Rehabilitation,"* Kansas City, Mo.: Community Studies, Inc., 1961. Unfortunately this study neglects the effect of the illness episode itself. This topic is better covered in an old but excellent study: Barker, R. G., Wright, B. A. and Gonick, M. R., *Adjustment to Physical Handicap and Illness*: A Survey of Social Psychology of Physique and Disability. N. Y.: Soc. Sc. Research Council, Bull. 55, 1946. The issue is also widely discussed in the literature on psychosomatic illnesses.

5. Lemkau, Paul V. *"Prevention in Psychiatry." Am. Journal of Public Health*, 55: 554-560, 1965.

6. *"A Proposed Program for National Action to Combat Mental Retardation,"* President's Panel on Mental Retardation, Washington: U.S. Government Printing Office, 1962. Although the results of adequate early experience and, in particular, experiences implied by the term "maternal care" have been stated earlier by John Bowlby in *Maternal Care and Mental Health* (Geneva, WHO, 1952) and by Erving Goffman in *Asylum* (N. Y. Garden City, 1961), the Commission report applies the findings to mental retardation in forceful statements.

7. *Diagnostic and Statistical Manual*, American Psychiatric Assn., Washington: American Psychia. Assn., 1952.

    The older nomenclature began with a division of the mental illnesses into acute and chronic brain disorders and behavior disorders not known to be accompanied by brain pathology of a structural or toxic type. The new nomenclature abandoned this distinction as a part of reaching the goal of finding an internationally acceptable nomenclature for psychiatry.

8. The issue of agency collaboration and coordination has only recently received frank discussion although the problem has been recognized at least as early as 1945, the date of the Platt and Gunn Report, Gunn, S. M. and Platt, P. S., *Voluntary Health Agencies, An Interpretative Study*, N. Y.: Ronald Press, 1945.

    One of the best recent discussions, including an analysis of the dynamics involved in agency collaboration, is to be found in Sasser, Mervyn, *Community Psychiatry: Epidemiologic and Social Themes*, N. Y.: Random House, 1968.

9. *"Guidelines for the Federal Grant-in-Aid Programs to Support Mental Health Planning."* In Digest, *State Mental Health Planning Proposals*, National Institute of Mental Health, Bethesda, Maryland, 1965.

10. Halpert, H. P. *"Communications Aspects of State Mental Health Planning."* Thesis submitted to the School of Hygiene and Public Health, The Johns Hopkins University, June, 1966. (Unpublished.)

This thesis study deals primarily with the issues of communication between agencies and the extent of agency inclusion in mental health planning. While in many instances the establishment of communication was inadequate, it is clear that efforts were made in most states' plans to encourage collaboration.

11. *Health Is a Community Affair*, National Commission on Community Health Services. Cambridge, Mass.: Harvard University Press, 1966.
12. Rutstein, D. D. *The Coming Revolution in Medicine.* Cambridge, Mass.: Inst. Tech. Press, 1967.
13. Lemkau, Paul V. "Methodological Problems in Evaluating Follow-up Services to Psychiatric Patients." (Paper read at I.V.N.A. Conference, Annapolis, Maryland, published in abstract, 1962, I.V.N.A., Baltimore, Maryland.)
14. Hilleboe, H. E. and Lemkau, P. V., *General Health Administration and Mental Health.* Prepared for the National Conference on Mental Health in Public Health Training held at Airlie House, Warrenton, Virginia, May 27-30, 1968. (To be published.)

Part IV

PSYCHIATRY'S COMMITMENT IN THE WORLD

Hope is the dream of a waking man.
—ARISTOTLE

Psychiatry has its dreams—not idle ruminations, but conscious, active strivings for a better world. So the growth of hope is a healing element in the clinic, a motivating factor in the process of discovery, and a force for change in the human community. Thus hope provides a blueprint for the future.

This part of *Hope—Psychiatry's Commitment* is dedicated to that vision. Because psychiatry is committed to hope, it has an ever-expanding awareness of the vision of man and (as Dr. Farnsworth states) "responsibility for taking the leadership in building up those conditions, attitudes, and practices which enhance the dignity of man." Judge Bazelon writes of the reevaluation and reform of criminal law in the light of our expanding knowledge of the causation of human behavior. Doctor Kubie considers the contribution of psychiatry to basic but unsolved problems of human existence. Doctor Salk forecasts the application of biological principles and concepts to the problems of human behavior. And Doctor Menninger analyzes our vision of hope for change in the face of the strongest opposition—the character of man.

24

DANA L. FARNSWORTH, M.D.

It is difficult to be objective about Leo Bartemeier. The composite of all his qualities forms the image of a man who always rises above any shortcomings he may have in specific situations. His positive qualities of character are so massive that were he to make a mistake of judgment no one would believe it—or one would be sure that he was given the wrong facts. His influence upon all his friends and contemporaries has been a solid source of strength for American psychiatry and for a society which now more than ever needs such men. I am proud to be his friend and colleague and to have the opportunity of honoring him.

Psychiatry's Response to Social Change

AT THE CENTENNIAL CELEBRATION (in 1946) of the first public demonstration of ether's use in surgical anesthesia, Raymond Fosdick gave an address on "The Race With Chaos," devoted primarily to the dangers inherent in the fact that we were learning to control nature before learning self-control. He commented that the complexity of the revolution in our physical environment was so vast and so rapid that our minds could hardly cope with it, but unfortunately neither could our social ideas, our habits of life, or our political and economic institutions. In his view, "the fundamental issue of our time is whether we can develop understanding and wisdom reliable enough to serve as a chart in working out the problems of human relations; or whether we shall allow our present lop-sided progress to develop to a point that capsizes our civilization in a catastrophe of immeasurable proportions."[1]

Fosdick made a strong plea for the development of the social sciences and the humanistic studies, as a ballast to keep civilization afloat. He noted the disdain of many Congressmen for the social sciences—just "various kinds of ideology," as one of them expressed it. He wanted research of a high order in these fields, by men of disciplined minds, high integrity, and objective scholarship.

During the ensuing 24 years, events have progressed along the lines predicted by Fosdick but possibly even more rapidly than he foresaw. Not only are our political and economic institutions under attack but our churches, colleges and universities, and our various disciplines as well. The purpose of this chapter is to look at the forces eroding confidence in our established institutions, and at the idealism struggling for expression, largely in terms of how they concern psychiatry and psychiatrists. That our society is fraught with turmoil is beyond dispute; that it also offers promising and feasible vistas of change is likewise undeniable—though the latter view is by no means so widely promulgated as the more pessimistic estimate of contemporary trends. A careful scrutiny of both adverse and favorable elements in our society may, hopefully, conduce to that kind of realistic optimism essential to social progress.

In the United States the disparity between the "haves" and the "have-nots" is apparently increasing (at least the impatience of the poor with their plight is increasing), and in the total world the gap between the Western industrialized societies and the under-developed countries is also increasing. Thus the United States is a favorite target for hostility from the economically underprivileged, both at home and abroad. It is important, while realizing this, to remember that rapid social change may signify either decay or renewal, depending upon the values upheld by the society. Hoffer has pointed out that "drastic change, under certain conditions, creates a proclivity for fanatical attitudes, united action, and spectacular manifestations of fanaticism and defiance; it creates an atmosphere of revolution."[2]

In an era in which many improvements are possible and the energy and knowledge to bring them about are available, it is not surprising that hope and idealism may bring much turmoil and conflict. This country's commitment to the ideal of education for all its citizens (to the extent to which they are capable of acquiring it) has resulted in a paradox—opportunities for some of its citizens unparalleled in modern history *and* an extremely vulnerable state. Unless a state espousing universal education is comprised of citizens who are all willing to work for social justice at the same time, groups with conflicting interests may resort to force to back their demands. de Tocqueville implied the hazards of a lack of economic opportunity when he said, "If, then, a state of society can ever be founded in which every man shall have something to keep and little to take from others, much will have been done for the peace of the world."[3]

The late 60's have been, and the early 70's promise to be, a time of great turmoil within the world-wide social system. Various revolutionary movements have been occurring in nearly all parts of the world, notably Latin America, the Far East, the Middle East, and Africa. Previously, Americans saw these as having certain common characteristics—they were far away, they concerned other people, the issues were obscure. Now it is different. The revolution is here, the participants are our own people as well as those of other nations, and they are not solely the under-privileged, the oppressed, the downtrodden; they include large numbers of students and other young people who come from affluent families and who have had every possible economic advantage.

The revolution, both here and abroad, may be called a "revolution of unfulfilled expectations" and a struggle for power by groups of people who have not previously been able to act. Not only is there a revolt against faulty distribution of material goods, but a persistent questioning of the apparent priorities established by society's policy-makers. Behind all these questions lie the spectres of the population avalanche, nuclear war, increasing environmental pollution, and the manipulation of large numbers of people by the mass media to influence buying habits, tastes, and opinions.

The speed with which revolutionary ideas spread is far greater than ever before because of world-wide instant communication, particularly by television. Good ideas and destructive ones are spread more or less in-discriminately. Action is often stimulated before there can be a thoughtful discussion of the issues in dispute. What might appear to be a centrally-organized revolutionary conspiracy is more likely to be a rapid series of acts that imitate the methods and successes of quite disparate groups in distant places, a kind of serendipity in reverse.

All this has resulted in what might be called a crisis in values through-out society. Many members of the protesting groups, in their idiosyncratic ways, seem to be professing a higher ideal than is customarily practiced in such matters as war, human dignity, meeting basic human needs, and good education. But the methods they use are frequently contradictory to their professed ideals. This inconsistency confuses many persons who forget the ideals motivating the protestors, and focus instead on their disruptive methods. Thus the points at issue become obscured by the strong negative feelings aroused.

The intensity and violence of the students' role in protest has become more and more noticeable in the late 60's. These young people have de-clared themselves to be against: the Vietnam situation, failure of the civil rights movement, the many gaps between the "haves" and the "have-nots," air and water pollution by industrial leaders who ignore the needs of others and of the ecological balance itself, the growing impersonalization of organizations, the cult of "built-in obsolescence," the threat of nuclear or biological war, and the lack of frankness (to the point of deception) practiced by government and institutional leaders.

Legitimate though these accusations may be, the value of student criticism has been vitiated by the fact that some of the more vehement protestors have used methods previously considered unacceptable. Violence, obscenity, denial of esthetic standards, and attacks on the family, education, religion, and moral standards—all of these are in the armamentarium of student protest. The idea of deferred gratification has been repudiated, and many persons feel simply that their every demand, social and personal, is entitled to immediate fulfillment—a concept which John Murray has called "narcissistic entitlement." Even those bending their energies toward the right goals sometimes use "wrong" methods; they have become fanatics. (Santayana once defined a fanatic as a person who redoubled his energy after he lost sight of his aims.) "The danger in fighting against hypocrisies," as Professor Paul Freund of Harvard has warned, "is that the righteousness of the cause gives way to self-righteousness about means."[4]

To add to the confusing elements in an already complex situation, several groups—some of the more radical student organizations among them—have taken as their avowed aim the destruction of society (and in particular the capitalistic system), hoping that something better will arise from the ruins. The colleges and universities are considered to be the agents of "the system," of being in complicity with the wrongdoings of society, and hence as early targets for destruction. Their openness, their atmosphere of freedom, and their extreme vulnerability to violent tactics make them ideal targets.

Professional and religious groups have also come under attack by various groups who view these agencies of society as supporters of a value system which should be destroyed or at least drastically changed. Disruption of professional society meetings with peremptory demands, and of church services to insist on payment of reparations for past injustices, has become almost commonplace. Society itself, as well as its various discrete institutions, is being attacked by those whose idealism is expressed in demands for instant and far-reaching corrections of all existing injustices.

In Western society, particularly, more spectacular progress has been made during the last 150 years in the physical sciences and in technology than in the social sciences. And the latter have perhaps overemphasized theoretical research and statistical analysis, concerning themselves with *how people live* rather than with *how people ought to be able to live.* Learning how to control the environment has appeared to have a much higher priority than learning how to control self. We are just beginning to realize that learning how to master the environment, even to the point of interplanetary travel, is an easier task than raising the standards of living and the aspirations of great masses of people. This applies not only to the "underdeveloped" or "emerging" countries such as those of Latin America or Africa, but also to the task of upgrading the quality of living in the deteriorated urban sections and remote rural areas of this country.

Thimann has called attention to the paradox of science being under fire because its successes, dramatic as they are, have been partially but not totally successful in raising the quality of living of all citizens.[5] Indeed, some idealistic and thoughtful persons see science as a destructive force. He suggests that science teachers might do well to stress the role of science as an instrument of service and as a means of helping to cure mankind's ills, rather than relying on the more theoretical approach of the fascination of science and the power of the scientific method. Psychiatry suffers from the same handicap; whatever it does well raises so many added expectations which are unrealizable because of insufficient resources that its critics appear to be increasing. Such criticism should be welcomed rather than regretted so long as it remains within constructive limits, stimulating improvement in methods of treatment and encouraging more young people to enter the specialty.

An analysis of the academic interests of student protestors and their young adult compeers often reveals that the most ardent are those concentrating in social sciences and the humanities. Relatively few come from the ranks of those specializing in the physical sciences. We may hazard a tentative explanation: that the student working in the physical sciences has already made up his mind as to what he wants to do; his activities are more "relevant," the focus of his study is more specific, and both his goals and the steps necessary to achieve them are fairly clear in his own mind. The student of humanities or social science, however, unless he is interested only in statistical and quantitative factors, is involved in a vast range of human and social problems. In a sense, everything that happens to him, everything that he sees, pertains to what he is studying. He lacks the specific focus of the chemist or the structural engineer; his attention is more dissipated, and because he does not have specific facts to be learned, steps to be followed, and goals to be mastered, he is much less sure of what ought to be done with the knowledge he acquires.

The chemist, the mathematician, the engineer are one step removed from the direct involvement with the human situation which is the daily confrontation of the social scientist. The task of the social scientist is to analyze the problems of society, suggest ways of solving them, and set up some of the machinery of social change and social action, but for many of these changes he needs the help of specialists in other fields. A sociologist may be able to tell that new low-cost housing is needed, but he cannot create it himself. He must have the specialized knowledge of many other people—for example, of an architect who knows of structural stresses and building regulations but who also shares the sociologist's concern with putting his knowledge to use in order to effect social change.

Psychiatry is in a peculiarly advantageous position of bridging the gap between "what ought to be" and "how it can be brought about." As the science which knows man at his most intimate, it sees most clearly what is wrong; and it can see how environmental factors cause mental illness and can in many cases suggest or even effect a cure for many of these problems. But there have been uncovered vast, previously unknown needs for health services. Nearly all people now want what only a small percentage could receive previously. These unmet needs are being discovered at a time when there are not enough funds and not enough trained people to do all that is expected; this means that a very much larger share of our national wealth will have to be devoted to the maintenance of health, the training of new health workers, developing new modes of treatment, and working out new methods of funding.

These problems are especially crucial in psychiatry. State Hospital care has been inadequately supported, and has too often been of a merely caretaking, rather than rehabilitative, nature. Private hospitals are still much too expensive for most people. Community Mental Health Centers have not increased in number so as to meet community needs in minimizing the effects of emotional conflict at the point of origin and developing techniques for resolution of crises. Treatment by drugs, electroshock, and other physical modalities could be adapted to large numbers of people, but by themselves these treatments only relieve symptoms, they neither resolve the underlying conflict nor improve substandard environments. Psychotherapy is so time-consuming that there will probably never be enough therapists to treat all those who need help; and some persons, especially the psychologically unsophisticated, receive little benefit from this technique. Group psychotherapy has been effective to some degree, but it has also lent itself to various kinds of exploitation which tend to discredit the procedure as well as the whole profession of psychiatry.

Thus it is understandable that psychiatry, like other branches of medicine and most of the other institutions of our society, should be under attack. This fact in itself is not new, for the profession has always had its critics, and always will have if it lives up to its responsibilities. But the present series of attacks comes from so many sources, both within and without the discipline, that it behooves all psychiatrists to give as much effort to preserving the crucial functions of their specialty, and to emphasizing the bonds which all psychiatrists share, as is now being devoted to discrediting them.

From various quarters psychiatry is not only blamed for not doing enough; its basic principles are under attack. Although many are self-contradictory and based on misunderstanding of the discipline and its aims, these attacks can do serious damage to the profession unless they are met and resolved.

Much of the suspicion comes from those who, misunderstanding the essential nature of psychiatry, see it as a manipulative technique rather than a search for self-understanding, inner freedom, and ways to improve the quality of living. Psychiatrists have been attacked as moralists (or, by others, as anti-moralists), as manipulators of society, as persons who protect weak individuals from the consequences of their mistakes, and as agents of spreading middle-class attitudes and values. The right-wing political activist sees psychiatry as an attempt to erode morality and patriotism. The Black resident of an inner-city ghetto says, "How can a white psychiatrist possibly understand my problems and my life?" Persons with deep religious faith are disturbed by psychiatry's refusal to endorse specific religious beliefs and its unjustified reputation as a destroyer of faith in spiritual values. A hippie says, "How can a psychiatrist care anything about me if he insists on asking that I pay for treatment?" And all manner of the dispossessed see psychiatry as a middle-class luxury, an agency of the Establishment, and a force which will destroy whatever cherished identity or autonomy they feel.

A more subtle attack, and one which will yield less readily to education, comes from those who do understand what psychiatry is but reject its basic premises of scientific methodology, logic, interpersonal responsibility, and rational approaches to irrational situations. Thus many physicians distrust psychiatry and try to fit emotional disorders into their familiar medical models of disease, ignoring those aspects that do not fit. Adherents of extreme right-wing political groups may understand the nature of psychiatry but see it as a threat to their doctrines. Adherents of the radical left may view psychiatry as a rival, a competitor, and attack it with the same sort of ferocity, and for many of the same reasons, as they attack liberals. Hence the paradox that criticisms of psychiatry come with equal intensity from those who view it as a defender of the established order and those who see it as an agent for social change.

Some persons fear psychiatry because they believe that it might uncover some of their own rigid but inadequate ego defenses, and they have considerable justification for this fear. Many strong movements for social change or for a continuance of the status quo are based on complex mixtures of personal convictions and psychopathology. Thus the observation that "some people and organizations cannot tolerate being thoroughly understood by large numbers of other people."

Infighting within psychiatric organizations has weakened the profession and its stance toward the outside world. A variety of attempts have been made to politicize the discipline. Those who are particularly enthusiastic about community work have attacked those who continue in private practice as being selfish and rejecting their duty to society; private physicians counter that their colleagues in community work are trying to destroy private practice and bring in socialized medicine. There has been a strong tendency for some practitioners to evolve special techniques of their own. Some of these are good and some not so good; but many tend, as do deviant instances in other disciplines, to create faction and to dissipate the potential for good inherent in the science. It is not the advocacy of new approaches that invites loss of confidence, but the derogation of older schools of thought.

In all too many instances, psychiatrists are neither diplomatic nor articulate spokesmen for their profession; this fact may be due to a reluctance to take sides for fear of alienating others. While this is often a necessary stance in individual psychotherapy, it is an inappropriate one for the psychiatrist as a citizen—and for psychiatry as a social science. Unless psychiatry becomes associated in people's minds with ethical stances or with honest attempts to attain a high level of ethical behavior, it will be rejected. There is a crisis in values throughout society, and psychiatry, with its unique ability to see problems, to evaluate causes, and to counsel, cannot sit idly by. Neither can it become involved in special kinds of social or political manipulation. Whatever action is taken must come about through the development of sound attitudes on the part of individuals in an atmosphere of the greatest possible freedom.

Patients often interpret the tolerance of psychiatrists toward illegal, immoral, or unesthetic behavior which is exhibited during psychotherapy as exhibiting a lack of any standards. Although this tolerance is necessary during psychotherapy, people can (and must) come to understand that the therapeutic technique of complete tolerance does not represent the psychiatrist's actual belief; and psychiatrists must see that psychiatry as a profession can and should endorse responsible standards of behavior. The college psychiatrist, for example, when treating a patient who has problems in respect to drug abuse or promiscuity, does his best to help the patient toward self-understanding and self-control without moralizing. But in papers published on these subjects college psychiatrists can quite properly, without any violation of privacy, expose their concern about these forms of behavior which erode the individual's integrity and self-image.

Before discussing the contribution psychiatry can make to the amelioration of social problems, it would be well to mention one thing it should not do—and that is to become involved in premature political pronouncements. Many organizations, especially universities and professional societies, are being pressured to take specific stands on a wide variety of political and social issues—the war in Vietnam, involvement in secret government research, programs to deal with unsatisfactory conditions both at home and abroad. Institutions should be very much concerned with social and political issues and should alert their members as to the exact nature of the issues involved, but the members cannot all agree with one another. In fact, institutions which do have a high consensus are probably going to be regressive in their thinking, because, within them, dissent is discouraged and progress is made unlikely. Any particular stand which is taken by individuals or groups should plainly be identified as *not* being held by the organization. To pretend that there is a consensus when there is not is only to divide the membership of any organization. As Goethe said, "Opinions divide, sentiments unite."

This will at least partly answer the question of whether the profession of psychiatry, as it is represented by the American Psychiatric Association, should become political or take stands on social issues. It must, by its very nature, be concerned; but it should not try as an organization to take stands on such issues unless there has been full discussion by, and a consensus obtained from, the appropriate task forces, councils, and committees. These in general should stress concern about those factors which worsen or improve the quality of living; only in very rare instances should they become political, in the sense of endorsing one of several competing policies where any one of the policies may be very beneficial.

What then *should* be psychiatry's role in current social issues? It must remember its dual nature as a physical and a social science. Although psychiatry is the practice or science of treating mental disease, psychiatrists are students of human behavior in all its aspects. It must concern itself with disturbances in the physical, psychological, and social background of individuals which give impetus to the development of mental disease. Almost by necessity a psychiatrist (if he believes in the possibility of prevention) must become involved as a citizen in community issues that concern human dignity, standards of taste, ethical behavior, and ways of reducing isolation and developing a sense of meaning and purpose in people's lives. He must therefore be sensitive to all manifestations of racism; of any unfair discrimination; poverty; factors which can impair life, freedom, thoughtfulness, creativity, individuality, sound approaches to problems, and all those measures which give meaning and purpose to an individual's life. Particularly he must be concerned about developing conditions which give children a chance to develop optimally in mind and body.

At times there appears to be conflict between those who insist that the problems of the mentally ill must be dealt with in terms of more intensive treatment, and those who feel that the problems are most effectively approached through improvements in the social system. This conflict is probably unnecessary. Many persons, possibly most, feel that both approaches are needed and that neither should receive undue emphasis over the other.

This realization of psychiatry's double role in individual treatment and social change has come about slowly. During the decade after World War II, many leaders in American psychiatry, notably Kenneth Appel, Harry Solomon, and Leo Bartemeier, became very much concerned with the inadequate resources which the psychiatric profession had to attack the problem of mental illness. Through their efforts and those of their colleagues, the Joint Commission on Mental Illness and Health was developed; its report was completed in 1961. Subsequent reports detailing the problems of the mentally retarded have followed, as well as the report by the Joint Commission on Mental Health and Illness of Children.

One of the main suggestions of the Joint Commission on Mental Illness and Health, the development of Community Mental Health Centers throughout the country, was implemented in 1963 with the message of President Kennedy to Congress and the passage of special legislation. Although the highly idealistic and complex program has met considerable difficulties, notably lack of personnel and lack of funds, it is becoming well-known throughout the country.

The report of the President's Commission on Health Manpower, completed in 1967, revealed that health services of all kinds were grossly inadequate for the increasing demands made by practically all segments of the population. The Joint Commission on the Mental Health of Children still further increased awareness of the discrepancy between health resources and health needs in its 1969 report, attempting to make the American people realize that a much larger proportion of their interests, efforts, and resources must go toward the appropriate nurturing of the physical, mental, and emotional health of children.

For as long as recorded history has existed, no one has seemed particularly optimistic about any improvement in the institution of the family; observers have been commenting for thousands of years on the signs of its weakening influence. Certainly at the present time, family stability appears to be decreasing. Parents are confused about their role in relation to their children, social planners are not particularly effective in developing procedures that strengthen the family, and the various agencies that minister to families' needs are fragmented and frequently difficult of access. There is an acute need for sound and reliable information, readily available to parents, which would aid them in achieving a higher degree of self-confidence in dealing with their children. Obviously such a publication should not be a recipe book, a how-to-do-it volume, but one which deals with attitudes and practices of parents. This should be particularly directed toward the topics of discipline, spending time with children, sexual education, openness of emotions, ways by which love and affection are expressed, handling of negative emotions, and so on. Parents need help in understanding the kind of privacy that is desirable for them to have and for their children to have.

They also need to know more about how to be appropriate role models. Many try to ingratiate themselves with their children by aping their children's behavior, and this is not particularly appealing or convincing to young people. Some parents can view and act toward their children only as extensions of themselves rather than as separate individuals. They should know more about the interplay between permissiveness and firmness, indifference and rigidity. The various forms of exploitation of children and their parents through advertising and manipulated fashions and fads should be scrutinized. Likewise the role of television, both as an educational instrument and as entertainment, could be profitably discussed. On all these matters psychiatrists should have something to say to parents that would help them approach problems with their children in a sound way and without feelings of guilt. All parents should realize that most of their problems are the norm and that any time a child is not active enough to assert his own individuality, his development is being impeded.

Psychiatrists have an unequalled vantage point from which to appraise ideas and develop new ones that will enable parents to perform their functions with confidence, flexibility, competence, and a minimum of guilt and maximum of satisfaction. Unfortunately, advice or information that is relevant to the middle or upper classes may not be at all relevant to those who live in urban ghettos. Consequently psychiatrists must cut through the cultural barriers and seek to develop ways to communicate with, and influence the attitudes of, families in those areas, either through living in the ghetto or from other modes of obtaining particular awareness of the problems of black people and other minority groups.

Psychiatry might well concern itself with trying to separate out the goals which seem consistent with the development of a more just society and expressing them in a form which is clear enough for a national consensus to be reached. If this were done, those who are trying to attain such goals might not find it necessary to become violent in order to make their views heard and appreciated. What is at stake here is channeling the great energy of many diverse groups into working toward common solutions of problems, rather than wasting their energies in fighting one another. In the resolution of such problems, persons whose specialty makes them particularly knowledgeable about the subtleties of human behavior should be of considerable help.

Through a number of stages, beginning with the care of those who have become so ill that they cannot care for themselves in an open society, psychiatry has progressed to the point where some of its practitioners are trying to enlist its principles to cure collective as well as individual ills. Likewise, many persons outside the discipline look to it to achieve miracles comparable to those performed by surgeons, microbiologists, and public health workers. The fact that present resources are inadequate, and that emotional and mental illness is widespread in our society, has led psychiatry (and other medical disciplines) to explore ways to work constructively with members of the other caretaking professions concerned with human behavior. These include fellow physicians of all specialties, educators, lawyers, members of the clergy, community leaders, and (in a very special way) parents.

In most instances of such collaboration, psychiatry and psychiatrists can probably be most effective by working with the professional individuals themselves. They can educate teachers in methods to increase the possible level of mental health among their students. Clergymen can be taught how to be better counselors for those who come to them in trouble and given more confidence in their own ability to deal with human problems. Businessmen can be instructed in ways to increase employees' morale, pride in their work, and human dignity. One large and particularly neglected area is that of the psychology of crime and punishment. The previous belief was that punishment was the way to prevent crime, and this idea is still predominant in the minds of many law-enforcement personnel. Rather than using our institutions to make individuals who have committed crimes still more alienated, new ways must be found by which individuals who have committed crimes can be taught to regain their place in society.

In spite of occasional evidence that my confidence may be unfounded, I am firmly idealistic about psychiatry and psychiatrists. No other group of observers has such an intimate view of man, and, because of this, so much responsibility for effecting change. The psychiatrist, in his office and in his consultations with members of other caretaking professions, is concerned largely with individuals—how to aid them in working toward sound solutions of their emotional conflicts. The psychiatrist as a citizen, and psychiatry as a profession, must assume responsibility for taking the leadership in building up those conditions, attitudes, and practices which enhance the dignity of man.

REFERENCES

1. Fosdick, R., "The Race With Chaos," *Harvard Alumni Bulletin*, Vol. 49, No. 4 (November 9, 1946), pp. 171-174.
2. Hoffer, E. *The Ordeal of Change*, New York: Harper and Row, 1963, p. 4.
3. de Tocqueville, A., *Democracy in America, Part II*, Vol. IV, London: Saunders and Otley, 1840, p. 185.
4. Commencement Address, Tufts University, June 1, 1969.
5. Thimann, K., "Science as an Instrument of Service," *Science*, May 30, 1969, Vol. 164, No. 3883, p. 1013.

25

HON. DAVID L. BAZELON

Men of science, religion, and law sometimes seem to offer simple solutions to the problem of fault and individual responsibility. But within each of these great disciplines there are rare men with humility and wisdom enough to know how much we do not know, and to seek enlightenment wherever it may be found. Dr. Leo Bartemeier is one of the least dogmatic men I have ever known. As a deeply religious man and a psychiatrist he has given me constant encouragement in my own effort to open the legal system to include modern insights into human behavior. He is not only a great psychiatrist but also a great friend, with an extraordinary capacity for love.

The Future of Reform in the Administration of Criminal Justice

A man was going from Jerusalem to Jericho and he fell among robbers who stripped him and beat him and departed leaving him half-dead.

This passage describes a celebrated case of assault and robbery. Its melancholy echo rings through today's newspapers:

. . . a 42-year-old watchmaker was found brutally beaten Wednesday in his shop . . . , police reported.

Literary style changes but not the substance of tragedy:

I weep to think of what a deed I have to do
Next after that; for I shall kill my own children.
My children, there is none who can give them safety.
And when I have ruined the whole of Jason's house,
I shall leave the land and flee from the murder of my
Dear children, and I shall have done a dreadful deed.

The Medean drama recurs in our time:

A Montgomery County mother shot and killed her three teen-age children yesterday, then ended her own life with a single shot from the death weapon she had bought only Wednesday, apparently with murder in mind.

THE 20TH CENTURY increase in crime has not brought great changes in the nature of the crimes. The future lies not in preparing to meet new and ingenious crimes but in fresh approaches to old problems.

The crimes which most concern us are those that threaten us in our streets and homes. We do not feel so threatened by the organized crime associated with political and economic corruption. We feel that the war against organized crime can be handled by the generals, and indeed the Department of Justice is now giving it effective attention. Sanctions are ineffective not because they are inappropriate but because the professional gangster gives himself long odds against being convicted.

The public is relatively unconcerned also about white-collar crimes, such as income tax evasion and stock frauds. We feel that the criminal law can curb such crime. Exposure is often punishment enough. No doubt the Benthamite notion that the criminal calculates pain against pleasure has some validity in this area. Bentham's system was a middle-class device more or less applicable to many middle-class crimes. But the law's deterrent effect is far removed from the juvenile delinquent who risks years in jail by grabbing a woman's purse. Calculation of potential pleasures and pains is not for him.

So our current concern is with crimes of violence. There is a feeling that we are really losing control in this area. The Chief of Police in Washington recently despaired that 1969 had started with another phenomenal rise in crime, despite the fact we have many more men on the streets than we had when the upsurge began a dozen years ago.

We are beginning to realize that the rising crime rate is not caused merely by weak law enforcement. Poverty in all its manifestations—lack of basic necessities, family breakdowns, mental disorders, unsupervised youths, school dropouts, alcoholism, drug addiction, and so on—is the chief factor producing anti-social behavior. From my own experience, I know that most defendants convicted of crimes of violence in the District of Columbia are indigent. A successful war on poverty would come close to solving the crime problem. But eradication of poverty seems only a little more likely than abolition of crime.

With respect to procedural matters, the criminal law is today facing the effect of poverty. The Report of the President's Commission on Law Enforcement and Administration of Justice is comparable to the Wickersham Report in the significance of its recommendations. It follows two decades in which the bench and bar have reformed first one and then another area where the law delivered less than it promised to the indigent defendant. But reform was undertaken piecemeal, as attention focused first on problems associated with the right to counsel, then on arrests and searches, then on coerced confessions and illegal police behavior. Now the wheel has come full circle and we have a renewed awareness of the crucial nature of the right to counsel. We are beginning to recognize that the assistance of competent counsel is required to safeguard the indigent's constitutional rights. Courts in the vanguard are suggesting that counsel ought to be present not only at formal proceedings but at every point at which the case may be won or lost. The Supreme Court has already guaranteed the arrested man the right to a lawyer when interrogated or placed in a lineup.

Procedural reforms are essential for initiating substantive reforms. Under our adversary system, no reforms—procedural or substantive— are likely without the effective assistance of counsel. The President's Commission recommended:

> The objective to be met as quickly as possible is to provide counsel to every criminal defendant who faces a significant penalty, if he cannot afford to provide counsel himself. This should apply to cases classified as misdemeanors as well as to those classified as felonies. Counsel should be provided early in the proceedings and certainly no later than the first judicial appearance. The services of counsel should be available after conviction through appeal, and in collateral attack proceedings when the issues are not frivolous. . . .

We have a long way to go before this goal is met and the wealth or poverty of a defendant makes no difference to his chance of a fair trial. The process is under way. But even if we enforce all procedural safeguards and all constitutional rights, we shall *not* have gained humane and rational criminal law. We mock justice by assuming that procedural safeguards are equally available to all people accused of crime, but we mock it more cruelly by assuming that all are equally free to choose or refrain from illegal behavior. The Task Force on Law of the President's Panel on Mental Retardation put it this way:

> Sometimes it is apparent that some specific factor is needed to provide equal treatment for the unequal. . . . If height is an advantage, the

short man may at least be given a box to stand on. But bolder and more far-reaching supplements may be needed where intellectual stature or social adaptability lies far beneath customary standards. To give a person liberty to choose between alternatives of which he can have no appreciation is to defeat and mock the concept of liberty.

Equality of *rights* before the law does not have as a correlate equality of *responsibility* before the law. People are not equally endowed, either personally or socially. In the past the criminal law has dealt chiefly with our disappointed expectations. In the future it must deal with the inequalities in natural endowment and opportunity of the people who stand charged before it. This goes to the core of criminal law—the concept of responsibility.

We have begun to realize that society must recognize its responsibility for individual inequality. Pope Pius XII forcefully asserted the relation between slum housing and delinquency. He said:

> Enough cannot be said about the harm that these dwellings do to the families condemned to live in them. Deprived of air and light, living in filth and in unspeakable commingling, adults and, above all, children quickly become the prey of contagious diseases which find a favorable soil in their weakened bodies. But the moral injuries are still mortality, juvenile delinquency, the loss of taste for living and working, interior rebellion against a society that tolerates such abuses, ignores human beings and allows them to stagnate in this way, transformed gradually into wrecks. . . .

"Society itself," the Pope said, "must bear the consequences of this lack of foresight."

Strange though it may seem, the notion that the law must recognize the facts of social life is sometimes regarded as immoral. It is argued that if we recognize reasons for failure to meet our expectations, this destroys the expectations and lowers the moral standards of society. I suggest that the opposite is true. We reenforce the validity of the expectations when we strip away the pretense that all can meet them. We have a *moral* duty to avoid the trap of Sunday morality—of ignoring the realities in order to maintain the facade.

There is also a more sophisticated objection to the law's recognizing the gulf between expectations and reality. Many people assume that morality is served by condemning and punishing those who disobey legal fiats. I suppose we punish others partly to overcome our own fear of losing self-control—to shore up our own defense mechanisms—and partly because of misguided religious notions. Religion emphasizes the accountability of the individual to God. In secularizing this concept, we have too often retained strict accountability while overlooking its divine corollary of forgiveness and compassion.

I am certainly no theologian but I recently discussed this idea with a friend, Father O'Doherty, who is head of the Department of Psychology and Logic at University College, Dublin, Ireland. The priest in the confessional, he pointed out, is a judge (he is called "judex") and the confessional is called the sacred "tribunal." He is acting for God in a very literal sense. He is concerned with accountability but accompanies it with divine forgiveness. In the secular world, we borrow the idea of holding people accountable. But we forget that in the religious view of accountability the individual assuming it is rehabilitated—he is forgiven and absolved. In the secular world we use accountability to justify retribution. We seem to be unconcerned with forgiveness and mercy—we even verbalize our lack of concern by instructing the jury not to be swayed by sympathy for the defendant.

I suggest that this is "doing God's work" in a totally misguided, if not presumptuous, fashion. Father O'Doherty gave a historical explanation for "the erroneous notion that the judge should 'do God's work' in the sense that as judge he should be concerned with 'sin,' or the 'internal state of the individual's conscience.'" He said it is a survival of the confusion in medieval society where the responsibilities of church and state were closely intertwined. Yet in a real sense, he argued, our notion of justice should be a reflection of Divine justice—although not with the Divine concern for the internal state of the accused's soul.

I would not abolish the concept of moral responsibility, or necessarily abandon punishment. But we must fashion them to our needs as a human society. Society cannot dispense with its expectations of its citizens. To recognize the difference between our expectations of other human beings and the realities of their behavior does not deny that expectations affect behavior.

The criminal law cannot fulfill its function as a social tool if it continues to ignore the complexity of causation. Courts should not assume responsibility where there is reason to believe that the defendant's actions were inspired by something other than abstract evil in the Miltonian arena where God and Lucifer eternally contend. Though there are great gaps in our knowledge about the causation of behavior, this does not mean that we have no such knowledge from psychiatry, sociology, anthropology, physiology and other disciplines. We are not morally justified in ignoring what we know. We often seem so intent on punishing that we do not want to be confronted with information which might make punishment seem inappropriate. We ignore so much scientific and common sense data as to causation in order to catch and punish the rat—always assuming that there is a rat. We are content with a vast superstructure of codes, trials, prisons and so on, and do not look to see how it fits its base.

Yet we have not been able to bury all our doubts. We are worried for instance about the recidivism rate—about the fact that harsh punishment seems to be an ineffective deterrent. But we look to simple remedies within the system: probation and parole, sentencing institutes, more and more policemen. There is much to be said for each of these palliatives—but not for our timid approach to them.

Take our approach to sentencing itself. We spend much money on sentencing institutes for judges whose efforts are directed toward obtaining uniform sentences. Of course it is wrong for one person to spend 25 years in jail and a similar offender who committed a similar crime to spend five. But isn't it more important to inquire how much good the prison can do in either case? And while these sentencing institutes ponder which factors make probation or parole more appropriate than prison, should they not examine the quality of the probation service itself? Such an examination would, I think, be very disquieting.

To my mind the Federal Probation System ought to be a model for the country. Yet it is short on help not only from psychologists and psychiatrists but also from competent, devoted probation officers—who are often the product of chance rather than a rational selection system. The power of appointing and promoting probation officers rests in each district court. A probation officer can be removed by the court "in its discretion." There is no "in-service" transfer as a matter of course. Perhaps as many as ten per cent of our probation officers do not meet even the *minimum* qualifications recommended by the Judicial Conference of the United States 27 years ago, in 1942. One judge has appointed a former used-car salesman.

It has been asserted that the power to appoint probation officers must be vested in the district judge so that he will have confidence in them and their recommendations. One of my colleagues who served for many years as a United States District Judge has pointed out the fallacy of this idea:

> Most probation officers serve in metropolitan areas. In these areas there is no atmosphere of intimate confidence. The relationship is one of impersonality. Those who suggest that this intimacy of relationship is required in order for probation to function are those who

want to keep the probation officer under the judge's thumb. If we are to avoid abuses such as using the probation officer as a personal flunkey, we must provide him with some degree of independence from the judge, particularly in rural areas where the federal judge is king.

It is difficult to conceive how we can insure the probation officer's independence of thought while he remains dependent upon the judge for his appointment, tenure and promotion. If we are to have a national probation service of trained professionals, they must be selected by and responsible to a unified central authority rather than responsible to all of the district judges with varying attitudes and practices. This would also encourage standardization of sentencing procedures—along with probation procedures.

It is another depressing reflection that the experienced head of the Federal Bureau of Prisons has to plead with Congress *not* to fix minimum mandatory penalties of five years for second-degree burglary and twenty years for first-degree burglary in the District of Columbia. James Bennett pointed out that "these Draconian penalties almost without parallel elsewhere in the United States are self-defeating . . . they will not have the intended effect of deterring this type of offense."

Somewhat to my amazement, a few theorists of the criminal law have now come out into the open and argued that besides its two generally accepted purposes—reformation and deterrence—a third rationale of the criminal law, vengeance, is also valid. Most of us still prefer to clothe our retributive instincts in the garb of deterrence. But we are told that, since retribution is a "natural" human instinct, it is right and necessary for society to vent its feelings on the defendant. All agree that the *individual* must not give way to these feelings; he may not personally avenge a murder or even take his own life. A life for a life is acceptable, it seems, only if we all join in the taking. I hope the law has a less emotional, more rational and more moral base. True, we all have aggressive, punitive urges. But should the criminal law carry them out? Many people believe that international conflict begins with and feeds upon our aggressive impulses, but few would advocate war. Awareness of our aggressive instincts should help us to refrain from aggression—not commit it collectively.

We should be more likely to avoid useless punishment if we reflected on *why* we punish and what we expect from punishment. We shall not know what punishment is useless unless we inquire *why* the wrongdoer acted as he did. Once we know why—or even begin to ask why—we shall better understand how to treat him, and how to deter others.

The common law purports to inquire into the causation of conduct when the insanity defense is raised. It has not ploughed deep. You are familiar with the *M'Naghten* rules and with the controversy which has surrounded them for more than a hundred years. I sometimes think we approach that controversy in too academic a fashion. We rarely get to what actually happens—what actual verdicts are based on what actual testimony. I think you would be shocked, as I have been, to read the records in cases where convictions under the *M'Naghten* rule have been sustained. Let me tell you about a murder case in which the defendant was sentenced to death. On appeal, the Washington State Supreme Court affirmed the conviction and the United States Supreme Court declined to review it. The facts were this. At the age of twenty-two, Don White beat an old woman to death in a laundry room. He raped her, took her ring and watch, which were of little value, then spent an hour in the room, folding laundry, placing some of it under the head of the dying woman, and chatting with the unsuspecting people who came into the laundry. Later that day, he killed a longshoreman, whom, like the old woman, he had never seen before. He stabbed him with a knife, then wandered a little distance away to drink wine and watch the police come and go. At trial, expert witnesses on both sides testified to the accused's serious mental disorder. Consider his background. He had never lived with his mother—who was only thirteen at his birth. When he was four months old, a red cap at a railway depot hailed the woman who became his adoptive mother to ask if she wanted a baby. Despite his superior intelligence—his IQ was about 130—he was expelled from every school he attended. Nine times he was in state institutions, with a growing record of violence and delinquency. When White was only eleven years old, a child psychiatrist said he was suffering from "a very malignant mental illness," that "institutionalization is absolutely necessary," and that "he will almost certainly wind up in prison or in a state mental hospital."

I will not discuss all the evidence, but it is apparent that, whatever the cause, the defendant was terribly sick, that his sickness was of long duration, and that it had been brought to the attention of the authorities time and time again.

The Washington Supreme Court squarely faced the issue: "The question before us is whether we, as the majority of jurisdictions, should refuse to extend absolute immunity from criminal responsibility to persons who, although capable of understanding the nature and quality of the acts (the ability to distinguish between right and wrong), are unable to control their own behavior as a result of mental disease or defect. . . . One argument for such change," the court noted, "is that we must take advantage of new developments in psychiatry. [But] there is nothing new about the idea that some people who know what they are doing still cannot control their actions." In other words, the court recognized that no new knowledge was necessary to see that White was grossly disordered. But the court *held* that the insanity defense "is available only to those persons who have lost contact with reality so completely that they are beyond any of the influences of the criminal law. . . . [T]he *M'Naghten* rule," the court concluded, "better serves the basic purpose of the criminal law—to minimize crime in society. . . . [W]hen M'Naghten is used, all who might possibly be deterred from the commission of criminal acts are included within the sanctions of the criminal law."

I am reminded of the 19th century English judge, Lord Bramwell, who quaintly expressed his approval of *M'Naghten* in these terms: "I think that, although the present law lays down such a definition of madness, that nobody is hardly ever really mad enough to be within it, yet it is a logical and good definition." William H. Seward, as defense counsel urging the insanity plea to a jury in 1846, said that we seem to demand

> entire obliteration of all conception, attention, imagination, associa-
> tion, memory, understanding and reason, and everything else. *There
> never was an idiot so low,* never a diseased man so demented. You
> might as well expect to find a man born without eyes, ears, nose,
> mouth, hands and feet, or deprived of them all by disease, and yet
> surviving, as to find such an idiot or lunatic, as the counsel for the
> people would hold irresponsible.

It seems to me now, as it seemed to me in 1954 when we abandoned *M'Naghten* in the District of Columbia, that a test of responsibility which allows Don White to be sentenced to death is no test at all. I think that when we broaden the test—by allowing the jury to consider whether the accused's mental disorder was such that he should not be thought responsible—as a criminal to be punished—we go a long way toward developing a useful courtroom inquiry into causation. I hoped that *Durham* would result in treatment rather than punishment for the mentally disordered. In this, it has been only partially successful. In the District of Columbia the last decade has seen an increase in acquittals by reason of insanity, but this has been largely offset by a decrease in the number of defendants found incompetent to stand trial, so that the total number of persons charged with crime who are eventually hospitalized instead of imprisoned has not changed very much.

In most cases, of course, the insanity issue is not raised. But when it is raised, expert testimony is usually given in conclusory diagnostic terms so that the jury is not really informed as to why the accused behaved as he did. We do not yet know what the results would be if the accused's mental and emotional condition and the dynamics of his behavior were explained to the jury in detailed, understandable language.

In other jurisdictions, the mentally disordered are acquitted even more rarely than they are in the District of Columbia. The test of criminal responsibility is an area for experimentation, and one in which there is probably no single correct solution, whether the *Durham* rule, which other jurisdictions have not adopted, or any other. But it is deeply distressing that fifteen years after *Durham* and more than a hundred years after *M'Naghten*, we in the United States still punish by imprisonment and death many offenders who are seriously disordered. In this sense *Durham*, and all our thinking on responsibility, has failed.

It is fallacious to argue that it would be "unsafe" to liberalize the insanity defense. Some argue that it would leave too much discretion in the hands of psychiatrists, particularly with respect to release. "I am not willing," said one judge, "to let the security of society depend upon a science which can produce such conflicting estimates of probable human behavior." But as Havelock Ellis said at the end of the last century:

> To seek for light in the fields of biology and psychology, of anthropology and sociology, has seemed to many a discouraging task. The results are sometimes so obscure; sometimes, it even seems, contradictory. . . . But if the path lies through a jungle, what is the use of the best and straightest of roads that leads astray? If a critic were to point out to a biologist . . . the limitations of the microscope, he would be entitled to reply—But excuse me, however imperfect the microscope may be, would it be better to dispense with the microscope? Much less when we are dealing with criminals, whether in the court of justice or in the prison, or in society generally, can we afford to dispense with such science of human nature as we may succeed in attaining.

I submit that nothing could be less safe than isolating a disturbed offender in prison, without treatment, for a fixed time and then releasing him without inquiring into his mental condition. Our experience in the District of Columbia shows that relaxation of *M'Naghten* does not produce chaos: it does not release dangerous, disordered people into the community. Nearly all states have some provision, comparable to that in the District of Columbia, for detaining and treating a mentally ill but dangerous offender who has been acquitted by reason of insanity. Of course, compulsory hospitalization has its dangers too—but from the standpoint of individual liberty, not public safety.

The compulsory hospitalization of acquitted offenders raises difficult problems of civil liberties which will tax the conscience and judgment of judges, prosecutors, defense counsel and hospital officials. Even at best, compulsory hospitalization is only a partial solution. Although some mentally disordered offenders are so dangerous that they must be confined in institutions, others are not. The treatment of those who require help but are not dangerous challenges our resourcefulness. We should not think in terms of either/or—prison or hospital—but should tailor dispositions to fit individuals. What we must avoid is becoming so overwhelmed by the complexities of the caretaking process that we do nothing at all.

Some experts have argued that if we go beyond *M'Naghten,* if we allow a jury to weigh the responsibility of one who, though sick, has some sense of wrongdoing, and invite psychiatrists to explain how mental illness affected his behavior, we might as well let him tell us how factors other than illness produced anti-social conduct in other cases. Why not let expert witnesses tell us whether physiological, economic, social or other factors contributed to deviancy? The distinguished British sociologist Barbara Wootton sees the same implications and asks: If we excuse the "mad," why not also the "bad"? She says:

> The creation of the new category of psychopaths is the thin end of what may eventually prove to be an enormously thick wedge: so thick that it threatens to split wide open the fundamental principles upon which our whole penal system is based—undermining the simple propositions . . . as to tbe responsibility of every sane adult for his own actions, as to his freedom to choose between good and evil and as to his liability to be punished should be prefer evil.

For, she continues,

> Once the grossly and persistently anti-social can claim to be treated as medical, and not as moral, cases, it is surely only a question of time before the mildly anti-social claim the same privilege. . . . To say that A must be judged guilty and punished because the doctors do not yet know what to do with him, while B must not be held responsible for his actions because he can be reformed by medical attention, is really to dig the grave of the whole concept of responsibility: for A, poor soul, is being punished not for his offence but for the limitations of medical knowledge. In a year or two's time, when medical science has advanced a little more, people like him also will rank as psychopaths and be treated as sick, not as wicked.

Lady Wootton concludes that, once we go beyond the limitations imposed by *M'Naghten*, there will be no logical stopping place short of abandoning the concept of criminal responsibility. She is content to allow the concept to "wither away." Other students of the insanity defense, just because they fear and foresee this outcome, would cling to *M'Naghten*.

But these experts are sympathetic to the needs of mentally ill offenders. They urge psychiatric treatment after conviction. Their argument is that the proper place for the consideration of complete psychiatric evidence is in and after sentencing, not in the determination of guilt. Hold the man responsible on the basis of *M'Naghten*; then remove the gag from medical testimony to decide what treatment he needs. There is sweet reasonableness in this view. And it has the added attraction of being easy. It withdraws from the community a difficult and troubling issue. But that issue, in my judgment, is one which the community has not only a right but a duty to consider. If we first find guilt and then promise to provide treatment for the person in spite of his guilt, we turn away from the question which should concern us most—the causes of criminal behavior. That is the question toward which *Durham* is directed. Even if our prison system were transformed, I should still be opposed to finding guilt regardless of moral responsibility on the theory that the accused would be "treated" in prison. I think the success of efforts to treat the individual offender depends on the community's awareness of his needs—of how he came to act as he did. And the best available means for generating such awareness is to provide as much of this information as possible to the community, or at least to its representatives on the jury, who will be forced to consider it seriously if they are required to assess the defendant's responsibility. I want the public, and not just the professionals, to know what caused the accused's behavior, so that they can have some idea of what is required not only for treatment but for the prevention of like cases.

Durham deals with defendants suffering from mental disease or defect. Whether we choose to stop there or go further, I think we should abandon the alleged "safety" of *M'Naghten*. It is a know-nothing—and learn-less—safety. But if *M'Naghten* is unacceptable, we need not go to the other extreme, abandon the concept of responsibility, and largely abolish the criminal law. While no purpose is served by holding people to standards they could not attain, the existence of standards and their enforcement in appropriate cases has clear social utility.

In moving away from the classical legal concept of criminal responsibility, *Durham* does not embrace the mechanistic interpretation of human behavior which seems to be generally accepted by modern biologists. So it is open to attack from opposite directions. I think *Durham* revealed —but did not create—complex and hidden philosophical as well as administrative issues. I think the criminal law cannot avoid the riddle of responsibility. The future is in confronting it, with whatever resources the law may have or may acquire.

The genius of the common law is its capacity to assimilate new knowledge and adapt to new needs. It has not used this capacity in the area of criminal responsibility. Recent decades have witnessed tremendous advances in relevant knowledge about human behavior. But legal thinking about "criminal insanity" has scarcely shifted in over a century.

I would urge that the criminal law abandon the myth of total individual responsibility and adapt to the realities of scientific and psychiatric knowledge. This cannot be accomplished by a single decision of any court or in any single jurisdiction. The process will be slow and continuous. New and unsuspected difficulties will appear as we move forward. But the flexibility of the common law provides the tool for meeting them as they arise. What the common law cannot do, while remaining true to its tradition, is stand still while the world is in flux.

26

LAWRENCE S. KUBIE, M.D., D.Sc.

*It is both an honor and a privilege to share in this cele-
bration of the 75th birthday of Leo Bartemeier. His rare
capacity for affection includes a tolerance for disagreement even over important issues. Consequently, differences
of opinion never divide him from his fellow men. By his
spirit he brings opponents together and replaces hostility
with loyalty. In this he is almost unique among scholars,
including scientists and especially psychiatrists and psychoanalysts. Sometimes his great confidence in human good-
ness leaves him vulnerable to deception by others; but he
can accept even this without losing confidence in man's
basic integrity and generosity. This is why he has been
entrusted with posts of high responsibility in the councils
of the American Medical Association, the American Psychiatric Association and the American and International
Psychoanalytic Associations. It is this same quality that
gave him the inner strength to accept uncomplainingly
the two great personal tragedies, the death of his only son
and the death of his wife. While still in practice in Detroit, his concern for the general cultural implications of
psychiatry expressed itself in the organization of "The
Cornelian Corner." Later it was expressed again by his
leaving practice to take charge of the Seton Psychiatric
Institute in Baltimore.*

The Cultural Significance of Psychiatry

THE PROBLEM which concerns me here is both complex and subtle.
It will not involve me in the current bickering among different schools of
psychiatry and psychoanalysis, nor in a correction of premature and

* This paper is published with the permission of the Friends Hospital of
Philadelphia, as a slightly expanded and revised version of the paper presented at the annual meeting of the Friends Hospital in May, 1965, and

excessive claims for therapeutic miracles with drugs and/or the application of techniques derived from the conditioned reflex. Nor will I bog down in discussions of premature efforts to evaluate therapeutic results. I will attempt rather to consider the significance of modern psychiatry for our whole culture. Such a search will of necessity include some passing reference to its therapeutic and preventive functions, because of their general cultural and sociological importance. Implicit here is also the question of whether a higher percentage of us need psychiatric help today than was true in the past. About this too I will only note in passing that there is no evidence that percentage-wise the neurotic process is more prevalent today than it ever was. Of course there are more human beings, and of these a larger percentage are at the two vulnerable ends of life. This has increased the absolute number of those who need and seek help but not the over-all percentage. One may wonder whether our increasing readiness to seek psychiatric help means a greater dependency, or a greater humility, or a greater honesty, or some change in the abstractions called "human weakness," or in the potential health or sickness of our whole culture. A consideration of the cultural significance of psychiatry cannot evade these questions. Yet they are not basic to the issue which I will ask you to consider here. I will take as my thesis that, if we and our culture are to survive, we must find answers to three basic, unsolved and interrelated problems of human life.

1. Either man must learn how to bring himself up wholly without those early neurotic distortions which have always been universal, but which we have overlooked or dismissed as unimportant; or else, if this is impossible, then he must learn to resolve them in such a way as not to leave in the human child accumulating residues of distortion, out of which the neuroses and psychoses of adult life are later generated.

2. Man must learn how to transmit to succeeding generations whatever wisdom about living he acquires through living. This vital ability to pass on to the child the wisdom of age has eluded every human culture.

3. Man himself must learn how to become free to change, to change in such a way as to insure to himself the possibility of future and continuing change. (Until today, man has learned how to change almost everything in the world except himself and his own nature.)

The ultimate attainment of these three goals will bring to man the

subsequently published and distributed by that hospital. Copyright © 1965, Lawrence S. Kubie, M.D.

only freedom which really counts—namely, freedom from those rigid psychological mechanisms which keep him enslaved.

These are the three challenges which human culture faces, and it is to these that psychiatry must contribute, if it is to have any permanent and basic impact on human culture. These have always been important; but today, as our whole culture is turning back to Methuselah, these needs are even more pressing. The longer we live, the more urgent does it become that we learn to live wisely—and free of the ubiquitous, masked neurotic distortions of that which we euphemistically call "normal" human nature. Longevity gives us some reason to hope that we may find a solution to this. Yet longevity does not guarantee wisdom, although it does give us more time to struggle for it; more time to learn from our errors. For we must face not only the fact that dying is going to become an increasingly difficult and elusive achievement, but also that the aging process will come later and later and progress more slowly, until ultimately it may disappear entirely from human life and from human culture. Therefore we have no option. We must do something about learning to live more wisely ourselves and to pass on that wisdom to successive generations. It is not enough to be as old as Methuselah, unless added years mean added wisdom and added maturity, and not merely increased power to be destructive. Only a major cultural breakthrough will make this possible. In fact this is why I chose to discuss the ultimate cultural significance of psychiatry, rather than its immediate practical relevance to medicine, health, industry, and so forth. What I have in mind involves all of these but extends beyond them.

In spite of the fact that some may think this a pessimistic position, it actually originates in a fundamentally optimistic assumption. After all, the only true pessimistic was Pollyanna, who was so afraid to face any of the realities of life, so convinced that if she ever faced them they would overwhelm her, that she had to sugar-coat everything. Is this not the ultimate in pessimism? The optimist on the other hand has confidence that if we acknowledge first that things are wrong, very wrong, and then set out to define what is wrong, we will have at least a chance to find out how to set things straight. Is this not precisely how medicine has grown? And is there not then a profound optimism in facing tough facts, such as the fact that we have been at the business of being human beings for quite a long time, yet have not made a very good job of it, nor learned as yet how to do it better? Clearly the search for how to do a better job requires first a willingness to face the reality of human failure, then the pursuit of a high degree of technical knowledge, and finally the courage to experiment with basic cultural changes. Lamentations and exhortations have no place in this program.

Many philosophers and many religious sects have assumed that they knew the ultimate solution. Yet none has had either the techniques or the dedication to devote itself to a slow, painful, humble search for the answer. Actually we are just beginning to realize that the study of our failures as human beings and the search for better ways to *be* human constitute the most important challenges with which we can confront human culture. In fact, study and research must precede even the advocacy of any assumed solutions. Modern psychiatry is just the beginning of such a search.

Please note that I do not say that psychiatry can pretend to hold the answers. What it may lay claim to are methods for seeking answers. Its significance to human culture and to human life is its dedication to the process of search, to the effort to find out why being a human being, even under the most favorable of circumstances, is such a difficult assignment; and why in spite of the eons of time that we have been at it, we have not yet been able to find out how to make a better job of being human.

Not only does psychiatry have no ready answers; even its techniques of search are still fumbling and inexact. But imperfect though they may be, these techniques represent progress in the long trek toward man's mastery of himself and his environment.

How do universal neurotic distortions of human development come about? They arise out of certain universal human vulnerabilities. First among these is the fact that early in life things happen to us which impose a fixed emotional pattern (what might also be called a "central emotional position or potential"), which thereafter becomes the center of emotional gravity for an entire life. In some, this is depression; in others anxiety, anger, or elation. In many it is mixed. Throughout life we tend to return to this central affective position, being precipitated back into it either suddenly or slowly and insidiously. To experience such a feeling is normal only as long as it arises in response to appropriate and adequate circumstances. The affective state becomes distorted and has in turn distorting secondary consequences only when the affective pattern becomes fixed and obligatory and repetitive and/or is touched off by inadequate and inappropriate circumstances. The basis for this sort of affective distortion is usually imposed very early in life. It has something to do with why children have nightmares before they have ever been exposed to danger. Like so many things in life which seem simple, this phenomenon actually is subtle and complex. Had it been simple, it would have been solved many years ago.

Related to this is the fact that impaired emotional patterns are sensitive to the impact of "triggering" experiences which can explode them in extraordinary ways. We are familiar with this in the familiar form of phobias: e.g., terror in the presence of something harmless—a butterfly, a high building, a crowded room, or wide open spaces. As we walk along the street, we may pass a familiar but unimportant figure, perhaps a doorman at a hotel. Suddenly he wheels around, turning his back on us to look the other way, perhaps to pick up some bags. At that moment something may happen in one of us. As a reality the man himself and his gesture mean nothing; but this sudden whirling, this turning of the back, may be a symbol which triggers rage in one person, panic in another, a drop into depression in a third. Depression, panic, rage and even elation can be precipitated by just such unimportant episodes. Furthermore they may show up as delayed imprints on our later fantasies or dreams, or at the next encounter with a stranger. Such tiny episodes happen to all of us every day as we walk along the street, as we sit at home and read and think, as we drift off to sleep, or as we wake up. They are unimportant in and of themselves; but of utmost importance for our understanding of human vulnerability.

The third component in the universal neurotic potential is even more inevitable and, if anything, even more complicated. This is the result of our dependence on the symbols by which we talk, communicate, and ruminate. Certainly if we could not do this, we would not be human; but the capacity to use symbols is the outcome of a developmental process which is also vulnerable to distortion. This development must include the capacity to make comparisons among different experiences so as to find similarities and dissimilarities among them and then the ability to make generalizations about them and to represent these generalizations by abstractions, and finally to represent the abstractions by symbols—visual, verbal, and paralinguistic, for example. Without this interlocking hierarchy of skills we could not deal with abstract concepts at all. Nor could we carry the images of experience out of the past to project them into the future. Therefore without them we could not anticipate or plan—nor bind into one continuum the near and far, the past, present and future of our own experiences. Without symbols we could not be lawyers, engineers, doctors, artists, philosophers, business men, teachers, writers, scientists, or theologians. Without symbolic tools we could not be humanly creative. The symbolic process is the tool which sets us apart from the subverbal animal. Unfortunately, however, this superb instrument, which enables us to communicate and create, is also extraordinarily vulnerable. It is at once an essential tool for our greatest creative potential and the focus of that special human vulnerability which is manifested whenever the component parts of the symbolic process become disassociated so that they become detached from one another: one part conscious or preconscious, another part inaccessible to conscious self-inspection. More strictly speaking, it is never the symbol which becomes unconscious, but its link to what it is supposed to represent. This link can be clouded or blocked or subjected to a process of substitution by which an emotionally innocuous object, event, or relationship is substituted for one which is charged with painful feelings. In this way the symbolic process can become a masking and misleading tool, instead of one which represents truly the flow of inner psychological experiences. Experiences which are buried, disguised, or masked in this way become sources of trouble; because so long as they remain inaccessible to any conscious approach they will remain inaccessible to corrective experiences. This is the process which introduces discontinuities into our psychological processes and creates an internal dictatorship of automatic, involuntary, insatiable, rigid, unlearning repetition. All of this occurs whenever "unconscious" components play a dominant role in the determination of human thought, feeling and purpose.

As a direct result of this dissociative process, our thoughts, feelings, hopes, plans, and purposes can all become enslaved to an internal dictatorship of unconscious processes: a dictatorship which is even more destructive than are the external dictatorships with which we have been struggling throughout so much of this century. These internal dictators (i.e., our buried unconscious processes) account for that which is rigid, insatiable, stereotyped, and unlearning in human nature. They limit our capacity to learn from experience, from success or failure, from rewards and punishment, from exhortation or reasons. They subject the ways in which we eat, drink, walk, dress, fight, play, love or create—indeed, every aspect of life—to patterns of obligatory repetition. All of us have seen this in children. Has any one of us ever known a child who did not have at least transient episodes of obligatory repetitiveness? This might show up first in tic-like movements, later in the way he dresses and moves, dawdles or rushes, in his orderliness or disorderliness, in his eating and sleeping. Even when these patterns of repetitive behavior alter or disappear spontaneously, as they may do, the underlying sources remain uncorrected. Thus they contribute to future patterns of obligatory behavior, sometimes reappearing in increasingly serious forms, until they become destructive ingredients in the structure of the whole life and personality. This may turn the normal rebelliousness of adolescence, which is under the voluntary control of the adolescent, into blindly compulsive rebellion which can no longer be turned on and off. It can make out of the normal impulse to be "good" an equally compulsive and involuntary submissiveness. Its influence can distort studying and learning, the capacity to develop new ideas or to acquire new information. It underlies the complaints of many of our best graduate schools that they get the best brains in the world but do something to destroy them. They declare that they must find out why so many of their ablest youngsters are dropouts; and why even those who survive the grind (in the sense that they get through their exams) emerge with their creative potentials crippled. This seems to be outstandingly true in engineering—and less true in medical education. It occurs in the law as well, and in theological seminaries where theological educators are concerned about it. And, according to teachers of the humanities, it happens to their students too. And why not? If the classics and the humanities did not solve life's problems for the ancients, why should we expect them to do so for us today?

Here it is evident that we are facing more unsolved problems. It is because of this incessant and costly interplay among the neurotic and the learning processes that, as I mentioned above, we do not yet know how to pass wisdom on from one generation to another. The consequence is that whole generations of man, whole cultures, repeat the same mistakes without learning from them. This is a fantastic state of affairs for a race or culture which pretends to be mature, sophisticated and wise.

Also this is why we do not yet know how to enable human nature itself to change. We can change everything in the outside world; but we have not yet learned how to make it possible for man himself to change.

As I indicated at the outset, these are the three stigmata of our cultural failure; and we must face with humility the fact that our greatest cultural instruments have not succeeded in solving these problems. To point this out is what some people label "pessimistic." Yet unless we face this painful reality, unless we acknowledge its existence, we will never even attempt to find ways to prevent it.

Modern psychiatry is very young. Traditional psychiatry on the other hand (i.e., the psychiatry of those psychoses which come at the end of the road) is not young. For countless years, people have recognized psychotic breakdowns, and the need of such patients for hospitalization in order to protect both the individual and society. What is new is the study of the process by which psychosis evolves out of neurosis, and by which neurosis arises in the first place as an early deformation of normal development. This study, which had to wait on the evolution of the techniques which modern psychodynamic psychiatry and analytic psychotherapy have brought to human culture, does not insure the success of analysis or yield final answers to the great unsolved problems of human culture. But it has resulted in the development of analysis as an essential exploratory instrument without which a full understanding of the process by which we fall ill is impossible.

For the studies of the failures in human living which are produced by the neurotic process we have an impressive medical model—the conclave of doctors around the autopsy table. Medicine has even developed a special discipline called "pathology" for the study of its own failures. Medical schools and teaching hospitals have a solemn rite called the "clinical pathological conference," where the internists, surgeons and pathologists gather together *in the presence of their students* to study their own failures. I know no other discipline in which professors study their failures openly in the presence of their students. This is why it was an enormously important moment in human culture when doctors first had the honesty, the humility, and the courage to do an autopsy. And guided by this precept, psychiatry now is trying to study the experiential, sociological, intrapsychic and biological conditions under which human beings fail, not in dying but in living. To understand failure in living is surely as important as it is to understand the biochemical failures which lead to death.

I will add just one further point. It concerns a fallacy which has permeated our every institution, including our most pretentious educational and cultural instruments and establishments, throughout history—namely, the illusion that each addition to ourselves is in and of itself valuable. All of us surely know the definition of a rich man, that he is just a poor man with money. Similarly a man who is stuffed with facts like a Strasbourg goose (preferably facts that someone else does not have) may be just a fact-collector, a poor man with unusable facts. The fact-collector is not unlike many art or stamp collectors. Frequently and unfortunately the most erudite man in any field may be immature and unwise; and the relationship between erudition and wisdom today remains purely accidental. The most important goal that education can pursue is to find out how to close this gap. These considerations circle back to the necessity to understand the subtle, neurotogenic, psychological mechanisms which keep men from maturing. It is because of them that only a few of us acquire the degree of wisdom and the kind of maturity which can make knowledge creative rather than destructive in human life. This is why the psychic autopsy is essential, i.e., the autopsy of our failures in life, through the analytic study of the neurotic process and of its psychotic disorganization, so that psychiatry can make its spiritual contribution to human culture. This is the goal to which all of our cultural instruments today and tomorrow must be dedicated.

27

JONAS SALK, M.D.

Leo Bartemeier's geniality, optimism, and hope have nourished not only his confidence and courage but that of others as well—to walk where angels fear to tread. His deep convictions, both religious and intellectual, and his magnanimous and generous spirit, have been a force for good and an inspiration to others. He has made a meaningful mark upon the profession for which he himself is so richly gifted. To him I offer this small contribution—with respect and admiration.

Man's Biological Potential

MAN HAS NOT always been. He had a beginning, and we may assume that he will have an end. But, for us, the question of his beginning or end is not of as great importance as that concerned with his present. This does not imply a lack of interest in the past or in the future; on the contrary, the present has meaning as part of a continuum. It is from this point of view that we will reflect upon man—and to justify my interest in what is regarded as a philosophical question I have chosen to speak of "Man's Biological Potential." These words in themselves convey the idea of time, and change, and evolution.

We are all interested in the question implied in this title, and from more than an academic point of view. We are aware not only of man's problems but each of us, in his own way, professionally addresses himself to one or another aspect of this large question. Until such time as they are answered, questions continue to create fields of force toward which we are drawn, and toward which we drive ourselves.

A lecture presented 14 December 1961 before The Maryland Psychiatric Society meeting at the Seton Psychiatric Institute.

This statement in itself says something about man. It says that ideas have power and that man possesses a mechanism that responds to the impelling force of ideas. Man is interested in the mind of man. His curiosity is based not only upon a desire to know for the sake of knowing, but also for the reason that it will be useful to know. This means that curiosity is a property of the mind of man. Associations are made, concepts are developed, and man eventually sees how his knowledge may be used to solve the problems he recognizes. Recognition of a problem comes when one can imagine a situation different from that which exists; man's ingenuity is then applied to influencing the order of nature and trying to create a world closer to his heart's desire.

Since the order of nature includes man himself, it was inevitable that man's attention would turn eventually in the direction of himself and his mind when threats to physical survival, which at one time were of more immediate and individual concern, became less pressing. It was inevitable, too, that the development of a critical level of basic knowledge would bring about the realization of hitherto unrecognized powers and that this would permit and encourage realistic thought about problems, the recognition of which might otherwise continue to be avoided.

It is difficult for most to face questions that seem to defy solution, and it is all too easy for some to accept answers that block further inquiry. But this is not the way of science.

SCIENCE AND MAN

When I use the term *science*, I think of it as the art by which we inquire and explore. There is an art to all human activities—to hunting, navigation, painting, writing, and to managing, administering, practicing law and medicine, etc., etc.

Science is man's most recent way of addressing himself to the very questions that have occupied him since he developed this kind of awareness, and since he developed the equipment with which to deal with sensations and reactions evoked by awareness. By virtue of the fact that science exists, we must say, of course, that its emergence and development were inevitable, just as we must acknowledge that the existence of man is testimony to his inevitability (even though I doubt that a sentient human being, if present in the universe ten million years ago, would have been able to forecast the inevitability of man or of science).

THE MEANING OF MAN'S POTENTIAL

Let us look at our own lives and inquire as to the point in time when it became apparent that the pattern would unfold as it did. I do not want to get into the arguments about pre-destination but, rather, to establish a sense of the limits of predictability, when as biologists we address ourselves to the question of man's potential.

As I speak now of man's biological potential I have in mind man's capacity for change—and man's own influence upon himself in this regard. As a point of departure I introduce the question of man's view of himself, since this depends upon the premises he chooses and the assumptions he makes. I will proceed on the basis of assumptions and premises that derive from biology. In the interest of condensation, I will make a large leap and say that man not only incorporates the history of physical and biological evolution, but, in man, a new nodal point in evolution occurred, analogous to the first emergence of life, or the first appearance of animal life as distinct from vegetative life. Many other nodal points occurred in evolution such as the "invention" of the cell membrane and of the nucleic acids which make up the coding and decoding information system for heredity.

The brain has evolved to a point where we are aware of the question with which we are confronted and the brain even contains equipment with which to deal, at least in part, with such questions. Imaginings are the product of that organ. Is this not a situation analogous to that which existed when potentialities in the first forms of life were coupled with structures as well as opportunity for the development of still more complex structures, and for self-replication that led ultimately to man? If contemplation, abstract thought, and technology have appeared in man for the first time, then what is the nature and meaning of this potential?

BASIS IN BIOLOGY

So that we not leap off the deep end, into the realm of science fiction, nor become victims of the morbid pessimism that is perennially prevalent, nor become intoxicated by the optimism of those who ignore certain facts of life, I would like to draw attention to a few interesting phenomena that have been discovered by biologists in recent years. I will cite the view of a distinguished mathematician and administrator of science who recently made some profound observations on "The Emerging Unity of Science." This scientist is Dr. Warren Weaver who summarizes these discoveries as follows:

. . . At the recent Cold Spring Harbor Symposium on "cell regulating mechanisms" there were beautiful reports on our present knowledge of the 1000-2000 enzymes, all contained within a single cell and simultaneously controlling the chemical reactions occurring there; on the synthesis of RNA by DNA, the material composing the genes; on the subsequent role of RNA as an intermediate conveying genetic information from the genes to the ribosomes in the cytoplasm, thus dictating the structure of the protein enzyme being synthesized; on the feed-back whereby the products of an enzyme-activated reaction inhibit the enzyme activity; on the "enzymatic adaptation phenomenon" whereby certain regulator genes control the synthesis of the enzymes.

The contributors to these fundamental pieces of knowledge have not been classical biologists but, for the most part, are chemists and physicists who have addressed themselves to biological questions. The basic character of the questions upon which they have focused has had a unifying effect upon the physical and biological sciences, just as earlier physics and chemistry became united indistinguishably as the physical sciences. We speak now of the natural sciences, including biology, and we may soon come full circle to the term *natural philosophy*.

The phenomenon of unification in science encourages me to describe certain of the phenomena discovered by those biologists whose interest, at the molecular level, is in the relationship between structure and function in living systems. I am prompted to do this because I believe that there may be analogies between molecules and men. Rather than a tendency to regard anthropomorphic explanations as reflecting man's egocentricity, this may be a recognition that man is an aggregate, at a higher order, of complex systems, and that any given effect or characteristic may be analogous to a simpler, but still very complex system either at the cellular or sub-cellular level. (I know the pitfalls of over-simplification, but bear with me for a moment longer for this brief excursion.)

When I speak of "Man's Biological Potential" using the biological metaphor, I express thoughts about some of the attributes and behaviorisms of man. Earlier I referred to science as one form of the art of inquiry. This is another way of saying that the scientist is a particular kind of thinker who expresses questions and thoughts in ways that are different from those of other kinds of thinkers. But the development of science is part of the continuum of evolution of ideas and methods of thought, and of the equipment for this process, i.e., language for symbolic expression. Another large liberating evolutionary step was the appearance and development of the opposable thumb, manual dexterity, and technology.

The liberation of man's potential for thought and for technology rests on the development of language and manual dexterity. The potential possessed by man's central nervous system at an earlier stage of evolution can be thought of as having been developed further, or educed, by the potential that existed for language and for manual dexterity and their further development. Test this yourself by noting the difference in the condition of your mind or your thoughts both before and after you have expressed yourself on any subject. How often is it that you realize the substance in your mind only *after* you have expressed yourself? Science, which uses language, is a disciplined way of thought and inquiry which has developed special rules and technical skills and is liberating man for further evolution as did the basic changes that resulted in language and manual dexterity.

The sharp distinctions between different classes of thinkers and doers tends to limit the interaction between people and disciplines. I am just as disparaging of biologists who evade complex and difficult questions about man as I am of "behaviorologists" who look askance at the introduction of relatively simple biological concepts intended to suggest the possibility of simplification as a working basis for thinking about very complex functions.

Before introducing a few such over-simplifications as possibly useful analogies, I would like to describe what may be certain basic bio-molecular phenomena that appear to have some analogies to more complex immunologic and even psychologic phenomena.

ENZYMATIC ADAPTATION PHENOMENON

I will introduce the technical portion of this discussion by describing the "enzymatic adaptation phenomenon" in which the synthesis of enzymes is controlled by certain regulator genes. Mention was made earlier of feed-back effects whereby the products of an enzyme-activated reaction inhibit further enzyme activity, as would an "enzymostat" if such could be constructed. These revelations, together with the knowledge that more than a thousand enzymes exist in a single cell, simultaneously controlling the chemical reactions occurring therein, serves to justify the comment by Warren Weaver, "that we are at last beginning to get some real understanding of the total economy of cellular metabolism" and the further remark that, "It would be hard to imagine an example more clearly exhibiting organized complexity, nor an example more basic and universal."

It is because of its general character that I want to call attention to one particular aspect of the "enzymatic adaptation phenomenon" as an example of a simplifying thought that derives from biology. I will illustrate the point by the following instance taken from microbiology. Bacterium (B) that does not contain a particular enzyme (E) for a specific substrate (S) will, upon the addition of substrate (S) to a culture of (B), begin to synthesize enzyme (E). Bacterium (C) which is also free of enzyme (E) will not synthesize this enzyme even under the conditions favorable for (B). Thus (B) and (C) are different with respect to their capacity to make enzyme (E) and to act upon substrate (S). The capacity to make this enzyme and to carry out the particular functions of digesting substrate (S) is genetically determined. However, this is not the fact I want to illustrate, but rather do I wish to emphasize the fact that Bacterium (B) does *not* make enzyme (E) *until* it is exposed to substrate (S). Thus, the potential of the microbe to produce the specific enzyme is "educed" by the substrate. It is as if the organism does not reveal its potential for making this enzyme until exposed to the challenge—or, stated another way, until it is under the specific environmental influence in which the cause is the target of the effect. The mechanism is such that it cannot be said that the bacterium has "learned" to digest the substrate, but rather that the capacity of the bacterium to perform in this way was "educed." Those who first discovered this phenomenon described it as "induced" enzyme synthesis. Perhaps we can reconcile the use of the two different words by saying that the substrate "induces" the enzyme synthesis and that the potential of the bacterium to do so is "educed." Neither "induction" nor "eduction" can occur in the absence of genetically determined competence on the part of the bacterium. In passing I want to mention a matter of still further interest, which is that the inducing substance operates through the suppression of an inhibitor.

It should be evident that, when a simple substance such as galactose is introduced into a reactive bacterial culture, a whole series of highly complex events are set in motion, and a series of rather precisely programmed events occur which represent, in a way, the cumulative heritage of this particular organism. The ritual of this complex reaction is well established and occurs in a way suggesting a cultural heritage and great knowledge on the part of the bacterial cell. However, its *anticipatory biological potential* was not revealed until challenged.

ANTIBODY FORMATION

Let's move now to a more complex system such as antibody formation in any vertebrate—and man is as good an example as any. It is believed, in accordance with at least one theoretical formulation, that, in the same way that the capacity for a bacterium to form an enzyme pre-exists, simply waiting to be subjected to test, the capacity of man to form antibody pre-exists and simply awaits contact with the suitable antigen; i.e., cells "programmed" to form antibody are activated to do so by contact with a specific antigen. It is of particular interest to note a fact that has been demonstrated—but the acceptance of the interpretation of which is still questioned by many—that continued antibody production does not require the continued presence of the antigen. The facts suggest that the antigen-induced cell, and even its progeny, persists in remembering the initial experience, as if the cell had "learned a lesson," and continues to exhibit the trick it had learned in performing the feat of producing antibody.

You are all familiar with the effect of a second antigenic stimulus, given at a later time, which is referred to as the phenomenon of "recall" or, as it is commonly called, the "booster" effect. This exaggerated, seemingly "learned" response is the consequence, in part at least, of an increase in population of cells competent to form antibody, multiplication having occurred under the stimulus of contact with the challenging antigen. Proof does not exist for the many gaps in understanding the specific intermediates in the process of antibody synthesis; however, the effects observed are quantitatively compatible with explanations on a molecular level. In this example of antibody formation we have touched on a phenomenon analogous to memory; we have related this to the enzymatic adaptation phenomenon. I have chosen to juxtapose these seemingly unrelated phenomena and now I want to mention another.

CONDITIONING IN PLANARIA

I want to mention some observations recently reported by investigators working with the flatworm planaria. They have noted that a conditioned response to light can be induced in this primitive worm, and that when cut in half, the regenerated halves, to which tail and head regenerate respectively, when full grown, both possess the same conditioned response. It is as if there is a replicating substance in the worm that is responsible for the memory or retention of the conditioned response. It has also been reported (by Corning and John, of the Center for Brain Research, at the

University of Rochester) that the enzyme ribonuclease, in contact with the tail-half, will prevent retention of the conditioned response in the worm regenerated from the treated tail-half but will have no effect upon the continued presence of the conditioned response in the full worm regenerated from the head-half. This leads to the tentative conclusion that "memory" in the worm is important and when RNA is digested by RNAse (ribonuclease) this property disappears, as in the tail-half when so treated. The persistence of memory for the conditioned response persists in the head-half which is believed to be the ultimate source of the molecules in which memory is recorded, perhaps by a mechanism as in the formation of "adaptive" enzymes and in antibody formation.

The findings and ideas here mentioned are in keeping with the results of studies by Holger Hyden and his colleagues at the University of Goteburg, in Sweden, which suggest an important role for RNA and for glial cells in memory.

IMMUNOLOGIC TOLERANCE

These facts from analytical biology are cited because they may have some relevance to the question of man's biological potential. Let us now return to a further phenomenologic inquiry which may, at first, seem to add to the confusion but which I hope will, in due course, help simplify. Let us examine the immunologic phenomenon of skin-grafting with which you are familiar. The point I wish to make by the immunologic example is that during the long period of maturation before adulthood (but very likely principally in early childhood), events impinging on the CNS can conceivably have an effect, corresponding not merely to the memory-related effects in simpler systems just described, but to the effects of antigens which result in induced immunologic tolerance. I will try to explain what I mean by this by referring to the classical experiment of Medawar and his colleagues with in-bred mice.

As you know, in-bred mice are produced by continuous brother-sister matings, resulting essentially in all mice being immunologically identical, as are identical twins. A mouse of in-bred line A will accept a skin graft from another line A mouse but will reject, as foreign, a graft from a line B mouse. If a mouse from in-bred line A is injected, before birth and while still in utero, with a suspension of cells from an in-bred line B mouse, it will, after it is born, accept a skin graft from line B. Thus, mouse A, which normally rejects a graft from B, was made tolerant to B by treatment, before birth, with cells of B. A similar injection of cells from a line B mouse into an A mouse after (rather than before) birth would result in an accelerated rate of rejection, or increased intolerance to a graft. It would seem that, depending upon the relation to a critical point in time in development, a given experience will result either in a state of tolerance or intolerance, and at bottom this is an immunological reaction based upon the formation of a particular kind of antibody.

ANALOGY BETWEEN RES AND CNS

This makes one wonder whether, in the early years of life, attitudes and behavioral reactions of many kinds may not be constructed in a similar way. It makes one wonder whether, depending upon the point in time when an incident occurs, or attitude is presented, it would result in one or another effect. If this were so, it suggests a reason for fixation of attitudes and prejudices once established.

Carrying the analogy between the central nervous system (CNS) and the immunologic system (RES) one step further, and recalling the phenomenon of "adaptive enzyme synthesis," the idea suggests itself that the mechanisms by which learning takes place may conform to that suggested by the "selective" rather than the "instructive" theory of antibody formation. I should explain that the instructive theory implies that all antibody-forming cells are essentially similar in that each antibody-forming cell can be instructed by any antigen (a particular multivalent vaccine, for example) to form antibody to all antigens. The selective theory implies that each individual antibody-forming cell possesses the capacity to react only to certain antigens while the host as a whole will react to a very wide range of antigens. By analogy, this would mean that there pre-exists in the different learning cells of the brain, for example, a latent capacity for the development and expression of the characteristics, or reaction patterns, that are later exhibited; these genetically determined patterns exist in the protoplasm and are not expressed until impinged upon by circumstances in a way that would develop the skills, thoughts, actions and total personality that eventually characterize the individual.

The idea of a selective theory of learning, if we may call it that —meaning that the potential for what is learned is pre-determined, rather than that at the beginning there is a clean slate with unlimited potential in all individuals—and the realization that learning is an unfolding process bears on the question of man's potential and on the possibility of educing what might generally be referred to as the "more desirable" human attributes and capabilities.

The foregoing may be summarized by saying that man goes through a plastic stage of development, during a prolonged period after birth, during which his mind and emotions can be shaped by the experiences and ideas to which he is exposed. This will influence his character, his values and his choices and, in turn, determine the causes and goals to which he becomes committed. The limits of possibilities within him are genetically determined and exist in his protoplasm as if anticipating demands that will arise. Education and experience bring out the pre-existing possibilities that would otherwise remain latent, or would never be expressed, unless opportunity occurred to develop the potential that emerges.

FIELDS OF FORCE

It is evident that each individual is different from all others and, individually, requires discovery of his own special attributes. For evolution, in its broad meaning, including non-genetic or cultural evolution, cultures and societies may be said to create fields of force for change. In the same sense, an individual creates a field of force upon himself and contributes to the field of force that acts upon others. If we then speak of such fields of force, and of the effects induced thereby, we observe a directional influence upon human potential induced by environment—whether this be physical, social, or personal.

Enough has been said to convey the idea that men exist not only as separate and contiguous individuals with others but also as units or cells of the multi-cellular organism that we refer to as "mankind." Therefore, man, the individual, is simultaneously under the influence of two separate fields of force, the center of one of which is in himself and the center of the other is in society, or the culture of which he is a part. If, for one reason or another, he becomes alienated from society or from himself, it is likely that he will become alienated from the other as well, because his humanity depends upon contact with the centers of both, and it is from these his motivation springs.

NATURE OF MAN'S NEEDS

Heretofore, we did not know enough of the workings of biological systems to be able to deduce principles which might conceivably be applied toward our understanding of man and, particularly, of those activities of man in realms that have not been approached by scientists. Science, it is said, will not be able to explain everything. This is hardly the point. Is it not possible that even the comprehension of living systems, developed by those who practice the art of science, will help us understand more than we now do of man's creative, artistic, and esthetic needs and expressions, as well as his physical needs?

Even if we are regarded as no more than machines, it must be conceded that we are remarkable machines, able to produce ideas and able to respond to environmental influences that bring out unsuspected possibilities. Is this not analogous to the discovery, to which I have referred, of the existence within a micro-organism of a latent potential for enzyme function which is revealed only when the organism is exposed to an environment with which, hitherto, it had had no experience? Another example cited was the emergence of antibody in an organism exposed to an antigen to which it had not theretofore been exposed. And it seems that these effects involve the evocation of a response through the suppression of repressors that are part of the mechanism of homeostasis.

And so it is with man's artistic and humanistic expressions, which emerge under circumstances in which he is placed in an environment in which his talent or potential may be educed.

WHAT NEED WE DO?

How does man rise to the demand for a new level of integration and understanding?

We recognize the existence, in the rays of the sun, of elements which are essential for conversion of particular chemical compounds, that bones may be formed solidly. We recognize the influence upon our mood of sunshine and darkness, of the effect upon man of the seasons. We recognize the effects of atmospheres that are created by humans who are friendly or hostile. We see, in the expressions on faces, the way we or others feel inside. Such influences of external and internal human environments, which are all too evident, may be too readily dismissed because our understanding may be limited and, even more, perhaps, because we, too, are victims of the effects of these forces; in fortunate instances, we may be the recipients of the beneficence of the same forces. We may decline to be involved because we cannot be objective or, because of our subjectivity, we are involved in ways in which we should not be.

There was a time, before the effect—and therefore the existence—of vitamins was understood, when man discovered how to avoid scurvy, and then ricketts and, later, other nutritional deficiencies. Man also learned, even before he was aware of specific microbes, or of the scientific basis for specific prevention, to practice the art of living in ways that would avoid disease. Man also knew enough to stay out of areas infested with malaria, even though he erroneously attributed the "cause" to bad air.

Long before man understood the specific nature of the mechanisms that are operative, at the molecular, cellular, or organismic levels, he discovered, through observation and intuitive insights, ways and means of dealing with human problems which scientists later could explain.

It is magnificent to know the nature and role of nucleic acids in the life process, and it is difficult to imagine that there may be associated with certain nucleotides properties that have in the past led to war, and to the destruction of life on a vast scale, with the consequent influence thereof upon civilization and upon human evolution. Do we need to wait —for developing the practical means for fulfilling man's biologic potential—until the day of enlightenment when we can find the particular nucleotide related to each attribute, or characteristic, of man?

The Challenge

We continue to witness startling evidences of the enormity of man's inhumanity—even as its level is being somewhat reduced by measures that neither adequately nor appropriately match the problem because we do not yet fully or correctly understand its nature. As we see the successes that have been scored by an approach to man's problems through deeper understanding of the science of biology, we have reason to hope that our way into the future will be found by following the broad path of biology.

Man's view of himself and of the diseases that afflict him has only recently become biologically oriented.

His sense of security derives from the discovery and understanding of cause-and-effect relationships. What man now knows is but a small fraction of what he will know. His understanding will deepen as he accepts a realistic conceptual structure for the facts he learns. Therefore, biological explanations and models must be developed to encompass as broadly as possible the various manifestations of human behavior. The application of biological principles and concepts for an interpretation of behavior can revolutionize man's thought beyond anything that has yet been realized.

This is the direction of change, but how the new knowledge will contribute to man's control over himself individually and over the human condition remains to be seen.

28

KARL MENNINGER, M.D.

And now along comes this wonderful invitation to say something in a collection honoring Leo Bartemeier!

Brother Leo has always listened to my associations and outpourings. When I would tell him my wild ideas and dreams, long ago, he would listen and say, "Karl, that's good! You must develop that. Karl, that's great. Do that. I'll help." And then sometimes I did do it, and got all the credit and applause for its success. But back of me, as I always knew, stood Leo Bartemeier quietly smiling and saying, "Karl, that's wonderful!"

This is late thanks to give you and all too small, dear fellow, for all you have done for me these years. I don't know whether it was more faith or hope or love, but I know it was all three. And your friendship was of a very special and indescribable kind.

I want to say something not profound, not world shaking, but something I have been thinking about for a long time. I have not thought it through, but someone may pick it up and carry it further if it is worthy of it. I told Bartie about it on the phone and, as always, he said: "Karl, that is wonderful. Write that!"

So I will.

Changing One's Character

IN THE OLD DAYS psychotherapy was far from being the proud queen she is today. She was looked upon by the profession as a kind of permitted quackery, remunerative and often successful, but not very dignified and certainly not scientific. If, with the aid of a little brow-rubbing or faradic brush or Geissler tube manipulation or other forms of hocus-pocus, a patient could be "persuaded" to relinquish a symptom, the result was ascribed to suggestion and assumed to justify the means.

Sometimes the doctor tried to talk even himself into believing that there was a logical connection between the manipulation and the disappearance of the symptoms. Usually it was a clear case of "tit-for-tat": The patient had tried to "fool" the doctor with nonorganic symptoms and so the doctor could out-smart and "out-fool" the patient with manipulations and suggestions. The patient was cured of a symptom and the doctor got the credit (*and* the cash). Both the patient and the doctor saved face, and were benefited.

Psychotherapy has grown up since then, and risen greatly in prestige. Nowadays we concede that the patient is *not* deceiving the doctor, but himself; trying to fool the doctor is only incidental to getting some needed attention, some opportunity for protest. The good doctor will not treat him by further deception nor encourage self-deception; he will respond to the plea for understanding and try to *undeceive* him—that is, if he *wants* it enough.

The new psychotherapy gets much credit for some of these transformations, and its users believe that they occur more frequently and for more logical reasons than the "cures" of the old days. This is rudely disputed by some cold, calculating statisticians who claim that about the same number of sufferers recover no matter *what* the treatment method, or even with no treatment at all! But this is but the babble of scoffers and cynics!

There has always been some medical pessimism about the possibility of "changing" the nature or personality of patients. At the tail end of the era of therapeutic nihilism, about 1917, any "neurotic" or "neurasthenic" who got well was considered to have done so in some extracurricular way, or the recovery was a false one. To be "converted," as it were, to common sense and hence to resuming a rational, healthy way of life was less cure than re-education or reformation.

Freud described this transformation as the overcoming of unconscious resistance to recovery. He worked out a method of facilitating it which took a long time and much training, but it set a pattern and a model for scientific procedure. Freud also commented on a kind of change for the better which occurred without much help from the doctor. He called it a "flight into health"! Some people suddenly just seemed to turn over a new leaf and to need no more treatment. We all know people who "get religion" which seems to change their nature and behavior patterns. (See "Pathological Processes in Religion," by Philip Woollcott. *Int. Psychiatry Clinics* 5(4): 61-76, 1969.)

William James wrote what is perhaps his greatest book, *The Varieties of Religious Experience,* on this subject. Recently I reread it, and also Harold Begbie's *Twice-Born Men,* which appeared in 1909.[1] Begbie was inspired by James' book. James refers to Begbie's "twice-borns"—a prize-fighter, a robber, a burglar, a peddler and other such types. All lived in what the author depicts as an inconceivably dirty, vicious, poverty-stricken part of London (a ghetto?). Each of the ten characters Begbie described in detail was a desperate, abandoned, wretched character with years of drunken fighting, irregular employment, numerous prison sentences and much senseless beating and public abuse. Suddenly the fellow sees some hope of happiness in identifying himself with the Salvation Army!

Begbie had a simple explanation for this change of personality, this shift of identification and behavior patterns. Science, he asserted, cannot change a bad man to a good man but religion (faith) can! He stressed the loneliness, the new belief in something, the wish to belong, and the physical participation—marching and holding meetings or speaking to and for the group. Frequently he mentioned the pride of "self-victory" in the utterly different pattern of life when it is suddenly "elected" and followed, joyfully and consistently.

A typical case is that of a boy who ran away from a cold, miserable, dirty slum home at fourteen and joined a circus where he was ill-treated, underfed and overworked. By audacity, stealth and cheekiness he held on to his job, but his overuse of alcohol became so bad that he was finally discharged. He supported himself mainly by petty theft. Occasionally, utterly destitute, he would offer to eat dead cats for a bribe of twenty cents. Once, while sleeping in some bushes in a London park, he awoke to find a group of people gathered around him, and thinking he was about to be arrested, he charged out threatening to kill them. They told him they were having a religious service and invited him to join in it. He stood around and listened to them; gradually he "joined" this group and continued to work with the organization the rest of his life, marrying another Salvation Army worker and abstaining from all the drinking and other of his faults. A speck of hope, a surrender of willfulness and a resolute following in the way of Jesus.

Most psychiatrists would agree with Begbie, the Salvation Army workers and Alcoholics Anonymous that a man *can* change his ways, and that this conversion *can* be assisted by outsiders. We all agree that a man must *want* to change. Then, perhaps, even a considerably deformed and disorganized personality can restructure itself and become realigned with the requirements of social living. Such realignment does occur; we see others achieve it; we experience the thrill of accomplishing it ourselves.

It is from the confidence of this elation that we tend to venture further into new fields of "curing" or at least helping the unwilling sufferer.

We think we must find ways to circumvent the reluctance to accept our help. We must meet resistance and doubt and even hostility, not with promises (which the sufferer will suspect), not with deceit (which he will forever resent), and not—if it can possibly be avoided—with anything based on force. Yet the necessity must arise of preventing our prospective beneficiaries from leaving us. They must not leave us prematurely—physically, mentally, or by suicide. The inescapable conclusion is that we must, sometimes, overcome intractable self-destructive resistance by more than persistence and patience, but our techniques of insistence must be as skillful as the hand of the surgeon.

We used to be pretty stuffy about insisting upon our prospective patient taking a suppliant attitude if he wanted our help. His first payment on account had to be an unconditional surrender. The doctor knew what was best; the patient followed orders. It was a basic assumption that the doctor could do no wrong, could make no mistakes. Only some children the doctors expected to treat against their will—children and the mentally ill. The latter he generally avoided or sidetracked.

Today he still treats willing patients, but he is constantly reminded of the responsibility he has toward unwilling patients or potential patients. There are millions of people who ought to be helped but who reject his—or anyone else's—offer. Among the victims of alcohol addiction, that grievous phenomenon which affects five or ten million of our fellow citizens, there are many who partially want help but will not fully submit themselves to medical authority. They retain mental reservations, secretly or avowedly. The success of that worthy organization, Alcoholics Anonymous, is ascribed by many to the wisdom of its founders in requiring an applicant for help to completely and unconditionally surrender, freely admitting that he can no longer save himself. (See numerous studies by the late Dr. Harry Tiebout.)

Psychiatrists have demonstrated that *some* patients can be successfully treated even against their will. Indeed many have been treated and cured without *initial* cooperation. But in recent years the morality of undesired, unsought treatment has been questioned; the question asked is: *Should* sufferers be forced to receive treatment if they harm no one but themselves? Perhaps a patient is wise in choosing to remain ill, or at least to decline help from a doctor, but on the other hand this stubbornness and arrogance may be the very essence of the patient's illness.

One is reminded of Piet Hein's marvelous little gem:

> *The noble art of losing face*
> *may one day save the human race*
> *and turn into eternal merit*
> *what weaker minds would call disgrace.*[2]

The following words of Otto Will paraphrased by Ann Appelbaum are also wisely relevant:

> If the psychiatrist decides to treat an unwilling patient, for whatever reason, he must be prepared for certain hazards: the patient will resent and resist being forced into treatment, even though he may seem to invite and welcome the coercion or to ignore it. The psychiatrist inevitably loses any claim to neutrality or impartiality when he begins to treat another person against his will. He now cannot help but expose his reluctant patient to his (the psychiatrist's) goals and values. The psychiatrist assumes that his coercion of the patient will be vindicated by the outcome . . . in assuming responsibility for controlling another person, the therapist expresses great interest in that person and arrogates to himself powers one ordinarily does not have. The other person's response is influenced by memories of former experiences of being controlled, and he begins to attribute to the therapist the qualities of teacher, parent, guide. In the course of this, however, the person may begin to find the personality of the therapist attractive. He may begin to feel better in the context of a constructive human relationship, and gradually he may enter into a collaborative enterprise. . . .
>
> Meanwhile, the therapist needs to look closely at himself: Is he accepting the role of controller because it is natural for him, having been himself controlled by others for so long? Is it out of a desire for revenge against those who controlled him? Is it out of loneliness and a fear that he cannot have a relationship with another person unless he captures him by force? Is there a sadomasochistic pleasure for him in the exercising of power? Is there a wish to possess the patient? Perhaps the reluctant patient refuses to talk: Does the therapist begin to enjoy these silent hours of being alone with someone without any conventional interchange? Does the therapist want to act—to rescue someone in distress even against his will? Does he want to force a better life upon him? Does he want to convince others of his good intentions? Any such motives should be conscious. . . .[3]

We agree that human nature can be changed. We are almost to the point of agreeing that it can be changed even against the other person's will. But this is very dangerous because it makes us responsible for the direction in which the change is made.

Assuming this responsibility is a solemn task, not to be entered into lightly. The psychiatrist not only has the responsibility for making sure his own motives for change are disinterested and therapeutic; he also has the responsibility for determining whether his idea of a desirable change accords with the patient's needs and potentialities. With the unwilling patient, the psychiatrist becomes the sorcerer's apprentice. He has at his command miraculous powers for genuine amelioration or for bungling, well-intentioned "good." If he chants the wrong incantation, he may change an honest frog into a bogus prince, turning his patient into an unauthentic person doomed to grapple for the rest of his life with concepts and goals which are not truly his.

The psychiatrist has the obligation to keep abreast of the moral and ethical implications of every significant development in his society. And because society may well reject psychiatry unless it seems to work toward improving the quality of *all* men's lives, he must demonstrate concern for a whole culture—as well as the individual patient.

Effecting or assisting a metamorphosis in a human being is a difficult task which can be accomplished in many different ways; each of us has his favorites. Perhaps in another 100 years we will know which of these methods are the best and we will know more definitely their probabilities of success.

But until that time we must persist in study, self- and society-evaluation, and developing our "third ears" to detect the slightest vibrato of justified protest from the person or persons whose character we are trying to change.

REFERENCES

1. Begbie, Harold, *Twice-Born Men.* New York, Fleming H. Revell & Company, 1909. Also appeared under the title *Broken Earthenware.*
2. Hien, Piet, *Grooks.* Cambridge, Mass., MIT Press, 1966, p. 37.
3. Will, Otto: Address abstracted by Ann Appelbaum in "Transactions of the Topeka Psychoanalytic Society." *Bull. Menninger Clin.* 32:401-03, Nov. 1968.

Index